The Epidemiologic Study of the Elderly

The Epidemiologic Study of the Elderly

Edited by

ROBERT B. WALLACE

ROBERT F. WOOLSON

New York Oxford
OXFORD UNIVERSITY PRESS
1992

Oxford University Press

Oxford New York Toronto
Delhi Bombay Calcutta Madras Karachi
Petaling Jaya Singapore Hong Kong Tokyo
Nairobi Dar es Salaam Cape Town
Melbourne Auckland

and associated companies in
Berlin Ibadan

Published by Oxford University Press, Inc.,
200 Madison Avenue, New York, New York 10016

Library of Congress Cataloging-in-Publication Data
The Epidemiologic study of the elderly / edited by
Robert B. Wallace and Robert F. Woolson.
p. cm. Includes bibliographical references and index.
ISBN 0-19-506120-9
1. Aged—Diseases—Epidemiology.
I. Wallace, Robert B., 1942- . II. Woolson, Robert F. [DNLM: 1. Aged.
2. Epidemiologic Methods.
3. Health Surveys—in old age.
WT 30 E635] RA564.8.E64 1991
362.1'9897—dc20 DNLM/DLC
for Library of Congress 91-3003

9 8 7 6 5 4 3 2 1

Printed in the United States of America
on acid-free paper

Preface

As the number and population proportion of older persons increases, it has become clear that prior epidemiologic principles and field methods are inadequate for discovery, description, and analysis of the diseases and dysfunctions characteristic of these populations, and that new techniques are needed. This book is intended to summarize for health science students and practitioners the major conceptual and logistical issues of investigating the health problems of older persons in population context.

Most of the chapters are written for readers who have had an introductory course in epidemiology and biostatistics. However, the amalgamation of epidemiology and biostatistics with gerontology and geriatrics actually represents many disciplines, each with its own lore and methodologic approaches. In addition to epidemiology, biostatistics, and clinical geriatrics, contributing authors in this volume represent such disciplines as sociology, psychology, vital statistics, survey research, economics, health services research, demography, and psychiatry. Some knowledge of these disciplines will be essential for public health practice among older populations.

We wish to thank the many persons who contributed to the production of this volume. The contributing authors provided timely and thoughtful tracts in response to our requests. Particularly helpful were staff scientists of the Epidemiology, Demography and Biometry Division of the National Institute on Aging. The staff of the Department of Preventive Medicine and Environmental Health at The University of Iowa College of Medicine, particularly Ms. Terry Gray, contributed greatly to the production of the text. Finally, we wish to thank our families, whose forbearance and support is critical to all of our activities.

Iowa City, Iowa
October 1991

R.B.W.
R.F.W.

Contents

Contributors

Robert B. Wallace, M.D., M.Sc.
Department of Preventive Medicine
and Environmental Health
University of Iowa College of Medicine
Iowa City, Iowa

Linda P. Fried, M.D., M.P.H.
General Internal Medicine
Johns Hopkins Hospital
Baltimore, Maryland

George A. Kaplan, Ph.D.
Department of Epidemiology
California Department of Health Services
Berkeley, California

Mary N. Haan, Ph.D.
Division of Research
Permanente Medical Group, Inc.
Oakland, California

Richard D. Cohen, M.A.
Department of Health Services
Human Population Laboratory
Berkeley, California

Patricia L. Colsher, Ph.D.
Department of Preventive Medicine
and Environmental Health
University of Iowa College of Medicine
Iowa City, Iowa

Daniel H. Freeman, Jr., Ph.D.
Dartmouth Medical School
Family and Community Medicine
Hanover, New Hampshire

Martha L. Bruce, Ph.D.
Department of Epidemiology
and Public Health
Yale University School of Medicine
New Haven, Connecticut

Philip Leaf, Ph.D.
Department of Mental Hygiene
School of Public Health
Johns Hopkins University
Baltimore, Maryland

Lisa F. Berkman, Ph.D.
Department of Epidemiology
Yale University School of Medicine
New Haven, Connecticut

A. Regula Herzog, Ph.D.
Institute for Social Research
University of Michigan
Ann Arbor, Michigan

Willard L. Rodgers, Ph.D.
Institute for Social Research
University of Michigan
Ann Arbor, Michigan

Frank J. Kohout, Ph.D.
Department of Preventive Medicine
and Environmental Health
The University of Iowa
Iowa City, Iowa

Jay Magaziner, Ph.D.
Department of Epidemiology
and Preventive Medicine
University of Maryland School
of Medicine
Baltimore, Maryland

Jack M. Guralnik, M.D.
Epidemiology, Demography
and Biometry Branch
National Institute on Aging
Bethesda, Maryland

Andrea Z. LaCroix, Ph.D.
Center of Health Studies
Group Health Cooperative of Puget Sound
Seattle, Washington

Laurence G. Branch, Ph.D.
Department of Socio-Medical Sciences
and Community Medicine
Boston University School of Medicine
Boston, Massachusetts

Thomas E. Oxman, M.D.
Department of Psychiatry
Dartmouth Medical School
Hanover, New Hampshire

Teresa E. Seeman, Ph.D.
Department of Epidemiology
and Public Health
Yale University School of Medicine
New Haven, Connecticut

Dan L. Tweed, Ph.D.
Department of Psychiatry
Duke University Medical Center
Durham, North Carolina

Dan G. Blazer, M.D., Ph.D.
Department of Psychiatry
Duke University Medical Center
Durham, North Carolina

James A. Ciarlo, Ph.D.
University of Denver
Denver, Colorado

Daniel J. Foley, M.S.
Epidemiology, Demography and Biometry
National Institute on Aging
Bethesda, Maryland

Cynthia M. Taeuber
Bureau of Census
Washington, D.C.

Tamara B. Harris, M.D., M.S.
Office of Analysis and Epidemiology
National Center for Health Statistics
Hyattsville, Maryland

Mary Grace Kovar, Dr.P.H., M.S.
Office of Vital Health Statistics
National Center for Health Statistics
Hyattsville, Maryland

Richard J. Havlik, M.D., M.P.H.
Epidemiology, Demography
and Biometry
National Institute on Aging
Bethesda, Maryland

Harry M. Rosenberg, Ph.D.
National Center for Health Statistics
Hyattsville, Maryland

William S. Cartwright, Ph.D.
Health Economist
National Institute on Drug Abuse
Rockville, Maryland

Jersey Liang, Ph.D.
Institute of Gerontology
School of Public Health
University of Michigan
Ann Arbor, Michigan

Gina M. Jay
Institute of Gerontology
School of Public Health
University of Michigan
Ann Arbor, Michigan

Dwight B. Brock, Ph.D.
Epidemiology, Demography
& Biometry Program
National Institute on Aging
Bethesda, Maryland

Monica B. Holmes, Ph.D.
DMH Associates
Riverdale, New York

Douglas Holmes, Ph.D.
DMH Associates
Riverdale, New York

Kenneth G. Manton, Ph.D.
Research Professor of Demographic
Studies
Duke University Medical Center
Durham, North Carolina

Max A. Woodbury, Ph.D., M.P.H.
Professor Emeritus
Duke University Medical Center
Durham, North Carolina

Jon H. Lemke, Ph.D.
Department of Preventive Medicine
and Environmental Health
University of Iowa College of Medicine
Iowa City, Iowa

Greg A. Drube
Research Assistant
Department of Preventive Medicine
and Environmental Health
University of Iowa
Iowa City, Iowa

Peter A. Lachenbruch, Ph.D.
Department of Biostatistics
U.C.L.A.
Los Angeles, California

I

INTERDISCIPLINARY CONTRIBUTIONS TO THE EPIDEMIOLOGIC STUDY OF THE ELDERLY

1

Aging and Disease: From Laboratory to Community

ROBERT B. WALLACE

The purpose of this chapter is twofold: to provide a brief introduction to some concepts of the biology of aging and how they may relate to disease and to suggest how these notions may lead to better epidemiologic questions and methods. Although there is a rapidly growing body of biologic research on aging, extrapolation to population-based research must be largely speculative. As new biological principles and constructs emerge, it is likely that the propositions offered will need modification. The chapter will not consider aging from an evolutionary perspective, although this is of both theoretical interest (Woodhead and Thompson, 1986) and clinical relevance in terms of the emergence of some important chronic diseases.

AGING: WHAT IS IT?

Aging is often discussed but seldom defined. It may be defined broadly as the nature and determinants of the time-related changes in an organism's biological processes over the course of its lifespan. These processes are universal in living organisms and reflect importantly on their function and survival. If one accepts this definition, aging could encompass almost any process related to growth and development, adult physiology, and senescence, including disease pathogenesis. Thus, the study of aging is arguably among the most holostic areas of biological inquiry. Indeed, such holism is required. For example, the same growth-promoting genes that regulate growth and development may with altered function play a role in senescence. An analogous question, from an enivironmental perspective, is whether an untoward exposure during development might have adverse consequences on later aging processes.

From an experimental perspective, aging phenomena have been studied at many levels in both the plant and animal kingdoms, including in vitro molecular processes, cell function and survival, organ and tissue physiology, and the biologic behavior of whole organisms. Perhaps least well studied, because of both logistical and conceptual problems, is organismic aging in the ecologic and social context, and this is an area where epidemiology can offer important contributions. For example, how does living in a hot, tropical environment; working near electrical power lines; being poor; or not having enough social intercourse affect aging processes?

Along with the definition offered earlier, most research on the biology of aging involves observations of anatomic and physiologic changes in organisms over time or the survivorship of an organism or population. However, care is needed in utilizing time measures. For example, an hypothetical environmental intervention may delay puberty, and the relevant unit of observation of the effects of this intervention on adult function may then be time since puberty, not time since birth. Other major research paradigms employed to understand aging include comparing and contrasting aging processes (1) within subpopulation of a species (e.g., strains, ethnic groups, nationalities, or cultures) and (2) among species. As noted earlier, one of the most important ways in which aging processes are summarized is in terms of survivorship of a "birth cohort" or generation of a species. The survivorship curves have been observed and mathematically modeled and their shapes have been used to yield inferences about aging phenomena (Finch et al, 1990). Olshansky and his colleagues (1990) offer terminology to describe the survivorship phenomena, shown in Table 1-1. In general, the most important terms here are *life expectancy* and *active life expectancy,* both directly observable. As noted in the table, lifespan is a theoretical construct not directly observable, and only estimated. As discussed later, no lifespan can unfold in an environment "free of exogenous risk factors." Whatever the measure of survivorship employed, it should not be assumed automatically that patterns of mortality necessarily reflect all important biological processes during life, just as the causes of an individual human death do not necessarily summarize the conditions of health and disease during that person's life. In fact, exploring the relationship between the survivorship patterns of various human populations and the patterns and trajectory of functional status and disease throughout the lifespan of those populations could be an important issue in the epidemiologic study of older persons. In some experimental models, for example, altered longevity is associated with altered tumor occurrence (Weindruch et al, 1986).

In studying aging, it is generally assumed that complex organisms have finite lifespans, but in view of certain observations and experiments, this assumption should not be totally constraining. For example, connective tissue cells from animals are normally capable of only a finite number of replications in vitro, and this number correlates with the longevity of the species of origin (Hayflick, 1988). Under experimental

Table 1-1 Nomenclature of Survivorship in Aging Research[a]

Life expectancy	Average amount of time of life remaining for a defined population, all of a given age (or from birth)
Active life expectancy	Average amount of time of life remaining in a population of a given age, in a state free of a specified level of disability
Lifespan	Genetically endowed limit of life for an organism of a given species when free of exogenous risk factors; generally, a theoretical construct not directly observable
Average lifespan	The average of individual lifespans for members of a given birth cohort; because of cohort heterogeneity there is considerable variation; thus, this is also primarily a theorotical construct
Verified longest-lived individual of a cohort	A member of a species with the longest lifespan that is observed and verified

[a]Modified from Olshansky et al (1990).

conditions, however, some cells can become "immortalized" if infected with certain viruses. Also, DNA and its messages passed from one generation of a species to another are immortal in a certain sense. A more immediately relevant observation is the substantial inter- and intraspecies variation in survivorship, suggesting that there is pliability in aging processes and that either natural environmental variation or directed interventions may modify these processes. Perhaps the most dramatic experimental example of this pliability is the substantial prolongation of life in rodents with caloric restriction (Weindruch et al, 1986).

Whether in humans or in other species, inquiry into the nature of environmental factors in aging generally requires the assumption that, within a species, there is basic stability of the population's genetic makeup. This is because gene structure and function play an important role in the longevity of an organism. For example, the genetic manipulation of some organisms has increased longevity, one mutation having expanded the mean lifespan of the nematode by 65 percent (Johnson, 1990). Errors in the normal function of the genetic machinery that may occur during routine cell division, perhaps in association with mutational events, are posited to contribute to cell senescence and death (Goldstein, 1990; Kirkwood, 1989). Further, the conceptual distinction between genetic and environmental factors that alter biological processes is becoming blurred, particularly when an environmental factor operates by altering gene function. Conceivably, there are environmental mutagens that alter basic aging processes.

A frequently invoked concept in studies of aging, particularly in relation to environmental exposures, is *homeostasis,* the ability of an organism to maintain its function and integrity in the face of such challenges. This is important when exploring the role of environmental factors in health, because the ability to withstand some defined exposures, such as vehicular trauma, influenza viruses, or 100° F days, is demonstrably decreased at advanced ages. Homeostasis and the changing relation between host and environmental factors in disease causation may explain why some host risk factors for death decline with age and some environmental risk factors take on increasing prominence.

The increased susceptibility to environmental challenge among older persons has other implications for exploring the relation between an exposure and a disease. Suppose hot weather is associated with increased stroke incidence. If hot weather hypothetically also leads to sudden death from stroke in the frail "oldest old," then the relation between hot weather and stroke incidence may be obscured in that population, but not necessarily in the "younger old." This is because the environmental assault to the frail individual may lead more frequently to a sudden, unattended death, and the diagnosis of stroke is never made. While such phenomena require empirical verification, the presence of frailty and poor homeostasis may thus alter the behavior of clinical illness and the interpretation of environmental risks.

Since the environment probably has an important impact on at least some aging processes, it follows that inquiry into genetic factors in aging would be facilitated by maintaining a stable environment in which the genes are functioning. However, a stable environment is not always a safe assumption. Planetary climatic changes, dietary alterations, and other natural and unnatural changes are constantly occurring, and their impact on population longevity must be considered. On a more theoretical plane, residing on the earth's surface exposes us to environmental factors that may have potent effects on aging that are not readily perceived or altered, such as gravity or ambient gamma radiation. If these elements were changed, a given species might not have the same survivorship. Hypothetically, the "heritability" of longevity in a species might be quite different if it were raised in the weightlessness of outer space or in an environment free of natural plant toxins. It should also be remembered that the natural environment for most species includes other species, both flora and fauna.

Hundreds, perhaps thousands, of age-related anatomic and physiologic alterations have been observed in various species, from the level of molecular structure to the whole organism. Researchers have hoped some of these measures may serve to characterize the *general* state of an organism's aging, independent of its chronologic age, the so-called biomarkers of aging (Mooradian, 1990). However, no such measures have been convincingly demonstrated, for several reasons: (a) There is no agreement that any of the measures represent one or more fundamental, universal biologic processes that can be called "aging" (this is discussed further below); (b) the state or level of these markers has not yet been demonstrated in all organ systems and tissue types; and (c) few have been evaluated longitudinally to determine their relation to subsequent structure or function, or cellular or organismic survival. Combinations of physiologic measures have been used in theoretical models to calculate a "biological age" of individuals that is independent of chronologic age (Ruiz-Torres et al, 1990), and more work would seem to be profitable in this area. As noted later, this type of modeling requires that the physiologic measures do not also reflect disease processes, and this can be problematic.

If credible biomarkers of aging were discovered and validated—and the prospects are uncertain—they could be enormously useful to epidemiologic inquiry. They could be determined in defined populations and might serve as indicators of the general biological state of aging. To the extent that biomarkers serve this role and also reflect pathogenetic processes, they might be applied as predictors of disability and death, perhaps independently of currently recognized risk factors. It is obvious that in many current studies, multivariate predictors are dominated by chronologic age.

AGING VERSUS DISEASE

Leaving aside for the moment the distinctions between aging and disease, it should be noted that much of the elegant biological research on the determinants and processes of aging has been conducted on species in which conventionally defined diseases as conceived in humans either have not been studied or cannot occur. Fruit flies, yeasts, protozoans, and even many rodents usually do not serve as models of human disease. Diseases did not enter into most early biological research on aging, which was generally measured in terms of organism survivorship patterns. As noted earlier, many age-related changes in a species' structure and function have now been described. Examples in humans include altered organ function (e.g., maximum breathing capacity), metabolism (e.g., tissue insulin resistance), biochemical activity (e.g., speed of DNA repair after a standard chemical insult), and structural alteration (e.g., collagen cross-linking). In gerontology texts one can readily find graphs of declining respiratory function or renal creatinine clearance with age, changes that are attributed to "aging" largely because the observations were made in individuals who felt well and had no complaints or overt, diagnosed medical conditions.

The problem with this attribution is that there is no way to evaluate critically the subjects' tissues and organs to be certain that some or all of the population's functional decrements are not due to early stages of conventionally defined diseases. For example, decreased respiratory function may result from degenerative arthritis of the vertebrocostal joints, restrictive lung disease from past infections or inhalent exposures, or even subclinical congestive heart failure. An additional problem is that most of these inferences are made from cross-sectional data; one way to help assure that study subjects do not have nascent illnesses is to follow them for a few years after the observations are made and determine whether some develop. Thus, clinical or population surveys of health status may not add much insight into the biological determinants of that status.

With respect to the distinctions between aging and disease, the basic thesis promulgated here is that, from an epidemiologic and particularly an etiologic perspective, the processes of aging and the processes encompassing the pathogenesis of diseases should be regarded as a single category that contributes to ill health. The reason is that with the current state of knowledge, the infirmities and dysfunctions of older persons are due to combinations of processes that have been labeled "aging" in some disciplines and "diseases" in others, and for etiologic study this distinction is largely semantic and administrative. For example, if a 75-year-old is exposed to an environmental toxin that causes accelerated loss of nerve and muscle cell function and a concomitant but small increase in the rate of cell death with progressive muscle weakness, impoverished movement, and difficult ambulation, it is likely to be called aging. On the other hand, if the neurotoxicity leads to concomitant tremor or seizure, then it will likely be labeled a disease, possibly a "degenerative" one. If this putative toxin destroys genes that normally suppress cell growth, or the tissue undergoes substantial cell division in an attempt to regenerate, a neoplasm might result, and then it certainly would be called a disease. As another example, if cross-linking of connective tissue collagen fosters skin wrinkling, then it is labeled aging. If it leads to cataract, then it is a disease. Yet it is the same process.

Despite this plea for "lumping" rather than "splitting," it may be useful to consider the dichotomy between aging and disease. Table 1-2 suggests some of the observational differences between the two. Aging processes tend to be general and slowly progressive and to remain confined to their original anatomic sites. Diseases, on the other hand,

Table 1-2 Some Observational Differences Between Aging and Disease

Aging	Disease
Universal biological processes	Selective in species, tissues
Generally slowly paced but always progressive	Varying rates of progression; some regression
Ultimately deleterious	Varying harm to host
Emphasizes molecular, physiologic levels	Almost always anatomic disruption
Clinical impact often not easily discernible; rarely treatable	Impact usually discernible; often treatable

are more varied in distribution, tend to leave their original anatomic sites, and have varying rates of progression and regression. It is clear that the concepts and terminology of aging and disease can be useful in many spheres; however, in the effort to discover factors that lead to deteriorating function and health with age, the biologic distinction may be premature.

To restate this thesis in a slighly different way, it is likely that the factors that cause or accelerate "aging" processes are often the same as those that cause "diseases," and at least in some cases probably do so through similar biological pathways. If epidemiology is concerned with the discovery and removal of factors that contribute to dysfunction and poor health, then it may be useful to look beyond classical diseases to conditions or functional states that have been ignored because they have been considered immutable aging processes. This is not to deny the importance to health of conditions such as cancers or cardiovascular diseases, but only to plea for other kinds of "cases" in epidemiologic studies. One could envision case-control studies where a case is defined as extremity weakness due to muscle cell death and replacement with adipose tissue or as a lower level of cognitive function (not dementia) than would be expected from one's educational attainment. It is possible that risk factors for these "conditions" might be discovered and even eliminated.

CONCLUSION

The study of aging can be all-encompassing from a biological perspective. Aside from the inevitable gaps in understanding, conceptual issues need to be considered and clarified before pursuing scientific questions at the population level. But of course there has been substantial growth in biological knowledge in recent decades, and attention to this knowledge will yield better specification of research questions and research designs.

REFERENCES

Finch C, Pike MC, Witten M (1990). Slow mortality rate accelerations during aging in some animals approximate that of humans. Science 249:902–905.

Goldstein S (1990). Replicative senescense: The human fibroblast comes of age. Science 249:1129–1133.

Hayflick L (1988). The cell biology and theoretical basis of human aging. In Carstensen LL, Edelstein BA (eds), Handbook of Clinical Gerontology. New York, Pergamon Press.

Johnson TE (1990). Increased lifespan of *age-1* mutants in *Caenorhabditis elegans* and lower Gompertz rate of aging. Science 249:908–912.

Kirkwood TBL (1989). DNA, mutations and aging. Mutation Res 219:1–7.

Mooradian AD (1990). Biomarkers of aging: Do we know what to look for? J Gerontol Biol Sci 45:B183–B186.

Olshansky SJ, Carnes BA, Cassel C (1990). In search of Methuselah: Estimating the upper limits of human longevity. Science 250:634–640.

Ruiz-Torres A, Agudo A, Vicent D, Beier W (1990). Measuring human aging using a two-compartmental mathematical model and the vitality concept. Arch Gerontol Geriatr 10:69–76.

Weindruch R, Walford RL, Fligiel S, Guthrie D (1986). The retardation of aging in mice by dietary restriction: Longevity, cancer, immunity and lifetime energy intake. J Nutr 116:641–654.

Woodhead AD, Thompson KH (eds) (1986). Evolution of Longevity in Animals. New York, Plenum Press.

FURTHER READING

Johnson HA (ed), Relations Between Normal Aging and Disease. New York, Raven Press, 1985.

2

The Complexity of Chronic Illness in the Elderly: From Clinic to Community

LINDA P. FRIED AND ROBERT B. WALLACE

A dramatic change in the types of diseases that adversely affect health has occurred in the twentieth century. In 1900 the major causes of death were largely infectious diseases, but by midcentury they were supplanted by chronic diseases (National Center for Health Statistics, 1986a). As of 1978, among the 10 leading causes of death for persons 65 years and older, only two categories included infectious illnesses: influenza and pneumonia (ranked fourth) and bronchitis, emphysema, and asthma (ranked eighth) (Rabin and Stockton, 1987). Eight of the 10 leading causes of death in people 65 years and older are now related to chronic diseases, including diseases of the heart, malignant neoplasms, cerebrovascular disease, arteriosclerosis, diabetes, emphysema (as earlier), cirrhosis of the liver, and nephritis and nephrosis. One of the 10 leading causes is accidents (Rabin and Stockton, 1987).

In addition to this marked change in the causes of death, the causes of morbidity have shifted to chronic conditions. The absolute numbers of older adults with chronic diseases is high, as is the population burden. For example, 47 percent of people 65 years and over living in the community report prevalent arthritis, 43 percent report hypertension, 31 percent report heart disease, and 10 percent report visual impairment (National Center for Health Statistics, 1986b). The prevalence of chronic diseases also increases with age (Table 2-1). (National Center for Health Statistics, September 1986b), and the clinical consequences of chronic disease are usually long term. Overall, it is estimated that 80 percent of persons 65 years and over have at least one chronic disease (U.S. Senate, 1988).

These high-prevalence rates have several important implications for health. First, these conditions are associated with substantial population dysfunction and disability. Second, many chronic diseases are associated with high rates of health care utilization, including adverse outcomes, such as institutionalization. For example, circulatory disorders are strong predictors of institutionalization (Weissert et al, 1980), Third, the high prevalence of chronic diseases leads, with increasing age, to many older persons with more than one chronic disease, so-called co-morbidity (Guralnik et al, 1989).

Table 2-1 Increase in Prevalence of Selected Chronic Diseases with Increasing Age (United States, 1985) United States Civilian, Noninstitutionalized Population

	Age			
Condition	18–44	45–64	65–74	≥75
	(Number of chronic conditions per 1000 persons)			
Arthritis	52.1	268.5	459.3	494.7
Hypertension	64.1	258.9	426.8	394.6
Heart disease	40.1	129.0	276.8	349.1
Hearing impairment	49.8	159.0	261.9	346.9
Deformity or orthopedic impairment	125.3	160.6	167.9	175.5
Chronic sinusitis	164.4	184.8	151.2	160.0
Visual impairment	32.8	43.7	76.4	128.8
Diabetes	9.1	51.9	108.9	95.5
Cerebrovascular disease	1.9	17.9	54.0	72.6
Emphysema	1.6	15.2	50.0	38.9

*Source:*Seeman et al (1989).

Chronic disease is a major issue to be addressed in improving the health status of older adults, and thus a major focus of the epidemiology of aging. Although the basic premises of chronic disease epidemiology pertain in both older and younger adults (e.g., the multifactorial nature of risk factors for chronic diseases), there are issues of disease ascertainment and interpretation of special concern in studying older age groups. This chapter discusses these issues and some of their methodologic implications.

THE COMPLEXITY OF CHRONIC ILLNESS IN OLDER PERSONS

The overriding issue that distinguishes illness in older adults from that of young or middle-aged adults is the increased complexity of characterizing health status. Measuring and understanding this complexity of health status for epidemiology is a considerable challenge. This complexity derives from several sources: the presence of multiple chronic diseases, the increased risk of ill health associated with common environmental challenges, the higher proportion of persons at risk for adverse outcomes of diseases and their treatments, and the physiologic changes that come with increasing age.

Components of Illness in Older Adults

Part of the complexity of chronic disease in older adults is that the *types* of conditions that affect health status expand with increasing age, as degenerative diseases are superimposed on those that may occur at any age. As noted earlier, the prevalence of most chronic disease increases with age. For example, this is the case for arthritis, heart disease, diabetes, cerebrovascular disease, and visual impairment (see Table 2-1) (National Center for Health Statistics, September 1986b).

In addition to clearly defined diseases, many physiologic and anatomic alterations, both related to age and intrinsic to the individual, contribute importantly to health status. These changes associated with aging are linked with the additional appearance of chronic "geriatric conditions," such as hearing impairment (presbycusis), urinary incontinence, and unstable gait (Minaker and Rowe, 1985). Whether these are "diseases," dysfunctions, or physiologic alterations is a semantic issue; their overt clinical impact is detectable. Underlying these "geriatric conditions" and physiologic alterations is a set of vulnerabilities associated with aging that also puts the older adult at increased risk of worsening health and death. Examples include increased susceptibility to heat and cold exposure, decreased immune responses to infection, falls, altered taste and smell with undernutrition or toxicity from medications (Minaker and Rowe, 1985). The latter is especially important, since 12 percent of people 65 years and over purchase 25 percent of the drugs sold in the United States, and older adults have a two- to sevenfold higher incidence of adverse drug reactions than young adults (Vestal, 1978). In addition, up to one seventh of all hospitalizations are the result of adverse drug reactions, of which 50 percent are for persons 65 years and over (Minaker and Rowe, 1985).

Equally important, chronic conditions are associated with the development of disability. Forty percent of community-dwelling people 65 years and over report limitations in their activities due to chronic conditions; as a result, 10 percent are unable to carry on their daily activities (National Center for Health Statistics, 1986b). Sixteen percent of people 65 years and older who are living in the community report difficulty walking, with the percentage increasing from 13 percent of those 65 to 74 years old to 32 percent of those 85 years old and older (National Center for Health Statistics, 1987a). The more chronic the person's condition the higher the likelihood of functional difficulties (Guralnik et al, 1989).

Chronic conditions and age-related physiologic changes not only are important in themselves, but have a cumulative "secondary" morbidity of adverse outcomes (Fried and Bush, 1988; Guralnik et al, 1989). In addition, adverse social circumstances are more likely to occur with increasing age and to impact on health. The higher prevalence of adverse life events, such as death of a spouse, loss of friends, and moving from one's own home, the greater the detrimental impact on the person's physical and mental health (Evans, 1984).

Accurate ascertainment of these factors in an individual is complicated. A recognition of their presence and potential interplay is important to the epidemiologist for meaningful assessment of health outcomes and their associations with etiologic factors. In particular, many of these factors may both serve as effect modifiers of the risk status of the individual and be outcomes in themselves. Although the hypothesis being tested may not require the assessment of every important health dimension, if such factors are causally important and pervasive, it is important to ask whether they should be ascertained.

Changes in Physiologic Measures and Their Variances with Age

Textbooks on geriatrics often note that in older populations there are frequently increased variances of clinically relevant physiologic measures compared to younger populations. The types of measures sometimes include pulmonary function studies, muscle strength, measures of memory, or white blood counts. Although this "rule" is usually not rigorously proven or defended, the basic premise is that some older persons have maintained the values of youth, whereas more of the population has undergone decrements, whether due to aging or diseases. To the extent this is true, increased variance of selected measures may increase the requisite sample sizes or in some other way alter the design or analysis of a research project.

Perhaps more important, the *means* of many physiologic measures may change with age, and thus decisions about normal values and ranges need careful consideration. For example, many clinical laboratories do not alter normal ranges for values according to the age of the patient. Irrespective of the wisdom of such a policy, the investigator should always be aware of the basis for such ranges when making categorical decisions about subjects and values in an epidemiologic study.

Change in Illness Presentation with Increasing Age

Even ascertainment of common chronic diseases appears to become more complex with increasing age. There is increasing recognition that the symptom patterns associated with common diseases change with increased age (Irvine, 1984; Samiy, 1983). For example, the clinical presentation of myocardial infarction appears to change in older persons and follows a less "typical" or consistent pattern (Bayer et al, 1986). For other common diseases, classic symptoms can be absent (Irvine, 1984) or unrecognized in the presence of other syndromes or diseases (Fried et al, 1991), or they lose their utility as discriminants among disease status. These observations suggest that the potential for underascertainment rises with increasing age. Therefore, screening or diagnostic methods for ascertaining disease in the clinic or a population survey may require alteration for an older age group. The epidemiologist needs to verify that standardized questionnaires used to ascertain a disease are as valid in older persons as they are in younger persons. At the same time, clinicians need to raise their level of suspicion of an atypical presentation of a disease in an elderly patient because of the known prevalence of the condition in older age groups. In some instances, new criteria for incident or prevalent disease may be needed for older age groups in order to maintain adequate sensitivity and specificity for detection.

Accurate ascertainment is essential for valid estimates of the incidence or prevalence of disease or disability. Also, it is critical to the development of meaningful hypotheses and of biologically plausible models of causality to understand the change in physiologic and clinical issues that come with increasing age. Comprehension of the altered nature of health status in older adults is also necessary for defining at-risk groups and the interactions between the increasingly susceptible host and environmental exposures.

Health Outcomes

Another level of complexity in defining health status and goals for older adults is that, with increasing age, the number of health outcomes likely to be encountered expands along with the multiple types and high prevalence of illness. Health outcomes that appear salient to older adults include not just incidence of disease or mortality, but also functional alterations (physical, psychological, or social), patterns of co-morbidity, disability, quality of life, and adverse outcomes of health care utilization, such as institutionalization, hospitalization (often recurrent), or iatrogenic complications (Kane and Kane, 1981; McDowell and Newell, 1987).

The expanding number of health outcomes has implications for study design and analysis. There is an accumulating analytic experience, although not well documented in the formal literature, that as multiple dimensions of health status are measured in populations, these measures are often statistically associated with one another to varying degrees, whether or not such associations were hypothesized or make biological or clinical sense. For example, the following variables are all significantly related to each other in one cross-sectional study: depressive symptom levels, number of chronic illnesses, number of physician office visits, absence of an exercise program, higher alcohol consumption, and more physical dependencies. The dilemma is that this phenomena compounds the difficulty of assessing causal pathways or creating analytic models that can disaggregate these multiple associations.

There is clearly a large menu of possible health outcomes, and the choices often reflect the investigator's values. For example, few studies have been done to establish what older adults themselves see as primary health goals. However, there is a consensus that prevention of mortality carries less weight as a health status goal as individuals approach the biologic limits of the human lifespan. Quality of life and functional autonomy have assumed more importance as epidemiologic outcome measures, reflecting the perceived priorities of both older adults and their medical practitioners.

Co-morbidity

Co-morbidity, or the concurrent presence of more than one chronic condition, is highly prevalent in people 65 years and over and adds another layer to the complexity of chronic illness in older adults. In one recent U.S. national study, 49 percent of noninstitutionalized people 60 and more years old had two or more of nine chronic conditions surveyed; 23 percent had three or more, and 8 percent had four or more. These proportions increased with age, so that for those 80 years of age and older, 70 percent of the women and 53 percent of the men had two or more chronic conditions (Guralnik et al, 1989).

From an epidemiologic point of view, co-morbid conditions must be considered in interpreting causal models or associations. The presence of a co-morbid condition may modify the impact of an etiologic factor on the outcome. For example, assessing the role of coronary heart disease as a cause of physical disability requires knowledge of concurrent degenerative arthritis, which may also cause physical disability. Conversely, it may be important to ask, from the point of view of prevention, whether the adverse impact of heart disease on function is important only in the presence of co-morbid conditions.

The presence of a disease or its treatment can modify the manifestations and natural history of another. For example, one condition can worsen the symptoms of another. Arthritis of the knees or hips can lead to decreased mobility and decreased conditioning. These changes may cause individuals to expend more of their cardiovascular reserve to perform normal activities and thus increase the likelihood of clinical manifestations of coronary heart disease at that level of exertion. Also, the treatment of one condition may actually precipitate another. For example, diuretic therapy for hypertension can be a cause of incontinence and lightheadedness. Conversely, after the onset of coronary heart disease, a person with a history of hypertension may no longer have elevated blood pressure. This may be a result of altered cardiac function, or a result of medications for the coronary heart disease secondarily treating the hypertension.

Co-morbidity also needs to be considered in defining the population-based impact of etiologic factors. One risk factor can cause several different types of disease, exemplified by the etiologic role of smoking in both lung cancer and coronary heart disease (Jajich et al, 1984; U.S. Department of Health and Human Services, 1982) or the role of alcohol abuse in both cognitive impairment and injuries (Atkinson, 1988; Guthrie and Elliott, 1980). Each of these outcomes has a health impact of its own and joint, co-morbid impacts to be considered in association with the risk factor. Thus, the presence of co-morbid conditions complicates the process of establishing causality for one specific condition and of characterizing the risks associated with one etiologic factor.

Other possible scenarios regarding the association of co-morbid problems should be considered. For example, cross-sectional assessment of concurrently present illnesses may not reveal that one has caused the other [e.g., depression can be both an outcome of chronic disease(s) and a cause of physical symptoms of illness]. Cross-sectional analyses may establish an association between depression and a concurrent chronic condition but will be unlikely to clarify the direction of association (if there is one). Even if an association is identified, the possibility of confounding needs to be considered. Depression, for example, may result from a cause other than the condition of primary interest.

Co-morbidity is thus an important dimension of health status in adults, and it is therefore important to hypothesize and test for the role of co-morbidity in outcomes of interest. The complex interactions of co-morbid diseases need to be understood and taken into account in epidemiologic assessment of the causes of adverse health outcomes for older adults. Co-morbid illness may modify the primary factor of interest, and co-morbidity itself may also independently be a risk factor for adverse outcomes. Better understanding of the roles of co-morbidity in the health status of older adults could lead to unique approaches to prevention in this age group.

ISSUES IN POPULATION-BASED ASCERTAINMENT OF CHRONIC DISEASES AND SEQUELAE

The multifaceted aspects of ill health associated with older age groups thus have implications for the accurate identification of health status in the individual. Characteristics of the older population also can have great influence on findings of epidemiologic studies and need to be addressed, with implications for study design, implementation, and interpretation. Issues to be considered include the influence of the type of population on conclusions regarding frequency, impact, and etiology of a condition and the validity of self-report of health status.

Much more than for younger adults, the setting in which a problem is studied can influence findings regarding the importance of the condition or its consequences. Over 99.9 percent of adults under 65 years of age dwell in a community (National Center for Health Statistics, 1986c), and less than 11 percent are likely to be hospitalized in a given year, excluding those for deliveries (National Center for Health Statistics, 1986b). In contrast, older adults are more likely to be found in long-term care institutions and hospitals as well as in the community. Specifically, 1.4 percent, 6.8 percent, and 21.6 percent of people 65–74, 75–84, and 85 years and over, respectively, in the United States reside in nursing homes (Rabin and Stockton, 1987). In addition, 16 percent of people 65–74 and 23 percent of those 75 years and over report hospitalization at least once in a given year (Rabin and Stockton, 1987).

As a result of this difference in population patterns by age groups, estimated prevalence rates of disease or disability in older adults are likely to be highly influenced by population residence or health care utilization. Institutionalized persons have more chronic diseases and disability than community dwellers. As seen in Table 2-2, the prevalence of functional dependency varies greatly by the population assessed: Nursing home patients 65 years and older have five to 40 times higher rates of dependency in activities of daily living, compared to noninstitutionalized persons of the same age group (National Center for Health Statistics, 1987b). One consequence of this is that the population prevalence of disease and disability may vary among communities according to the availability and use of long-term care of home-based services.

As seen in Table 2-3, the prevalence of specific diagnoses, not unexpectedly, varies according to the site of ascertainment: the community, the outpatient ambulatory clinic, or the inpatient hospital setting. The severity of a specific illness and the type of treatment are major determinants of who will be hospitalized for a given condition. For example, persons with cataracts or arthritis are much less likely to be hospitalized than those with heart disease or pneumonia. Thus, the prevalent rates of disease are greatly affected by the setting as well as by the characteristics of the older population.

These differences in diseases by setting lead to other methodologic issues. As suggested earlier, severity of illness will likely be greater among those who are institutionalized or hospitalized, compared to those with the same diseases living in the community. Rates of co-morbidity and disability may also differ between these settings. There is also a higher likelihood of cognitive impairment in institutionalized persons compared to other populations, which can make historical data or self-report less valid. It is also possible that the generally better health among community-dwelling older adults reflects different risk factor exposures over their lifetime or other selection

Table 2-2 Percent of Persons 65 Years of Age and Over, Either Nursing Home Resident or Noninstitutionalized, by Type of Dependency in Selected Activities of Daily Living United States, 1984 and 1985

Type of dependency	Nursing home residents, 1985 (%)	Noninstitutionalized population, 1984 (%)
Requires assistance in:		
Bathing	91.2	6.0
Dressing	77.7	4.3
Using toilet room	63.3	2.2
Transferring[a]	62.7	2.8
Eating	40.4	1.1

Source: National Center for Health Statistics (1987b).
[a]Transferring refers to getting in or out of a bed or chair.

Table 2-3 Prevalence of Selected Diagnoses by Type of Population, Persons 65 Years and Older, United States

	Prevalence by self-report, noninstitutionalized persons (Health Interview Survey) 1985 rate per 1000 people[a]	Most frequent diagnoses of ambulatory patients 65–74 years, 1980–1981—no. of mentions as first, second, or third diagnosis per 1000 visits[b]	First-listed diagnosis at discharge from short-stay hospital, 1986—no. of inpatients per 1000 population[c]
Diseases of the heart	305	110[d]	77
Diabetes	104	78	6
Cataract	164	29	2.6
Cerebrovascular disease	61	[e]	23
Pneumonia	14	[e]	16

[a]Data from National Center for Health Statistics (1986b).
[b]Data from National Center for Health Statistics (1987a).
[c]Data from National Center for Health Statistics (1987c).
[d]Includes chronic ischemic heart disease, hypertensive heart disease and heart failure.
[e]Data not available.

biases that may impact on risk factor–disease associations. From an epidemiologic point of view, the population to be assessed has to be very carefully scrutinized.

Another clinical issue related to disease ascertainment in older persons is whether some patients, particularly those who are frail or who have multiple conditions, are treated with less diagnostic intensity when presenting with comparable signs or symptoms. For example, the likelihood of hospitalization after a stroke appears to decline with advancing age in some communities. Such clinical decisions may or may not be appropriate, but they may alter the rate at which full, verified diagnoses are made, and thus account for some interpopulation variation in the frequency or reliability of certain conditions. Diagnostic and disease ascertainment are also likely related to fiscal and geographic access to health services. In the United States, where economic access to hospital care is nearly universal when reaching 65 years of age, disease rates in that age group may appear, to some extent, artificially higher than among those below 65 years, who do not always have such access. Finally, elderly decedents are least likely to receive an autopsy, and thus will have less verification or addition of diagnoses to the death certificate that come with this procedure.

In view of the complexity of ascertaining health status in older adults, there has been concern about whether estimation of health status in this population is adversely affected by self-report, compared to physician diagnosis of disease. Recent studies, in fact, suggest that self-report of disease prevalence can be highly reliable and valid for common chronic diseases. For example, Bush et al reported a 76 percent to 98 percent agreement in persons 65 years and older between self-report and medical record report for eight common chronic diseases: angina, cancer (any), cataracts, diabetes, fractures, hypertension, myocardial infarction, and stroke (Bush et al, 1989). Seeman et al reported a high level of agreement between respondent self-report of conditions and/or symptoms and their medical records (Seeman et al, 1989). Therefore, the reliability of self-report of well-recognized chronic diseases appears to be high for older adults. (See further discussion in Chapter 6.)

The study of illness in older adults offers many challenges to the epidemiologist in terms of both accurate ascertainment of health status and its components and meaningful interpretation of findings. Development of better methods of ascertainment depends on epidemiologists appreciating the clinical aspects of disease and disability in older adults and how they differ from those of young and middle-aged adults. Utilizing this perspective, epidemiologists have an opportunity to understand incidence and prognosis of chronic diseases and their etiology and import in a way that clinicians cannot. Because of the slow, progressive nature of chronic disease, patients often present to a clinician for evaluation only when the symptoms become intolerable or when they become clearly ill. This may be particularly so for older adults, who are more likely to attribute symptoms to the aging process and not bring them to medical attention (Minaker and Rowe, 1985). Thus, the spectrum of many diseases, their functional deficits, and natural history remain to be determined in population-based studies. Etiologic factors identified in such studies will improve clinical understanding of effective interventions to improve the health status of older adults.

REFERENCES

Atkinson RM (1988). Alcoholism in the elderly population. Mayo Clin Proc 63:825–829.

Bayer AJ, Chadha JS, Farag RR, Pathy J (1986). Changing presentation of myocardial infarction with increasing old age. J Am Geriatr Soc 34:263–266.

Bush TL, Miller SR, Golden AL, Hale WE (1989). Self-report and medical record report agreement of selected medical conditions in the elderly. Am J Public Health 79:1554–1556.

Evans JG (1984). Prevention of age-associated loss of autonomy: Epidemiological approaches. J Chron Dis 37:353–363.

Fried LP, Stover DJ, King DE, Lodder F (1991). Diagnosis of illness presentation in the elderly. J Geriatr Soc 39 (in press).

Fried LP, Bush TL (1988). Morbidity as a focus of preventive health care in the elderly. Epidemiol Rev 10:48–64.

Guralnik JM, LaCroix AZ, Everett DF, Kovar MG (1989). Aging in the eighties: The prevalence of comorbidity and association with disability. Advance Data from Vital and Health Statistics, No. 170. National Center for Health Statistics, Hyattsville, MD.

Guthrie A, Elliott WA (1980). The nature and reversibility of cerebral impairment in alcoholism. J Stud Alochol, 41(1):147–155.

Irvine PW (1984). Patterns of disease: The challenge of multiple illness. In Cassel CK, Walsh JR (eds), Geriatric Medicine, Vol. 2, pp. 82–88.

Jajich CK, Ostfeld AM, Freeman DH, Jr. (1984). Smoking and coronary heart disease mortality in the elderly. JAMA 262:2831–2834.

Kane RA, Kane RL (1981). Assessing the Elderly: A Practical Guide to Measurement. Lexington, MA, D.C. Heath and Co., p. 63.

McDowell I, Newell C (1987). Measuring Health: A Guide to Rating Scales and Questionnaires. New York, Oxford University Press, pp. 23–26.

Minaker KL, Rowe J (1985). Health and disease among the oldest old: A clinical perspective. MMFQ/Health Soc 62(2):324–349.

National Center for Health Statistics (1986a). Advance report of final mortality statistics, 1984. Hyattsville, MD, September 26 (monthly vital statistics report, Vol. 35, No. 6, Suppl. 2) DHHS Pub. No. (PHS)86-1120.

National Center for Health Statistics, (1986b). Moss AJ, Parson VL. Current estimates from the National Health Interview Survey, United States, 1985. Vital and Health Statistics, Ser. 10, No. 160, pp. 13, 82–83, 106, 118. DHHS Pub. No. (PHS)8601588. Public Health Service, Washington, DC, September.

National Center for Health Statistics (1986c). Health, United States. DHHS Pub. No. (PHS) 87-1232. Public Health Service, Washington, DC, December, Table 64.

National Center for Health Statistics, Havlik RJ, Liu BM, Kovar MG, et al. (1987a). Health Statistics on Older Persons, United States, 1986. Vital and Health Statistics, Ser. 3, No. 25. DHHS Pub. No. (PHS)87-1409. Public Health Service, Washington, DC, June, p. 49.

National Center for Health Statistics, Hing E (1987b). Use of nursing homes by the elderly. Preliminary data from the 1985 National Nursing Home Survey. Advance Data from Vital and Health Statistics, No. 135. DHHS Pub. No. (PHS)87-1250. Public Health Service, Hyattsville, MD, May 14.

National Center for Health Statistics (1987c). 1986 Summary: National Hospital Discharge Survey. Advance Data from Vital and Health Statistics, No. 145. DHHS Pub. No. (PHS)87-1250, Public Health Service, Hyattsville, MD.

Rabin DL, Stockton P (1987). Long-Term Care for the Elderly: A Factbook. New York, Oxford University Press, pp. 6, 58, 123.

Samiy AH, (1983). Clinical manifestations of disease in the elderly. Med Clin North Am 67(2):333–344.

Seeman TE, Guralnik JM, Kaplan GA, Knudsen L, Cohen R (1989). The health consequences of multiple morbidity in the elderly. The Alameda County Study. J Aging Health 1:50–66.

U.S. Department of Health and Human Services (1982). Smoking and health: A report of the Surgeon General. DHHS Pub. No. (PHS)82:50179.

U.S. Senate Special Committee on Aging (1987–88). Aging America, 1988: Trends and Projections. U.S. Department of Health and Human Services, Washington, DC.

Vestal RE (1978). Drug use in the elderly: A review of problems and special considerations. Drugs 16:358–382.

Weissert W, Wan T, Livieratos B, Katz S (1980). Effects and costs of day-care services for the chronically ill. Med. Care 18:567–84.

3

Risk Factors and the Study of Prevention in the Elderly: Methodological Issues

GEORGE A. KAPLAN, MARY N. HAAN,
AND RICHARD D. COHEN

The striking changes in the age structure of the populations of most economically developed countries, particularly with respect to the proportion of older persons, have been widely noted (Rice and Feldman, 1983; Siegal, 1980). The reasons for these changes in the age structure of the population are not well understood, but they undoubtedly involve both decreases in the fertility of younger persons and increases in the survival of older persons. These increases in survival of older persons are striking.

Figure 3-1 compares the U.S. mortality rates for those 65–74, 75–84, and 85 or more years of age during 1950–1986 (NCHS, 1989). Over this period of 36 years, mortality rates declined by 43 percent, 32 percent, and 24 percent, respectively, in the three age groups. Ninety-three percent of the decline from 1950 to 1986 in all-cause mortality rates at ages 65–74 was due to declines in the rates of cardiovascular and cerebrovascular diseases (Figure 3-2). For those 75–84 and 85+ years old, the corresponding percentages were 87 percent and 67 percent.

These substantial declines in age-specific mortality rates provide the impetus to examine the role of primary and secondary prevention in improving the health of the elderly. So does the demographic imperative of increasing numbers of older persons. Preventive approaches traditionally have been based on interventions targeting factors previously identified as associated with increased risk for a particular disease outcome or event. Unfortunately, relatively few studies have been devoted to describing the role of risk factors among the elderly, and even fewer have involved controlled interventions aimed at risk factors.

Nonetheless, the evidence that does exist offers support for the idea that preventive activities can improve the health of older persons (Castelli et al, 1989; Kaplan and Haan, 1989; Stamler, 1988). In what follows, a number of important considerations in the examination and interpretation of risk factor associations in older populations will be discussed. These issues range from the consequences of time of measurement of risk factors to the choice of analytic techniques to the biological and social nature of the outcome being studied.

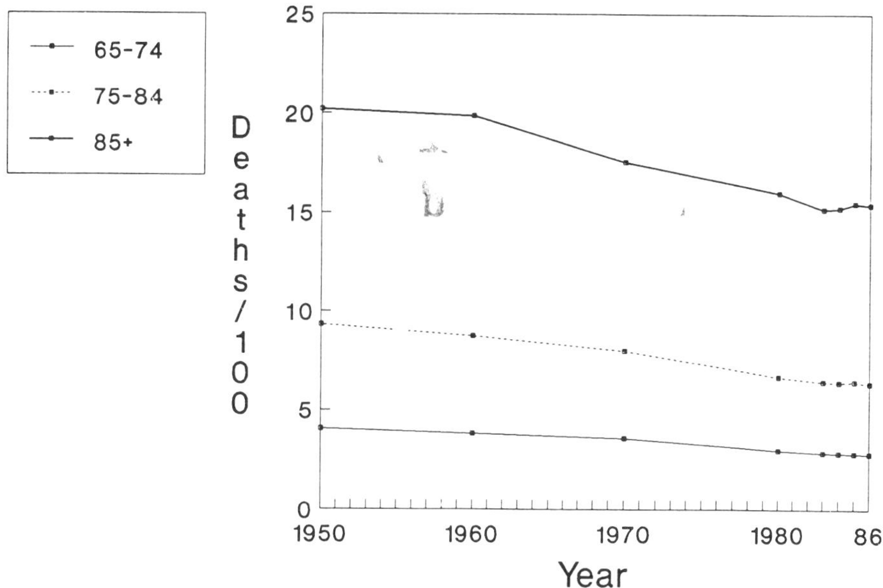

Figure 3-1 Mortality rates from all causes by age and year (United States, 1950–1986).

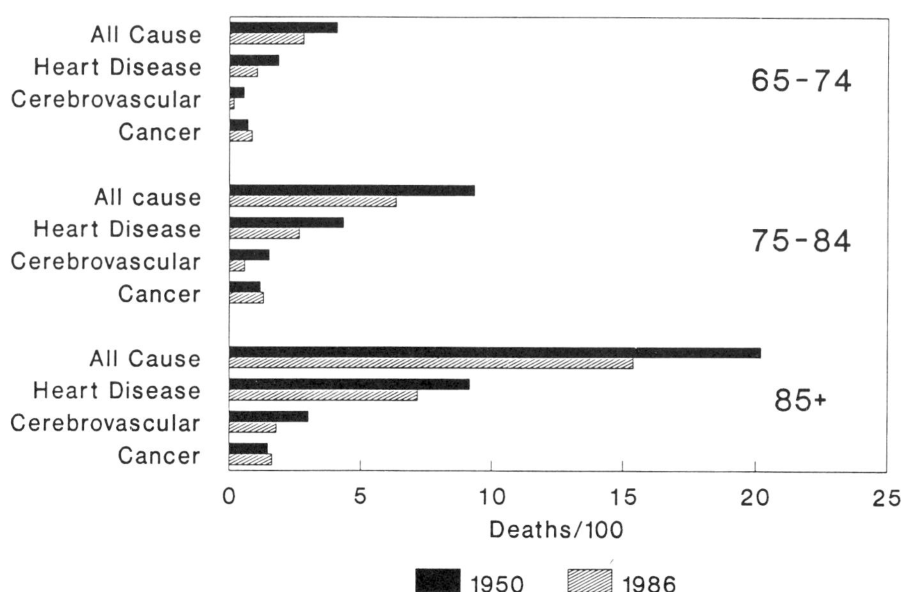

Figure 3-2 Mortality rates from various causes, 1950 vs. 1986 (United States, males and females).

A SCHEMATIC VIEW

To appreciate properly the complexities in the study of risk factors in older persons, it may be helpful to think of the disease process being studied as a stream with a particular course over time, paralleled by a road representing the aging process. With the passage of time the stream widens, indicating increased severity, and at some point there may be clinically significant events or death, which might be indicated by rapids or a waterfall. In some diseases, such as malignancies, it may be helpful to divide the course into periods of initiation, promotion, and progression (Farber, 1988). In some cases the disease may progress over long periods. For example, many cancers may have a latency period of 10–40 years, a time span also consistent with the development of many diseases of the cardiovascular system. For deaths associated with pneumonia, for example, the time course may be considerably shorter, although there may be a longer-acting process of nonspecific vulnerability, frailty, or otherwise compromised functioning that acts in the background. For most chronic diseases prevalent among older persons, there will have been a considerable period of disease progression before clinical recognition occurs, either because of the appearance of symptoms or because of a frank event. Routinely applied diagnostic tools may also result in clinical recognition without the occurrence of symptoms or events.

Also important to consider are the age-related physiologic and psychosocial changes, possibly unrelated to disease, that occur with the passage of time. This could be conceptualized as a road that moves parallel to but starts earlier than the disease stream. Although it is important to emphasize that disease effects need to be distinguished, whenever possible, from the primary, nondisease, manifestations of aging, it is also true that the development of clinically relevant disease needs to be considered in the context of aging. Aging-related changes may lead directly to alterations in disease risk, or they may interact with other factors to modify disease risk. For example, the older artery may be more susceptible to atherogenic influences (Hazzard, 1989), or age-related declines in pulmonary functioning, unrelated to disease, may lead to more severe consequences of acute bacterial pneumonias (Rowe and Wang, 1988). What is not clear is whether these age-related changes represent a "pure" aging effect or are inextricably intertwined with prior risk factor exposures and their pathophysiologic effects.

Finally, whether a prospective or retrospective study is being done, it is generally only possible to observe a limited portion of this unfolding process, ranging usually from perhaps months to a decade or so. Thus, the follow-up, or follow-back, time of a study will expose only a limited portion of the disease and aging processes to investigative scrutiny, and different parts of these processes will be exposed, depending on when the study starts. It is important to realize that the length of the study and where it begins and ends relative to both the disease and aging process may have a great influence on what is discovered with respect to risk factor–disease associations. Thus, there are three time-related processes simultaneously taking place related to (1) age-related changes not related to disease, (2) the development of disease and its consequences, and (3) the length of follow-up and the age range included in the study. Although there is currently insufficient information to understand the relationships fully between these three processes, consideration of many of the issues involved in studying risk factors among older persons will be facilitated by keeping these three processes in mind.

What Is to Be Prevented?

In chronic diseases manifested at older ages, considerable pathophysiologic changes may already have occurred. Therefore, risk factors in the elderly will be likely to accelerate transitions from preclinical disease to clinically significant disease. Most interventions traditionally focus on the prevention of pathophysiologic damage through risk factor reductions. In the elderly, although this still remains a goal, efforts may also focus on preventing or slowing the rate of disease progression and thereby influencing the rate of transition from preclinical to clinically manifested disease. Screening of asymptomatic patients and identification and prevention of risk factors that may precipitate such transitions are examples of such interventions.

To take atherosclerotic heart disease as an example, significant risk factors, such as smoking, at older ages, may be more closely related to precipitants of ischemic events than to the atherogenic process itself. Similarly, risk factors for osteoporotic-related hip fractures may be more closely related to endogenous factors, such as those related to balance and response to falling, and exogenous variables affecting the opportunities for falling, such as those related to physical hazards, than to the exact degree of osteoporosis.

Thus, the goal of prevention might be conceptualized, in the elderly, as the prevention or delay of the further progression of disease to a clinically significant event (e.g., the prevention or delay of the precipitants of such events). Such a view means that the notion of "pure" disease incidence in older persons may not be meaningful.

In addition to attention to the progression of chronic disease and their transitions, preventive approaches (and the associated search for risk factors) can profitably focus on many other aspects of the health of older persons. Foremost among these are those related to functional health. Functional health outcomes reflect the ability of individuals to perform activities and roles that are part of living independently and productively. These abilities strongly influence quality of life, which is so critical to the continuing health and well-being of older persons. Because functional health involves a complex mix of physiologic, behavioral, cognitive, and social factors, it is likely to be multifactorial in causation, and involve considerable interaction between determinants.

Some functional outcomes, such as urinary incontinence, may develop over shorter periods of time but are likely to reflect the influence of other long-acting chronic processes that increase vulnerability or susceptibility. In the case of infectious diseases, the same pattern holds, with susceptibility being influenced by the impaired functioning of damaged organ systems and compromised immune functioning (Garibaldi et al, 1988). In addition to being influenced by traumatic causes, functional changes often result from age-related physiologic limitations interacting with chronic debilitating disease. With respect to the "stream" metaphor, one might think of tributaries that join with other ongoing disease processes or exposures to precipitate additional clinical events.

Finally, there is a broad set of biopsychosocial outcomes that may be preventable to a significant extent. Examples of these include institutionalization, depression, frailty, social isolation, and cognitive declines. As with functional outcomes, these are likely to have several causes, reflecting complex admixtures of physiologic capacity; physical health; motivation; economic, social, and psychological resources; and social policy. Again, there is likely to be considerable interdependence and interaction between these different classes of risk factors.

Issues Related to Risk Factor Measurement

Time of Measurement

Ideally, one would like to have complete risk factor information for an individual, obtained by repetitive measurement and/or surveillance covering the total period of time relevant to the disease process being studied. This is seldom, if ever, possible. Without such a comprehensive evaluation, a series of tradeoffs must be made, the consequences of which have not often been studied. Risk factor levels obtained at older ages may not necessarily reflect characteristic values over the preceding years, having been influenced by changes in underlying function, by undetected disease, or by social processes. Thus, an 80-year-old who reports being physically inactive may have been active previously and changed because of poor health or for other reasons. Since this important issue of the correlation, or tracking, of risk factor levels over time has not been well studied in older persons, it is impossible to assess the extent of misclassification of risk factor levels that arises from lack of data on constancy or change in risk factor levels. Presumably, such effects are minimized if the follow-up period is short. However, the general impact of such misclassification is to dilute the magnitude of the association between risk factors and outcomes.

One possible solution is the retrospective recall of risk factor exposure levels. However, the validity of retrospectively reported risk factor information obtained from older persons is probably variable, and the collection of such data would be lengthy and complex, so such information will not necessarily help. Given the possible link between levels of cognitive functioning and underlying chronic diseases, unreliability and recall bias are likely to be introduced. Information on blood pressure, cholesterol, and many other laboratory measures is usually not available retrospectively.

In some cases such information is available, for example, for long-term participants in a study or for long-term members of a health maintenance organization. However, it is a complex choice to determine whether it is more accurate and effective to use information on risk factors collected earlier or later, an average level or a cumulative level, or measures of change or rate of change. Only a few studies have examined this issue in any detail, and few have studied older persons (Harris et al, 1985). The most important issues may involve consideration of which underlying disease processes and outcomes are being examined. For disease outcomes that involve chronic, cumulative processes it may be best to use as much information as is available, while recognizing at the same time that the current level may be more closely related to the triggering of clinical events. For example, if one were examining the impact of relative weight on development of osteoarthritis, it is probably more relevant to use measures that reflect cumulative exposure than it is to use current weight, particularly given the weight changes that occur with aging. On the other hand, current weight might be a stronger predictor than previous weight of current level of physical functioning.

To add complexity, it should not be assumed that exposures simply accumulate and "spill over" one day into a clinical event when some maximum tolerance has been reached. Although this may be true, it is also possible that that exposure may interact with endogenous susceptibility, which may change with age.

Quality of Risk Factor Measurement

Another area in which little information is available is that of quality of risk factor measurement. Although it has not been well documented, there is some reason to believe that, for some measures, there is an increase in within-person variability in some physiologic functions that reflects a pattern of increased "homeostenosis" (Besdine, 1988a). For example, it is believed that attenuated baroreflex sensitivity, perhaps related to arterial stiffening, may lead to increased lability in blood pressure in older persons (Rowe and Lipsitz, 1988). Without careful standardization, attention to repeated measurements, and control to reduce this variability, greater imprecision in the measurement of blood pressure in older persons would result.

Impact of Health Status on Risk Factors

The high prevalence of existing chronic diseases among the elderly (Irvine, 1990) means that the magnitude of risk factor levels may often reflect the impact of disease on the risk factor. For example, one would have to be very cautious in interpreting data for older persons that indicated that sedentary levels of physical activity were associated with decreased pulmonary functioning, unless it was possible to eliminate the possibility that low levels of pulmonary function led to reductions in physical activity. Similar problems would apply to a study that indicated that obesity was associated with greater risk of osteoarthritis, since osteoarthritis could lead to decreased levels of physical activity, which could lead to higher rates of obesity. Measures of weight, lipids, dietary intake, immune functioning, metabolic activity, hormones, depression, and many other risk factors can be influenced by diagnosed or occult disease. With diagnosed and treated disease, there may be considerable impact of medications on risk factor levels. In addition, behavioral changes associated with aging, such as becoming a widower, may alter risk factor levels as well. Where information is available on diagnosed diseases, several analytic strategies are available (cf. the later sections "Selection of Study Subjects" and "Issues Related to Analysis and Interpetation"); however, the high burden of preclinical disease at older ages leads to great difficulty in properly accounting for the impact of disease on risk factors. Information that suggests monotonic relationships between risk factor levels and disease severity can be helpful in this regard. For example, if information on the level of a risk factor is available for a population of older persons for whom a good deal of information on cardiovascular status is available and if the risk levels do not vary by cardiovascular status, then an association between that risk factor and some outcome is not likely to reflect the impact of cardiovascular disease on that outcome.

Issues Related to Study Design

Length of Follow-up

In a prospective study, the length of follow-up can have considerable impact on the observed association between a risk factor and an outcome. In fact, the assumption of a constant risk association over time, which underlies some of the currently favored analytic techniques such as proportional hazards regression (Cox, 1972), may not be appropriate. To the extent that information is only available on risk factor levels at the beginning of the study and the follow-up time is long, misclassification bias, as mentioned earlier, is a potential problem. Although the subject has not been carefully studied, it is logical to postulate that short follow-up periods, such as the two-year incidence periods used in many analyses of the Framingham study, may be more likely to reflect recent effects on late-stage pathophysiologic processes than long-acting chronic processes. Of course, if the risk factor "tracks" strongly over both the long and short term, it would be very difficult to distinguish between "early" and "late" effects.

There has been very little examination of these potential biases in studying risk factor–disease associations among older groups. In one study using the follow-up experience of 49–82-year-old members of the Framingham cohort, there was considerable diminution in the strength of the association between high-density lipoprotein cholesterol (HDL-C) and systolic blood pressure and the incidence of coronary heart disease when follow-up times of four and 12 years were compared (Castelli et al, 1986). The strength of the association between HDL-C and coronary heart disease incidence decreased by 36 percent and 22 percent for men and women, respectively, when the two follow-up periods were compared. For systolic blood pressure, the corresponding figures were 39 percent and 14 percent. These diminutions in the strength of the association, with increasing follow-up time, may stem from a variety of factors, including those related to lack of tracking of the risk factor, selective mortality of those at high risk (to be discussed later), changes in the physiologic impact of the risk factor, and changes in the clinical manifestations of the disease.

Selection of Study Subjects

It is commonplace in the design of epidemiologic studies to caution that choice of subject or patient population can have a major impact on whether associations are observed between a risk factor and an outcome. Such considerations become even more important in studies of the elderly. Foremost among these are concerns that involve inclusion or exclusion based on the health status of the study participants. Although it will be possible to find individuals free of a specific disease at older ages, disease-free persons represent an increasingly selected group, and the associations observed in such a group may not characterize the majority of individuals of that age. The impact of such selection on the observation of a disease–risk factor association could be considerable. Furthermore, there is substantial increase in the prevalence of co-morbidities among older persons. Persons apparently free of one disease may be likely to suffer from another that could have an impact on the risk factor–disease association being considered. Even those who have not suffered a clinically defined event may have considerable preclinical disease. Also, the existence of subclinical illness increases with age.

In short, prevalent illness and its treatment may confound the risk factor–disease association, if the study includes older persons with prevalent chronic disease. Carefully collecting illness history and treatment and assessing clinical and subclinical disease states can help mitigate this confounding influence. With such information, analyses can be stratified on health status information and/or risk factor–health status interactions can be examined. Where possible, it is also informative to conduct analyses on a series of graded outcomes. Thus, Guralnik and Kaplan (1989) were able to show that a set of risk factors was associated with risk of death, with low and intermediate levels of physical functioning, and with high levels of physical functioning.

Case-Control Studies

Although for a variety of outcomes, such as Alzheimer's disease, there may be no practical alternative to the use of case-control studies, there can be methodological problems in such studies. For example, Sackett (1979) identified a very large number of potential biases in case-control studies. Here we will only mention briefly some of the more important issues. Measurement of current risk factor levels in cases will always include the possibility of the disease affecting the risk factor. Assessment of previous exposure levels may be even more problematic among older populations because of age- and disease-related increases in memory problems, or the need to use proxies as a source of information. There does not seem to have been any direct examination of these issues with respect to older populations, although age-specific analyses of some studies would present such opportunities. In cases where the disease itself interferes with the ability to report risk factor information, proxy informants are necessary, and there is beginning to be an empirical base for evaluating the validity of such information (Magaziner, Chapter 8).

With respect to choice of controls, the usual controversies arise. The most important biases with respect to older populations are probably those related to the health status of the controls. Although it is tempting to use controls that are identified by virtue of their contact with the health care system, the high rates of morbidity in such groups and the fact that many chronic diseases share common risk factors and pathophysiologic processes will tend to bias the measure of association toward the null. With respect to population samples for controls, the choice of the population needs to be carefully considered. For example, inclusion or exclusion of age-eligible persons who are in nursing homes may affect the observed association. The issue of the representativeness of controls in an elderly population is more profoundly influenced by consideration of health status than it is in younger populations. Indeed, it may be difficult, it not impossible, for some studies to obtain older controls who are disease-free.

Issues Related to Analysis and Interpretation

Choice of Analytic Method and of Measure of Association

As in any epidemiologic study, the choice of analytic method and measure of association should be carried out carefully, mindful of the underlying assumptions. A number of such issues are particularly relevant to studies of older populations. High event rates in some studies of older persons, because of advanced age and/or long follow-up, will negate the useful approximation of the relative risk by the odds ratio. In mortality studies, high rates of competing causes will lead to substantial censoring. Thus, survival techniques that can accommodate such losses are preferable. However, the assumptions of survival techniques such as the proportional hazards model (Cox, 1972) should be tested whenever possible. For example, as noted earlier, the assumption by the proportional hazard model of a constant relative hazard over the entire follow-up period may not be appropriate when used with older groups and high event rates.

Because of the high rates of chronic conditions and medication use, careful consideration of confounding or effect modification by co-existing conditions and their treatment needs to be carefully considered. The structure of multivariate models used to assess the impact of potential confounders or effect modifiers needs to be considered. Analyses utilizing stratification of co-morbidity status or risk factor interaction with morbidity status may be useful. Although it is tempting to use indices that summarize the presence or absence of a large number of possible co-morbid conditions, such techniques can lead to an underestimation of the extent of confounding or effect modification due to these conditions. The use and construction of such indices should be informed by biologic and physiologic knowledge whenever possible.

The choice of which measure of association to use will follow from the selection of a study design and particular analytic tools. However, it should be recognized that different measures of association can reveal different age-related patterns. Figure 3-3(a,b) presents the results of six years of follow-up, by level of total serum cholesterol (<182 mg/dl vs. ≥182 mg/dl), for the over 350,000 persons who were screened for the MRFIT study (Stamler, 1988). As can be seen in Figure 3-3a, the six-year risk of coronary heart disease death rises monotonically as a function of age at entry into the study. Although the slope is steeper for the high-risk group (≥182 mg/dl), inspection of Figure 3-3b shows that the relative risk is decreasing, from 3.3 to 1.8, with increasing age for those over age 40. When the difference in risks between the high- and low-risk groups, the excess risk, is considered, the opposite pattern is seen. Excess risk rises, almost linearly, from 124.8 per 100,000 at age 35–39 to 705.0 per 100,000 for the oldest group. Thus, very different conclusions would be drawn concerning the association between levels of serum cholesterol and risk of coronary death, depending on which measure of association is used.

Both the relative risk and the excess risk can obscure potentially important relationships that are seen when the data in Figure 3-3a are examined. The interaction between age and the risk factor may be important information that would be missed if only the relative risk was considered. Since different approaches to modeling the interaction test particular forms of interaction, they should not replace actually inspecting the absolute risks. Therefore, it is important to consider the absolute risk levels. While the relative risk is lowest in the 55–57-year-old group, the excess risk is highest. This increase in the excess risk is of great importance from a preventive point of view, because it implies that for each 100,000 persons in a particular age group, more coronary deaths could be prevented by cholesterol control in the oldest age group.

The Meaning of Age

It is important to remember the fundamental interrelationships between age, period, and cohort (Kleinbaum et al, 1982; Susser, 1973). Exposure levels to a given risk factor

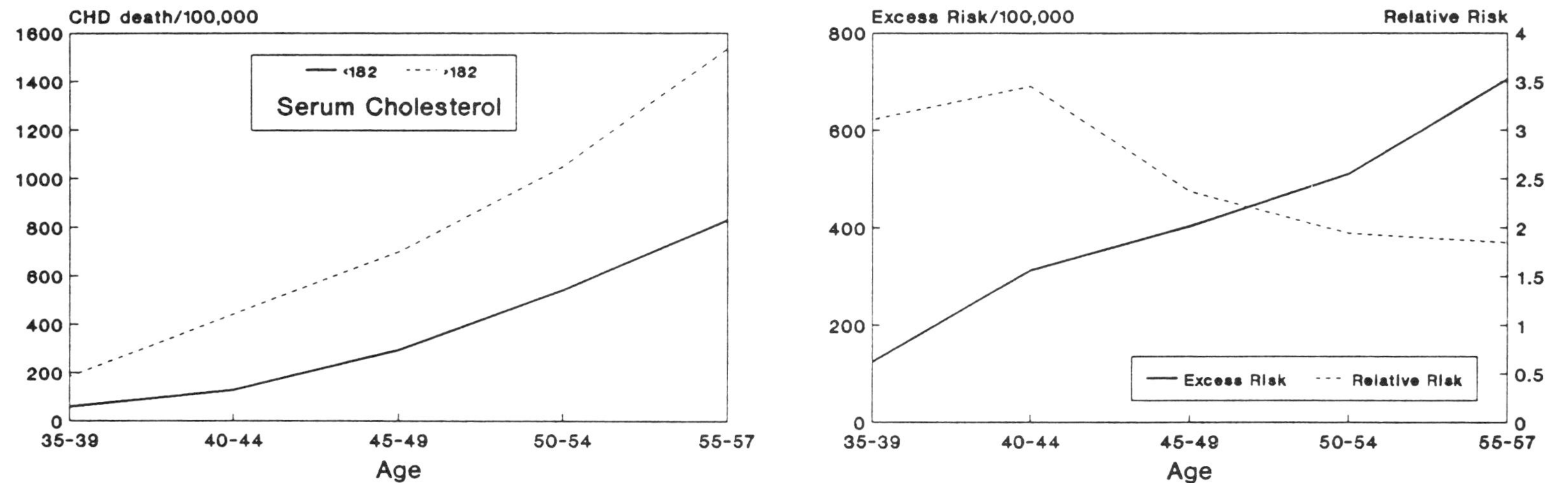

Figure 3-3 Absolute, excess, and relative risk of coronary death (6 yr) elevated serum cholesterol (356,222 MRFIT screenees, 35–57 years old).

in a given age group are also a function of the historical period and birth cohort to which that group belongs. Changes in the strength of an association with increasing age may be confounded by the effects of period and cohort. In general, any observation of one of the effects will involve confounding of the other two. Although various statistical techniques have been proposed to deal with these interdependencies, they are fundamentally inseparable because of the linear dependence of each variable on the other two. This can create problems in the interpretation of age-related changes in the association between a risk factor and an outcome because it is not known if a cohort or period effect is being observed. If there are period or cohort effects, then analyses based on the accumulated age-specific experience of a fixed cohort moving through time may misrepresent the nature of the association. For example, to accumulate enough persons in each age group, some analyses of the Framingham study data have examined biennial incidence of coronary heart disease accumulated for two-year periods starting when a person reached a particular age (Kannel and Vokonas, 1986). This means that someone who reached 70 years old in 1960 is considered the same as someone who reached that age in 1980. Interpretation of an age-related decline in the association between a risk factor such as smoking and coronary heart disease is clouded by the real possibility of cohort–period effects. Potentially informative approaches to this problem involve explicit modeling of period effects (Kleinbaum et al, 1982) or examination of age-specific risk factor–disease associations at different points during the extended follow-up. It also may be informative to compare period and cohort differences in exposure to particular risk factors, especially when considering changes in the strength of an association and outcome with increasing age.

Co-morbidity

With increasing age, there are increasing levels of co-morbidity. For example, in the Alameda County Study, 41 percent of those 60 years old or older reported three or more chronic conditions and symptoms (Seeman et al, 1989). Many symptoms and conditions were found to have substantial rates of co-occurrence. For example, although high blood pressure was reported by 26 percent of those over 60 years old in 1965, in 70 percent of the cases it was mentioned along with two or more other conditions or symptoms. These levels of co-morbidity have significant consequences. In the same analyses, those who were over age 60 and who reported three or more chronic conditions and symptoms, compared to those who reported none, had 25 percent higher risk of death over the next 17 years, 680 percent higher risk of reporting two or more additional morbidities nine years later, and 224 percent higher risk of reporting high levels of depressive symptoms nine years later.

These high levels of co-morbidity complicate the examination of risk factor associations with particular disease outcomes for a variety of reasons. Treatment of a co-morbidity can often have an effect on the morbidity under examination, changing its mode of presentation or timing. In addition, there may be disease–disease interactions (Besdine, 1988a; Korenchevsky, 1961). Also, a given risk factor may be associated with more than one outcome, and the presence of the co-morbid condition may influence the severity or progression of the outcome under study. The end result is that it is difficult to study the "pure" association between a particular risk factor and a "single" disease end point in older populations. Indeed, given these interconnecting patterns of morbidities, some of which are consequences of one another, it may be misleading to look for associations with single end points. For example, although it would be statistically possible to model the impact of a particular risk factor on functional ability while adjusting for the impact of various prevalent chronic and acute conditions, one would, in effect, be studying impaired functioning independent of many of the factors that simultaneously present themselves.

Related concerns apply to the examination of risk factors associated with deaths from particular causes among the aged. In one autopsy study of decedents older than 85 years old, no acceptable cause of death was found in 26 percent of the cases (Kohn, 1982). The reporting of co-morbidities on the death certificate is quite high and appears to have risen over time (Israel et al, 1986; Manton and Stallard, 1984). In 1979, more than one cause of death was mentioned on over 70 percent of U.S. death certificates (Israel et al, 1986). (This topic is discussed more fully in Chapter 17.) These patterns reflect the extensive amount of co-existing disease that make assignment of an underlying cause of death at the older ages so difficult. Risk factor associations based on analyses of multiple causes of death information or on all causes may more adequately reflect the nature of the terminal process in a substantial proportion of deaths in the elderly.

It may also be important to consider as an important outcome the co-occurrence of symptoms and conditions that may be indicative of a general systems breakdown leading to frailty and, ultimately, death. Studies of risk factor associations with systemic, overarching changes in functioning, across organ systems, might prove valuable.

Competing Risks

In any prospective epidemiologic study, the observation of an association between a risk factor and an outcome is potentially influenced by other outcomes that might remove (censor) the individual from observation. For example, an individual participating in a study of risk factors for lung cancer might die from cardiovascular causes and therefore not live long enough for an underlying tumor to be detected. Other sources of censoring include institutionalization or dementia, making the collection of data impossible. This problem of competing risks can be handled in a number of ways. If the risk of the competing cause is quite low relative to the risk of the cause under study, then the competing cause will have very little effect. Life table approaches to the competing risk problem have typically assumed, for computational simplicity, that causes of death are independent. In older populations, the high rates of interrelated co-morbidities make such assumptions unreasonable. Fortunately, other life table–based methods that do not assume independence of causes are available (Manton and Stallard, 1988).

The censoring of individuals from a study due to competing risks can be dealt with using other survival methods, such as the Cox proportional hazard model, which allow an individual to remain at risk so long as they have not contracted a competing cause. Thus, until the time of diagnosis or death from the competing cause, they contribute person-years of exposure to the analysis. Although this is a convenient solution to the problem of censoring, as mentioned earlier, the assumption of a constant relative hazard in the proportional hazards model may not be appropriate for some studies with older persons. If the overall risk level is high either because of age or because of long follow-up time, the assumption of proportionality will need to be formally or graphically tested (Kalbfleisch and Prentice, 1980).

Competing outcomes can also introduce problems due to what could be called "interfering risks." In these cases, which might be quite common among older populations, contracting another disease and/or treatment for that disease may have an impact on the relationship between the risk factor and the index disease under study. Analytically, this is a much more difficult issue. One solution is to use a form of the proportional hazard model that includes information on a potentially interfering cause and allows for time-dependent covariates. Thus, if and when the individual contracts the interfering cause, the value of that covariate is altered to reflect that change. Another possibility is to use techniques, such as the Grade of Membership model, that would allow various combinations of primary and competing or interfering causes to form separate sets (Manton and Stallard, 1988). Whatever approach is taken, it should be recognized that the interdependence of disease outcomes may be an important part of the chronic disease process in older persons, in itself worthy of study.

Reasons for Declines in Risk Factor–Disease Association with Increasing Age

A number of prospective studies have indicated that the strength of association between a risk factor may decline with increasing age. Although other patterns have also been found (Kaplan et al, 1987), the pattern is common enough to warrant discussion. There are four major reasons that such a pattern of declining strength of association with increasing age might occur. The first and most widely offered explanation one can call a "survivor" explanation. Figure 3-4 presents, schematically, the nature of this explanation. Consider two groups, one that is exposed to the risk factor and one that is not. Rather than viewing the exposed group, and for that matter the unexposed group, as homogeneous, they are seen as heterogeneous, composed of subgroups. In the simplest case, the exposed group is considered to consist of two groups, one that is "susceptible" to the risk factor and one that is not. The risk level of the nonsusceptibles in the exposed group is assumed to be equivalent to that of the unexposed group. Over

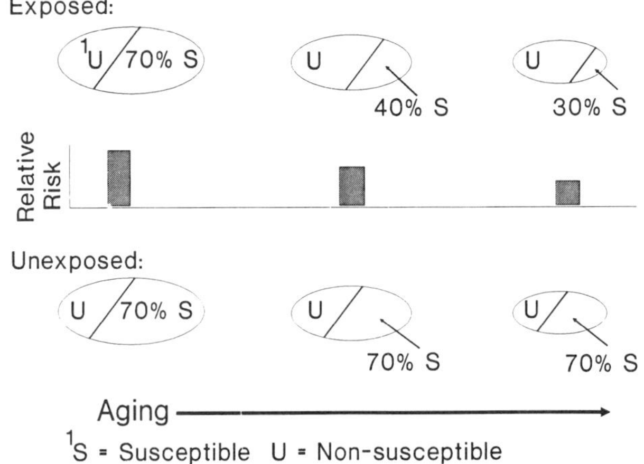

Figure 3-4 Reduction in relative risk with deletion of susceptible.

time, with aging, there is a progressive elimination of the susceptibles from the exposed group, leaving a group that becomes more and more like the unexposed group with respect to level of risk. As the two groups become more and more alike, the risk factor association weakens accordingly, ultimately reaching the null level if all the susceptibles are removed from the exposed group.

If a risk factor is associated with a fatal, or otherwise censoring, disease outcome, then over time, with increasing age, there will be a selective removal of the exposed from the population. However, this fact does not, in itself, account for diminished strength of association between a risk factor and an outcome with increasing age. The critical element of the selection explanation for decrements in strength of association with age is a postulation of susceptible and unsusceptible persons in the exposed group. Although factors related to susceptibility may exist, without their specification, the explanation becomes unprovable. That is, the lack of a risk factor effect in the exposed group is "explained" by postulating that the group comes to be composed more and more of persons who are not affected by the risk factor. What is needed to make the selection argument useful in understanding decreases in the strength of an association with increasing age is a specification of the genetic, biological, behavioral, social, psychological, and other factors associated with variations in susceptibility to a risk factor. This could be conceptualized as the identification of "risk factors" for susceptibility and can be studied using stratification or interaction approaches.

There are other possible explanations for declines in strength of association with increasing age. Figure 3-5 shows two situations in which the risk factor would have weaker association among older persons. In each of these, the risk level as a function of age for an exposed and unexposed group is presented. In Figure 3-5a, although the absolute level of risk is lower for the unexposed group, risk is rising faster with age in the unexposed group. Although it indicates a situation in which the risk factor effect declines with increasing age, this interaction with age could be interpreted as suggesting that the risk factor actually "protects" against the effect of aging. Figure 3-5b presents a common example of a ceiling effect that can be found when risk measures are used. If a high proportion of the exposed group is contracting the disease, then the ability of the risk level to rise further is severely constrained. In the extreme example, if everyone who has been exposed has contracted the disease, then the relative risk will have to decrease with increasing age, as more and more of the nonexposed persons get the disease. Depending on the age of the population being studied, the length of follow-up, and other factors, substantial death and event rates have been observed in prospective studies of older populations. For example, in a study using the Alameda

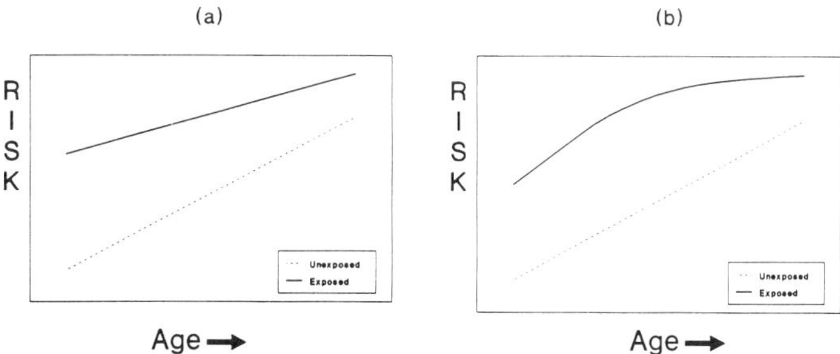

Figure 3-5 Hypothetical increases in risk in two groups.

County cohort, there was an 80 percent mortality rate in a 17-year follow-up of persons 70–94 years old (Kaplan et al, 1987). In the Framingham study, the eight-year risk of incident cardiovascular disease in 70-year-olds who smoked and who had a systolic blood pressure >195 mm, serum cholesterol >335 mg/dl, positive response to a glucose intolerance test, and evidence of left-ventricular hypertrophy was 82 percent (Kannel and Gordon, 1978). Inspection of the examples in Figure 3-5 should emphasize the importance of examining absolute levels of risk by age and risk factor status, rather than only ratio or difference measures of association. Without inspection of the risk or rate levels that contribute to such age-related measures of association, it is difficult to interpret changes in the measures.

Fourth, reductions in the strength of a risk factor's association with a disease end point with increasing age may also represent the changing impact of the risk factor on the progressing disease process. This changed impact may be related to progression of the diseases or concomitant aging. For example, a given risk factor might have a different effect on tumor promotion and progression. Similarly, the impact of factors that increase sympathetic activity on various disease outcomes may be reduced because of reduction in beta-adrenergic activity with aging (Weber et al, 1989).

When considering reductions in factors associated with increasing age, it is important to realize, as pointed out earlier in the example from the MRFIT study, that these trends may depend on the measure of association being used. Similarly, it is possible to have a decrease in the relative hazard with increasing age, accompanied by an increase in the odds ratio. Thus, the examination of age-related change in the association between a risk factor and an outcome needs to be seen as conditional on the measure of association chosen.

Choosing between these alternative explanations for observed declines in risk factor associations with increasing age is not easy. To the extent that no information is available to characterize the factors related to susceptibility, the "survivor" explanation needs to be seen as a heuristic to prompt a search for such factors. Inspection of the actual risk levels and how they vary by age and exposure group can help to direct attention to processes that are accelerating risk as a function of age in one group but not another, or can identify ceiling effects. However, few studies will have sufficient sample size to allow the calculation of stable age-specific and risk factor–specific risks. The third approach appears promising, although compromised by an inadequate understanding of both the pathophysiology of disease progression in older persons and the aging process. Given these limitations in our knowledge, interpretation of age-related changes in associations between a risk factor and an outcome should be carried out very cautiously.

Causal Interpretations

As in all analyses of observational data, great care is required in the interpretation of evidence for and against a risk factor being associated with an outcome in older persons. By far the biggest caution may be related to understanding the role of chronic conditions. Consider that urinary incontinence is an outcome that results from any number of acute and chronic diseases prevalent among the elderly. If a given risk factor is associated with one of these diseases, it is in part a risk factor for the development of incontinence. However, in the usual form of multivariate modeling, the disease might be detected as a confounder of the association between the risk factor and incontinence. Without a clear understanding of the mediating role of the disease, the risk factor would not emerge as an antecedent, causal factor (Susser, 1973). Thus, it is very important to bring knowledge of the potential pathophysiologic processes to bear on the interpretation of apparent patterns of confounding. Without such informed interpretation, a potentially modifiable risk factor related to the development of incontinence would be overlooked.

CONCLUSIONS

The substantial changes that have occurred in the mortality rates at the older ages suggest that there may be a considerable role for prevention among the elderly. However, the identification of associations between risk factors and disease outcomes in the elderly suffers from a number of methodological and conceptual challenges, some of which apply to epidemiologic studies in general and some of which are particularly germane to studies of the elderly. What little evidence there is supports a role for a number of modifiable risk factors in the health experience of older persons. However, this area of epidemiologic investigation is in its infancy, and much work remains to be done. Such work should be carried out with full awareness of the interrelationships between aging, pathophysiology and disease progression, and study design. Although the challenges are great, the impact of information gained from such studies could have a significant impact on both the duration and quality of life.

REFERENCES

Besdine RW (1988a). Clinical approaches to the elderly patient. In Rowe JW, Besdine RW (eds), Geriatric Medicine, 2nd ed. Boston, Little, Brown.

Besdine RW (1988b). Functional assessment in the elderly. In Rowe JW, Besdine RW (eds), Geriatric Medicine, 2nd ed. Boston, Little, Brown.

Castelli WP, Garrison RJ, Wilson PWF, Abbot RD, Kalousdian S, Kannel W (1986). Incidence of coronary heart disease and lipoprotein cholesterol levels. JAMA 256:2835–2838.

Castelli WP, Wilson PWF, Levy D, Anderson K (1989). Cardiovascular risk factors in the elderly. Am J Cardiol 63:12H–19H.

Cox DR (1972). Regression models and life tables. J Roy Stat Soc, Ser B 34:187–202.

Farber E (1988). Cancer development and its national history—a cancer prevention perspective. Cancer 62:1676–1679.

Garibaldi RA, Neuhaus EG, Nurse BA (1988). Infection in the elderly. In Rowe JW, Besdine RW (eds), Geriatric Medicine, 2nd ed. Boston, Little, Brown.

Guralnik JM, Kaplan GA (1989). Predictors of healthy aging: Prospective evidence from the Alameda County Study. Am J Public Health 79(6):703–708.

Harris T. Cook EF, Kannel W, Schatzkin A, Goldman L (1985). Blood pressure experience and risk of cardiovascular disease in the elderly. Hypertension 7:118–124.

Hazzard WR (1989). Atherosclerosis and aging: A scenario in flux. Am J Cardiol 63:20H–24H.

Irvine PN (1990). The challenge of multiple illnesses. In Cassel CK et al. (eds), Geriatric Medicine, 2nd ed. New York, Springer-Verlag.

Israel RA, Rosenberg HM, Curtin LR (1986). Analytical potential for multiple cause-of-death data. Am J Epidemiol 124(2):161.

Kalbfleisch JD, Prentice RL (1980). The Statistical Analysis of Failure Time Data. New York, Wiley.

Kannel WB, Gordon T (1978). Evaluation of cardiovascular risk in the elderly: The Framingham Study. Bull NY Acad Med 54:573–591.

Kannel WB, Vokonas PS (1986). Primary risk factors for coronary heart disease in the elderly: The Framingham Study. In Wenger NK, Furberg CD, Pitt E (eds), Coronary Heart Disease in the Elderly. New York, Elsevier.

Kaplan GA, Haan MN (1989). Is there a role for prevention among the elderly? Epidemiologic evidence from the Alameda County Study. In Ory MG, Bond K (eds), Aging and Health Care: Social Science and Policy Perspectives. London, Tavistock, pp 27–51.

Kaplan GA, Seeman TE, Cohen RD, Knudsen LP, and Guralnik J (1987). Mortality among the elderly in the Alameda County Study: Behavioral and demographic risk factors. Am J Public Health 77(3):307–312.

Kleinbaum DG, Kupper LL, Morgenstern H (1982). Epidemiologic Research: Principles and Quantitative Methods. New York, Van Nostrand Reinhold.

Kohn RR (1982). Causes of death in very old people. JAMA 247:2793–2797.

Korenchevsky V (1961). Physiology and Pathological Aging. New York, Basel/Karger.

Manton KG, Stallard E (1988). Chronic Disease Modeling: Measurement and Evaluation of the Risks of Chronic Disease Processes. New York, Oxford University Press.

National Center for Health Statistics (1987). Health, United States, 1986. Washington, DC, U.S. Government Printing Office.

National Center for Health Statistics (1989). Health, United States, 1988. Washington, DC, U.S. Government Printing Office.

Rice DP, Feldman JJ (1983). Living longer in the United States: Demographic changes and health needs of the elderly. Milbank Mem Fund Quart 61:363–396.

Rowe JW, Lipsitz LA (1988). Altered blood pressure. In Rowe JW, Besdine RW (eds), Geriatric Medicine, 2nd ed. Boston, Little, Brown.

Rowe JW, Wang S (1988). The biology and physiology of aging. In Rowe JW, Besdine RW (eds), Geriatric Medicine, 2nd ed. Boston, Little, Brown.

Sackett KL (1979). Bias in analytic research. J Chronic Dis 32:51–68.

Seeman TE, Guralnik JM, Kaplan GA, Knudsen L, Cohen R (1989). The health consequences of multiple morbidity in the elderly: The Alameda County Study. J Aging Health 1(1):50–66.

Siegal JS (1980). Recent and prospective demographic trends for the elderly population and some implications for health care. In Haynes S, Feinleib M (eds), Second Conference on the Epidemiology of Aging. Washington, DC, National Institutes of Health, pp 286–316.

Stamler J (1988). Risk factor modification trials: Implications for the elderly. Eur Heart J 9(Suppl D):9–53.

Susser M (1973). Causal Thinking in the Health Sciences: Concepts and Strategies of Epidemiology. New York, Oxford University Press.

Weber MA, Neutel JM, Cheung DG (1989). Hypertension in the aged: A pathophysiologic basis for treatment. Am J Cardiol 63:25H–32H.

II

ISSUES IN SURVEYING OLDER PERSONS

4

Ethical Issues in Conducting Surveys of the Elderly

PATRICIA L. COLSHER

There is a consensus that research should be done only with a vulnerable group if the same information could not be gained from a less vulnerable group (Annas and Glantz, 1986) and that investigators should make special efforts to protect the interests of potentially vulnerable research participants (American College of Physicians, 1989; Annas and Glantz, 1986; Boverman, 1983; Kendall, 1989; Riecken and Ravich, 1982; Warren et al, 1986). Because of the nature of their discipline, gerontologists and geriatricians may work with potentially vulnerable individuals and may be forced to confront the ethical issues associated with such research. It would be condescending to assert that all elderly persons are in need of special protection, and indeed such a belief might ultimately prove detrimental to them (Levine, 1986). Some elderly persons, however, have health, psychobehavioral, and social characteristics that may make them vulnerable. This chapter outlines some of the ethical issues that may be encountered in survey research with the elderly.

INFORMED CONSENT

The doctrine of informed consent is basic to the conduct of scientific research (Benson et al, 1985; Freedman, 1975). In cases where medical treatment is not involved, it requires that investigators disclose all relevant information, including but not limited to study purpose, procedures involved, and risks and benefits (Fletcher, 1983). Investigators are expected to insure that potential participants or their proxies understand the information, and participation is supposed to be voluntary and free from coercion (Fletcher, 1983). Although concerns about informed consent are by no means unique to research with the elderly (Cohen, 1984; Holder, 1988), competency, understanding, and voluntariness may sometimes be at special issue (Tymchuk and Ouslander, 1990), especially when doing research with frail elders.

Competency

Competency is a legal concept that is of ethical and legal importance to both clinicians and investigators. This discussion will focus on competency as it relates to the gross capacity to make decisions regarding specific actions.

In writing on consent for *treatment,* Drane (1985) proposed the use of a sliding scale of competency. When the potential benefits of the treatment clearly outweighed the possible risks, cognitive competency was defined as simple awareness of or orientation to the situation. When the risk–benefit ratio was more nearly equal, "understanding" was required, and when the proposed treatment entailed substantial risk, "critical and reflective understanding" were required. Some assert that in research with little possibility of direct benefit for participants, more stringent criteria should apply (American College of Physicians, 1989; Langley, 1989), even in population or survey research, when risk is usually quite low.

Appelbaum and Roth (1982) and Stanley and Stanley (1982) proposed similar, multilevel conceptualizations of competency to consent to research participation. The least stringent criterion requires simple evidence of a choice and is impaired only by severe cognitive impairment and psychosis. The most stringent criterion requires "appreciation" of the situation, which includes understanding the relevant information and its implications for the individual. Appelbaum and Roth (1982) have also suggested that there should be an "affective" component to the understanding.

The difficulty with many conceptualizations of competency, understanding, or even awareness, however, lies in their operationalization (Appelbaum and Roth, 1981; Appelbaum and Roth, 1982). When examined on a psychometric level, the notion of competency is complex and troubling (Morrison, 1987). The reliability and validity of tests used in neuropsychological evaluation have been questioned, and the utility of such tests for the elderly may be adequately investigated (Morrison, 1987). In survey research, if a formal evaluation of competency is included at all, it is likely to be a mental status screening examination. Although these tests may be suitable for detecting severely impaired individuals, they may be less useful when only mild or moderate impairments exist (Albert, 1988).

In addition, factors other than cognitive performance may affect competency (Appelbaum and Roth, 1981; Appelbaum and Roth, 1982). For example, cognitive function as measured by standard screening instruments may be intact, but if a potential participant has a psychotic thought disorder that impairs his or her ability to manipulate information rationally, competency may be affected (Appelbaum and Roth 1982). Lack of insight may also impair competency to consent to research (Appelbaum and Roth 1982).

When a potential participant has a cognitive impairment or mental disturbance so severe as to preclude any reasonable assumption of understanding, the issue of consent is often fairly straightforward. Under such circumstances, the initial contact with the potential participant may actually be with a family member who will inform the investigators of the potential participant's impairment. Similarly, when a potential participant is institutionalized, the institutional gatekeepers are likely to inform the investigator. Surrogate consent may then be sought, with the understanding that the surrogate should not consent if he or she believes the potential respondent would have refused to participate or if participation would not be in the potential respondent's best interests (American College of Physicians, 1989).

In addition, it is important to seek consent from the impaired individual. Even when the surrogate believes that the potential participant would be interested, the individual should certainly be allowed to decide not to participate (American College of Physicians, 1989). For example, Warren and colleagues (1986) reported that almost one third of surrogates who reported that they believed that potential participants would not want to participate actually consented to participation. Conversely, over 20 percent of persons who would not want to participate themselves gave consent for the potential participant. It should be noted that, in research with older persons, the surrogate consenter, often a spouse, may also be impaired. If so, it may be necessary to seek another potential surrogate.

The American College of Physicians' recent position paper on research with cognitively impaired persons (American College of Physicians, 1989) noted that it may be possible to obtain valid consent before an individual becomes incompetent (e.g., in studies of progressive dementias). They also suggested that such persons be asked to designate a proxy to be relied upon when the participant is no longer competent.

Understanding

Although sometimes viewed as distinct from competency, understanding is often dealt with as being on a continuum with or a component of competency (Levine, 1986), and it may be more troublesome than competency in research with the elderly. Persons with mild or moderate cognitive impairments, especially those with high premorbid functioning, may be competent (in the sense of being oriented to the situation) and consent to participation. Interviewers may note, however, that they perform poorly on mental status screening examinations or give inconsistent or inappropriate responses. Under these circumstances, it is difficult to know whether the participant genuinely understood the information presented in the consent process, and his or her consent may therefore be invalid.

Although not necessarily indicative of clinically important cognitive impairment, there may be qualitative differences in the way elderly persons process information. For example, the elderly may not process information as thoroughly or as systematically as younger persons (Reese and Rodeheaver, 1985), and this may result in a different understanding of the proposed study from what was intended. Because the elderly as a group have fewer years of formal education (Atchley, 1985), information summaries and consent forms, sometimes requiring college-level reading skills (Kendall, 1989), may be more difficult to understand. Finally, sensory impairments may interfere with understanding (Kendall, 1989). It is likely, however, that valid consent can be obtained if the investigators have anticipated and prepared for these eventualities.

Several studies have examined how well nominally competent research participants understand the information presented to them. In a clinical trial of propranolol after acute myocardial infarction (Howard and DeMets, 1981), 58 of the 64 participants (91 percent) were aware that they were participating in a research program, and 80 percent were aware of the purpose of the study. Although almost 90 percent of participants were aware that a placebo control group existed, fewer than half of them knew that control group assignment was random. Educational attainment, race, and age were all significant predictors of understanding.

Other investigators have reported less encouraging outcomes in potentially vulnerable groups. In a series of studies involving psychiatric patients (Benson et al, 1985), only 37 percent of depressed and 37 percent of schizophrenic research subjects giving informed consent demonstrated a good understanding of the purposes of the research.

The use of more intensive informational techniques, combining both in-person and videotaped presentations, improved understanding for depressives but not schizophenics. Rieken and Ravich (1982) found that 28 percent of patients (44 of 156) in Veterans Administration hospitals who had signed consent forms to participate in research were unaware that they were indeed participating in studies. Of those patients who were aware, only 10 percent demonstrated an understanding of the purpose of the research; 25 percent had little or no understanding.

Volition

Under some circumstances, older persons may be at particular risk of coercion. For example, if the caretaker gives proxy consent for participation, the potential participant may agree in order to avoid displeasing the caretaker. Studies done in nursing homes (Annas et al, 1986) or other institutions (Fletcher, 1983) may similarly be perceived as coercive. If a physician recommends participation in a study, elderly persons, who are less likely to question physicians (Haug, 1979), may participate in order to gain approval or out of fear that not participating might jeopardize their health care. Moreover, potential participants may misunderstand information summaries and consent forms and participate because they fear that their Social Security or other benefits may be at risk.

Elderly persons may be subject to more subtle pressures to participate, some of which might be conceptualized as potentially beneficial. For example, socially isolated persons may choose to participate in studies as a means of gaining social contact. Getting a letter from an "important" university or governmental agency may be flattering or provide an interesting diversion. The potential interpersonal importance of the interview is illustrated by the observation that vulnerable persons may contact the investigator long after their participation in order to ask for information or assistance unrelated to the study.

Related Concerns

Despite the best intentions of the investigators and the best efforts of the interviewers, difficulties may be encountered in obtaining consent. Some potential participants may skim or even refuse to read information summaries, saying they are certain that nothing inappropriate would be done. An individual may agree to participate but repeatedly interrupt or reschedule interviews, or otherwise cause his or her choice to be doubted (Langley, 1989). On occasion, a potential participate will want to be interviewed but will refuse to sign a consent form. Even after reading and discussing the consent form, the participant may remain concerned that he or she is consenting to something not explicity mentioned (e.g., a medical procedure or withdrawal of treatment) and may refuse to sign. Some persons may say that they never sign forms as a matter of personal principle and that their word ought to be good enough. It has even been suggested that the process of having an authority figure obtain the signature of a potential participant is inherently coercive (Brod and Feinbloom, 1990). Thus, even when an individual is competent and wishes to participate of his or her own volition, it may be difficult to satisfy fully the ethical and legal obligations (Levine, 1979) of the doctrine of informed consent.

Consent for Use of Data Bases

It may be useful to obtain additional information from medical or insurance records or other data bases established for purposes other than research. Obtaining informed consent for record review may be more difficult than obtaining consent for other types of research (Benbassat and Levy, 1988). Concern has been expressed that strict application of the doctrine of informed consent may jepordize retrospective epidemiologic research (Benbassat and Levy 1988; Waters, 1985). Appelbaum suggested obtaining a general consent at the time of admission, although a general consent would clearly not fulfill the obligations of informed consent (Benbassat and Levy, 1988; Appelbaum et al, 1984). Further consent may not be required if an appropriate review board determined that the research should be carried out, the proposed use of the data would not violate any conditions under which the information was collected, confidentiality would be protected, and the study would not have adverse effects (including unwanted contact, embarrassment, or liability) on the individuals whose records were to be used (Benbassat and Levy 1988; Holder and Levine, 1976).

RISKS AND BENEFITS

Although many of the types of questions involved in survey research may seem relatively innocuous, some may be troublesome for the elderly (Annas and Glantz, 1986). Persons may be upset by questions about illnesses and physical function limitations, because they highlight personal disabilities and losses. Questions about relationships with offspring, other relatives, or friends may also be disturbing. Persons who expect close family relationships may be humiliated by what they view as their own failure to develop and maintain closeness. Describing a network of friends that has been reduced because of death and institutionalization is understandably upsetting. Tests of cognitive function may be distressing to persons who have concerns about their own abilities. Other topics, including those relating to sexual function, alcohol consumption, and tobacco use, may be more bothersome to the elderly because of their attitudes toward them.

The use of performance tests of physical function (e.g., repeatedly standing from a chair, walking a timed course) raises special safety concerns. Even when respondents are given the opportunity to omit exercises they feel would be unsafe, some may decide to try tests that might be risky for them in order to please the interviewer or to "prove" that they are physically fit.

Regardless of the nature of the questionnaire, participation in a survey may be stressful, especially if the interview is lengthy. The interruption of daily routines and dealing with unfamiliar persons may be difficult for persons who are confused or frail. Even being contacted may be upsetting to some, who will want to know where the investigator got their names. Persons with unlisted telephone numbers may be upset when they are called in a study using random-digit dialing.

Protection of confidentiality is basic to the conduct of research. Untoward release of information is of special concern, however, in research with dependent elders. Family members or caretakers may be nearby during in-home interviews or may insist on being present, and privacy can be difficult to maintain in nursing homes and other institutions. When the information being gathered could affect the relationships between caregivers and the dependent elder, confidentiality is particularly important.

On the other hand, it is also possible that benefits may accrue as a result of participation in survey research. When screening instruments are included, it is possible that unsuspected illness may be detected. Although potentially coercive, the social contact and diversion involved in survey participation may also be enjoyable and interesting (Kaye et al, 1990). It is not uncommon for persons with chronic illnesses to indicate that they feel that participating in research may help other persons with their illness. Healthy persons may report similar altruistic motives (Holder and Levine, 1976). The satisfaction of these motives ought not to be dismissed as unimportant.

ACKNOWLEDGMENT

This work was supported by National Institute on Aging Grant AG-07094.

REFERENCES

Albert MS (1988). Assessment of cognitive dysfunction. In Albert MS, Moss MB (eds), Geriatric Neuropsychology. New York, Guilford Press.

American College of Physicians (1989). Cognitively impaired subjects. Ann Intern Med 111:843–848.

Annas GJ, Glantz LH (1986). Rules for research in nursing homes. N Engl J Med 315:1157–1158.

Appelbaum PS, Roth LH (1981). Clinical issues in the assessment of competency. Am J Psychiatr 138:1462–1467.

Appelbaum PS, Roth LH (1982). Competency to consent to research. Arch Gen Psychiatr 39:951–958.

Appelbaum PS, Roth LH, Detre T (1984). Researchers access to patients records: An analysis of the ethical problems. Clin Res 32:399–403.

Atchley RC (1985). Social forces and aging. Belmont CA, Wadsworth.

Benbassat J, Levy M (1988). Researchers' access to stored medical data: The Israeli experience. Institutnl Rev Bd 10(3):1–3.

Benson P, Roth LH, Winsdale WJ (1985). Informed consent in psychiatric research: Preliminary findings from an ongoing study. Soc Sci Med 20:1331–1341.

Boverman M (1983). Mental health aspects of informed consent process. In Berg K, Tranoy KE (eds), Research Ethics. New York, Alan R. Liss.

Brod MS, Feinbloom RI (1990). Feasibility and efficacy of verbal consents. Res Aging 12:364–372.

Cohen C (1984). Should prisoners be barred from volunteering from research? Medical experimentation on prisoners. In Levine C (ed), Taking Sides: Clashing Views on Controversial Bioethical Issues. Guilford CN, Dushkin.

Drane JF (1985). The many faces of competency. Hastings Center Rep 15:17–21.

Fletcher JC (1983). The evolution of the ethics of informed consent. In Berg K, Tranoy KE (eds), Research Ethics. New York, Alan R. Liss.

Freedman B (1975). A moral theory of informed consent. Hastings Center Rep 5:32–39.

Haug M (1979). Doctor–patient relationships and the older patient. J Gerontol 34:852–860.

Holder AR (1988). Disclosure and consent problems in pediatrics. Law Med Health Care 16:219–228.
Holder AR, Levine RJ (1976). Informed consent for specimens obtained at autopsy or surgery: A case study in the overprotection of human subjects. Clin Res 24:68–77.
Howard JM, DeMets D (1985). How informed is informed consent? The BHAT experience. Controlled Clin Trials 2:287–303.
Kaye JM, Lawton P, Kaye D (1990). Attitudes of elderly people about clinical research on aging. Gerontologist 30:100–106.
Kendall RE (1989). Comment on "Ethics of research with dementia sufferers." Int J Geriatr Psychiatr 4:239–246.
Langley G (1989). Review of "The clonidine test in patients with dementia." Int J Geriatr Psychiatr 4:241–246.
Levine RJ (1979). Clarifying the concepts of research ethics. Hastings Center Rep 9:21–26.
Levine RJ (1986). Ethics and regulation of clinical research. 2nd edition. New Haven, Yale University Press.
Morrison HL (1987). Neuropsychiatric assessment of dementia: Inadequacy of test protocols. In Rosner R, Schwarz HI (eds), Geriatric Psychiatry and the Law. New York, Plenum Press.
Reese HW, Rodeheaver D (1985). Problem solving and complex decision making. In Birren JE, Schaie KW (eds), Handbook of the Psychology of Aging. New York, Van Nostrand Reinhold.
Riecken HW, Ravich R (1982). Informed consent to biomedical research in Veterans Administration Hospitals. JAMA 248:344–348.
Stanley BH, Stanley M (1982). Testing competence in psychiatric patients. Institutnl Rev Bd 4(October):1–6.
Tymchuk AJ, Ouslander JG (1990). Optimizing the informed consent process with elderly people. Educ Gerontol 16:245–258.
Warren JW, Sobal J, Tenney JH, Hoopes JM, Darmon D, Levenson S, DeForge BR, Muncie HL (1986). Informed consent by proxy: An issue in research with elderly patients. N Engl J Med 315:1124–1128.
Waters WE (1985). Ethics and epidemiologic research. Int J Epidemiol 15:48–51.

5

Sampling Strategies for Studying Older Populations

DANIEL H. FREEMAN, JR., MARTHA L. BRUCE,
PHILIP LEAF, AND LISA BERKMAN

The emerging importance of the elderly as a segment of the population has captured the imagination of the popular press for a number of years. Simultaneously, scientists and demographers have given increased attention to this population. Various debates have been fueled in part by the relative paucity of data, a point noted by Dorothy Rice (1987) in her summary of "The Panel on Statistics for an Aging Population." She emphasized the importance of varied data collection activities to provide appropriate resources for planning and policymaking. Substantial progress in this area can be made by coordinating and focusing diverse data collection activities that are currently under way (Wallman, 1987), but it is unlikely that all the scientific requirements can be met with routinely collected data. For timely answers to emerging questions, survey samples will be needed for the foreseeable future.

A common tactic for surveys of population subgroups, such as the elderly, is to administer a special questionnaire to members of the subgroup as part of a general population survey. This was done in the Supplement on Aging to the 1984 National Health Interview Survey (NHIS) [National Center for Health Statistics (Fitti and Kovar), 1987]. The method is particularly attractive when sizable surveys are already in the field and accessible. Since the elderly represent only 11 percent of the general population, this approach is less attractive for smaller scientific and epidemiologic surveys. This chapter discusses two large studies conducted in the New Haven, CT SMSA that used different survey designs for essentially the same target population and frame.

The target population for these studies consisted of people ages 65 and over who were residents of either the New Haven SMSA or its central city. The total adult population of the greater New Haven area (the city of New Haven and 12 surrounding towns) in 1980 was 300,110 persons living in 150,371 noninstitutional households. The central city of New Haven has a noninstitutionalized civilian population of approximately 125,000 persons, of whom 12.3 percent, or 15,380, are 65 or older.

The two studies were the Epidemiologic Catchment Area Project (ECA) and the Yale Health and Aging Project (YHAP). The ECA employed a "nested sample" of the entire SMSA, whereas the YHAP oversampled age-restricted housing projects in the central city. Each study addressed problems that are typical of surveys of the elderly.

Table 5-1 New Haven Noninstitutionalized Population Age 65 and Over by Sex and Age Group[a]

	Age group					
Sex	65–69	70–74	75–79	80–84	85+	Total
Male	2074	1479	1027	604	439	5623
Female	3037	2528	2057	1244	891	9757
Total	5111	4007	3084	1848	1330	15380
Females/males	1.46	1.71	2.00	2.06	2.03	1.74

[a]Based on 1980 census.

The first problem is that after age 65, women tend to outnumber men by almost 1.7 to 1. Moreover, this differential increases with age (Table 5-1). Studies that must evaluate gender differences need to compensate for this differential.

The second problem is that the elderly tend to be heavily concentrated in age-restricted or age- and income-restricted housing. By age-restricted housing we mean housing, typically apartments or condominiums, that limits the age of residents. We exclude nursing homes and congregate living quarters from this definition. Preliminary estimates for New Haven indicated that at least 20 percent of the elderly population is concentrated in this type of housing (Table 5-2). The discrepancy between Tables 5-1 and 5-2 reflects the different projections of the New Haven Housing Office and the Bureau of the Census.

The final problem is that previous research had indicated that the prevalence of some conditions of interest, especially psychiatric disorders for the ECA, is rare in elderly populations. Since the elderly comprise only a small proportion of the general community, the number of elderly in an equal-probability sample (epsem) of greater New Haven would be too small for making precise estimates of prevalence and incidence rates or of risk factors of psychiatric disorders among the elderly.

In what follows the approaches of the ECA and YHAP for sampling the elderly will be discussed. Each approach solved the special problems of sampling the elderly in different and, it is hoped, valid ways. The implications of the survey method for analysis will then be discussed.

Table 5-2 New Haven Noninstitutionalized Population Age 65 and Over by Sex and Housing Type[a]

	Housing type			
Sex	Public	Private	Community	Total
Male	436	563	4584	5583
Female	909	1646	7259	9814
Total	1345	2209	11843	15397
Females/males	2.08	2.92	1.58	1.76

[a]Based on New Haven Housing Authority estimates.

NESTED SAMPLING: THE ECA

Rationale for ECA

The ECA was part of a larger study conducted in five communities. It was begun in 1980 and was sponsored by the National Institute of Mental Health. The purpose of the study was to estimate the incidence and prevalence of psychiatric disorders, describe the use of health and mental health services, and identify risk factors for specific psychiatric disorders. The ECA was a landmark study in psychiatric epidemiology, made possible by methodological advances in diagnostic nosology, instrument development, and survey design. Prior to the ECA project, studies of psychiatric diagnoses relied on clinically trained interviewers. The use of such interviewers is too costly and time-consuming for a large-scale community sample. As a result, large community-based studies generally assessed more global or less specific indicators of mental health.

ECA respondents were interviewed using the Diagnostic Interview Schedule (DIS) (Robins et al, 1981; Robins et al, 1985), a semistructured interview administered by lay interviewers. The DIS assesses the presence, duration, and severity of psychiatric symptoms and excludes symptoms due to physical illness or medication use. Computer algorithms use the data from the DIS to generate many of the more common psychiatric diagnoses as defined by DSM-III (American Psychiatric Association, 1980): major depressive disorder, bipolar disorder, alcohol abuse or dependence, drug abuse or dependence, phobia, panic disorder, obsessive–compulsive disorder, antisocial personality, somatization disorder, and anorexia nervosa.

The Design and the Utilities Frame

The design of the New Haven ECA had the dual features of a community survey of adults and an oversample of elderly residents living in the community. Data collection was designed to piggyback the collection of the oversample onto the design of the community sample. A full description of the study design is available elsewhere (Eaton and Kessler, 1985; Holzer et al, 1985; Leaf and Myers, in press). The goal was to contact approximately 4000 of these households, interviewing one person per household. With an expected response rate of approximately 75 percent, this approach would yield the desired 3000 community respondents.

Had the ECA been a simple random sample, these 4000 households would have been randomly selected from some population listing of all the households. This approach, however, would have generated a logistical and financial nightmare for the investigators who had to organize the interviewers' routes. Instead, the study employed a stratified cluster design. Each of Greater New Haven's 13 towns comprised a primary sampling stratum. The primary sampling units (psu's) were clusters of eight housing units (i.e., single-family homes, apartments, etc.), at intervals of 62 houses. These were picked within each town by following routes used by the local electrical company meter listings, supplemented by the City Directory and telephone book information. The first and fourth houses in each cluster were selected, for a total household sampling ratio of one in 31. One person aged 18 years or older was selected for interview at random according to the Kish grid method. Respondents aged 65 and older would be included in the community proportional to their numbers in the community.

The strategy for collecting the elderly oversample also was designed to minimize costs while making the sample as representative as possible of the actual community. The remaining six households in the clusters were screened for elderly residents. One elderly resident from each of the six households was interviewed if any resided there. If more than one elderly person resided in a household, a respondent was chosen by the Kish (1965:396–404) method.

Results

The first wave of interviews began in New Haven in July 1980 and was completed in one year. The response rate for the household survey was 77 percent, or 3068 interviews. The response rate for the oversample was 76 percent (of households with elderly residents), or 1966 interviews. Respondents came from a total of 2108 different clusters; 1201 of the clusters contributed to the elderly oversample. The number of elderly oversample respondents averaged 0.98 from each of the clusters, ranging from 0 to 6 (as many possible). Of the community sample residents, 610 were aged 65 or over, for a total of 2576 elderly respondents in the New Haven ECA sample.

Part of the sampling scheme included a strategy for weighting the data to adjust for several aspects of the sampling design. As collected, the ECA respondents were not strictly representative of the greater New Haven population. The sample deviated from the population both because only one adult was chosen from each household (thereby overrepresenting individuals who live alone) and because 23 percent of selected adults did not respond to the interview.

Selection weights were calculated for the household sample as the percentage of the population selected (i.e., 1/31) multiplied by the inverse of the number of adults living in the household. When the elderly oversample was added to the household sample, the selection weights for the elderly in the household sample were adjusted by 2/8, with the oversample representing the remaining 6/8 of selected elderly. The selection weights for the oversample were calculated by multiplying their selection factor by the inverse of the number of elderly living in the household (not total adults in the household).

Poststratification weights were calculated based on the 1980 U.S. Census population count of the greater New Haven area by age (12–24, 25–34, 35 –44, 45–64, 65+), race (black, nonblack), and sex: the number in each population cell was divided by the sum of selection-based weights for respondents fitting within the cell criteria (Hansen et al, 1953). With the addition of the oversample, the poststratification weights of all the elderly were adjusted to represent the elderly population.

The mean weight in the full sample was 59.61, ranging from 10.19 to 354.38. These weights allowed projection to the combined population of 300,069 individuals. The mean weight for individuals age 65 and over was 18.66, ranging from 10.19 to 98.45. For elderly respondents selected in the community sample, the mean weight was 21.05, ranging from 10.30 to 98.45. For respondents selected in the oversampling, the mean weight was 17.92, ranging from 10.19 to 54.44. When the sample and oversample were combined and weighted, 2576 elderly respondents represented 47,951 noninstitutionalized residents of Greater New Haven aged 65 and above. It follows that prevalence rates of psychiatric disorders estimated from the weighted data can be generalized to the noninstitutionalized adult community itself.

SUPPLEMENTED SAMPLING: THE YHAP

Rationale for the YHAP

The Yale Health and Aging Project (YHAP) was one of initially three and later four projects funded by the National Institutes of Aging under the *Establishment of Populations for Epidemiologic Study of the Elderly (EPESE) Program.* These projects were directed at ascertaining the general levels of physical and mental health in well-defined communities of older people. There was a particular emphasis on estimating the prevalence and incidence of certain chronic conditions, functional ability, levels of depressive symptomatology, and cognitive impairment. A second goal was to determine which behaviors as well as which biomedical, demographic, environmental, and psychosocial variables serve as predictors of declines in health, including the incidence of morbidity, hospitalization, institutionalization, and mortality among persons 65 and over (Berkman et al, 1986).

The Three Strata by Two Sex Design

The project goals required obtaining a sample that was generalizable to a "defined population." In the Yale project it was decided to undertake a probability sample of persons 65 and over residing in the central city of the New Haven SMSA. The sample would be used to obtain interviews with elderly persons so as to ascertain baseline information on health status, level of physical and cognitive functioning, socioeconomic status, and psychosocial resources and attitudes. All respondents were to be followed for several years and reinterviewed annually.

The YHAP sampling strategy was influenced by several factors. First, it was conducted after the ECA. Because of the intensity of the ECA sampling, it was clear that the YHAP sample should be drawn from the same frame. This would minimize the chance of recontacting an ECA respondent. Next, previous work in the New Haven area suggested residents of housing projects would be of special interest. Third, to obtain adequate numbers of male respondents, it was believed that as many males as females should be interviewed. Finally, budgetary constraints indicated that only about 3000 participants could be recruited.

These considerations led to the following sample design:

1. Sample 12/62 of non-ECA New Haven residences, excluding age- and/or income-restricted housing. All males and two thirds of females in this stratum were eligible for interviews.
2. Census non-ECA participants in public housing for the elderly.
3. Census non-ECA male participants in age-restricted private housing.
4. Sample 50 percent of non-ECA females in age-restricted private housing.

Table 5-3 Yale Health and Aging Project Sampling Fractions and Target Sample Sizes (*n*)

	Housing type			
	Public	Private	Community	Total
	Males			
Sampling fraction	54/62	54/62	12/62	–
n	380	490	591	1757
	Females			
Sampling fraction	54/62	54/62	12/62	–
Subsample	1.00	0.50	0.67	–
n	792	717	627	2450
Total	1172	1207	1218	4207

The subsampling of females was performed using computer-generated Kish selection procedures. This plan was adopted so as to produce stratum-specific samples of nearly equal size by sex. The selected sample sizes are shown in Table 5-3.

Results

All surveys have both good and bad surprises. Based on the experience of the ECA and other area projects, an overall response rate of 75 percent was expected for the YHAP. As can be seen (Table 5-4), this was reasonable in the community stratum. However, since age-restricted housing projects were to be nearly completely enumerated, intensive public relations work was undertaken, resulting in response rates between 80 and 90 percent.

Table 5-4 Yale Health and Aging Project Actual Sample Sizes, Response Rates, and Coverage

	Housing type		
	Public	Private	Community
	Males		
n	240	333	594
Response rate, %	87.2	81.1	78.8
Coverage, %	72.2	83.2	85.2
Mean sampling weight	1.8	1.7	7.7
Range: low, high	1,2	1,2	5,30
	Females		
n	488	535	622
Response rate, %	90.2	85.1	78.1
Coverage, %	68.5	88.0	84.2
Mean sampling weight	1.9	3.1	11.7
Range: low, high	1,2	1,5	7,62
Total	728	868	1216

The second surprise was a substantial shortfall of males in the elderly housing. This made it feasible to increase the total size of the community strata with a substantial focus on raising coverage rates. The second surprise emerged with the release of 1980 age- and sex-specific census data. The data indicated that substantially fewer elderly were residing in the public housing than originally expected. Taken together, the response and coverage rates are consistent with those obtained in most national surveys, particularly for the combined sample, which is dominated by the community stratum, where 77 percent of the target population resides. This made it possible to adjust the sampling weights with a process known as poststratification. Using these weights, it is statistically valid to estimate the number of elderly males and females on a stratum-specific basis. The final sample weight formula follows:

$$\text{Sampling weight} = \frac{1}{\text{CR}}\frac{1}{\text{RR}}\frac{1}{f_{\text{h}}}$$

where CR = coverage rate, RR = response rate, and f_{h} = sampling fraction (depends on housing and sex stratum).

ANALYSIS ISSUES

Although the ECA and YHAP used different strategies, both yielded probability samples from which means and proportions could be readily estimated. Difficulties arose, however, in estimating the variances of these statistics. One part of the problem is that by inflating the ECA or YHAP samples to the respective population of elderly, the effective sample size also appears to have been increased. The size of an estimated variance depends in part upon the size of the sample, with larger samples generally producing smaller standard errors. Many statistical software packages enable (either as the default or by options) the user to normalize the effective sample size used in estimation of variances to the size of the actual sample count.

Whether or not the weights are normalized, however, most statistical packages estimate variances under the assumption of simple random sampling. But the ECA and YHAP sampling strategies resulted in samples that were very different from a simple random sample. Rather than initially identifying individuals at random, people were identified from within clusters of neighboring households. Since neighbors are more likely to be similar than like people in the rest of the population, they cannot be considered "independent samples from the population." Furthermore, because different sampling weights are applied to individuals in the sample, everyone in the population is *not* equally likely to be selected into the sample. Both factors, clustering and differential weighting, are especially pertinent to samples of elderly respondents. Not only are the elderly differentially weighted, depending on whether they were drawn from the community or from an oversample, but elderly residents are very prone to clustering effects. As noted, many of the elderly in the New Haven ECA reside in elderly housing projects or in neighborhoods of long-term residents.

Statistical techniques that assume simple random sampling are not appropriate with these data or for many other data sets that were collected using any of a variety of stratification, cluster, or disproportional sampling survey designs. If simple random-sampling assumptions are used to estimate variances, it will appear that there is less variation in the whole population than there really is. Since most statistical software invokes the assumption of simple random sampling, the variances generated will be underestimated. The magnitude of underestimation is termed the *design effect* (i.e., the ratio of the design-based variance to the simple random-sample variance). By affecting variance estimates, design effects have implications for tests of significance and calculation of confidence intervals.

The problems in estimating variances that reflect complex sample designs have drawn considerable attention in the statistical literature. A number of approaches have been developed to calculate design-based variance estimates. The more common include Taylor series linearization (Shah and LaVange, 1981; Woodruff, 1971), balanced repeated replication (Koch et al, 1975; McCarthy, 1966), jackknifing (Fay, 1985), and bootstrapping (McCarthy and Snowden, 1985). A review of all but the last of these methods can be found in Cohen and Kalsbeek (1981).

Until recently, these statistical solutions often seemed too confusing, cumbersome, and costly for practical application to much community sample research. Most researchers ignored the inappropriateness of the simple random-sampling tests of significance that they reported. Some attempted to deal with the problem by adding to their statistical models variables used in the sampling design or weighting procedures. Others attempted to calculate a global design effect for the sample or subsample and then inflate all simple random-sampling variances in the sample or subsample by that constant (e.g., Hauser et al, 1975; Veroff et al, 1981).

In the past few years, however, a variety of commercial computer software has become available for use in estimating design-based variances of means, proportions, ANOVA, regression, and logistic regression models (see Cohen, 1983; Cohen et al, 1986; Francis, 1981, for reviews). Many of these programs are relatively easy to use and interpret. The cost of some of the procedures on mainframe computers is only somewhat more than simple random-sample runs; other procedures can be run on microcomputers. Evidence generated in using these software packages indicates that global or make-shift solutions to design-based variance estimation are inadequate and misleading. Global approaches tend to minimize the extent to which design-based estimates of variances deviate from those based on simple random sampling and ignore the variation in design effects across different parameters within a sample (Cohen et al, 1986; Freeman et al, 1985).

To demonstrate these points, we apply two widely available statistical techniques—Taylor series linearization and balanced repeated replication (BRR)—to the analysis of the ECA and YHAP elderly data. These design-based methods are both considered statistically valid and produce similar results (Bean, 1975; Frankel, 1971; Freeman et al, 1985). For all Taylor series estimates, we used the Research Triangle Institute's RTILOGIT (Holt, 1977; Shah et al, 1987) procedure. RTILOGIT is executed through the SAS software (SAS Institute, 1985) and uses SAS data sets. The code is very familiar to SAS users. BRR methods are also available commercially in software packages such as OSIRIS (Institute for Social Research, 1981). In this chapter, however, we report results from BRR programs that we wrote using SAS procedures (Bruce et al, 1987).

For both BRR and Taylor series techniques, the user must identify the sampling design in the program code. Variables that represent the primary sampling strata and psu's are sufficient for using the Taylor series linearization procedures. However, because BRR method replicates its analysis on unique half samples of the original data, 60 pseudostrata must also be identified in the samples by collapsing adjacent clusters or segments. Within each pseudostratum, two primary computing units were created. These pseudostrata and computing units can also be used with Taylor series models.

First, the ECA analyses are illustrated. Table 5-5 describes the sample characteristics of the New Haven elderly population. The first column lists unweighted sample sizes (i.e., actual number of interviews) and the second column lists the weighted percent of each category. The majority of elderly community residents are female, 37.8 percent are age 75 or older, and about half were married at the time of the interview. Almost 60 percent report a history of any of a number of chronic health problems (e.g., high blood pressure, cancer, stroke, heart disease), almost a quarter report their own mental health as being only fair or poor, and 6.7 percent met criteria for at least one of the psychiatric disorders assessed by the DIS within six months of the interview.

Recall that a design effect greater than 1 indicates that, compared to simple random-sampling estimates, an estimated parameter is less significant and has a wider confidence interval. Table 5-6 presents the design effects for variances estimated for logistic regression main effects of sex, age, marital status, chronic health problems, and self-reported mental health on the prevalence of any psychiatric disorder. The design effects are grouped by type of procedure (Taylor series or BRR) and, if Taylor series, whether the real strata or pseudo-strata were used. An important point about this table is that the estimated design effects range from 0.84 to 1.79. This means both that a global solution would be inaccurate and that, in the extreme case, the estimated design-based variance is 80 percent greater than what would have been calculated assuming simple random sampling. Only for the effect of age do we see an example of the design-based variance being smaller than the estimated simple random sample variance.

All procedures produce the same prevalence estimates, but the estimates of variances will differ. Although Taylor series and BRR do not produce the exact same estimated variance, the results are quite similar in most cases, especially when the same set of strata are specified. When the pseudostrata are used, the greatest difference in design effects between the two techniques is only 12 percent (0.91/0.84 for age and 1.36/1.21 for chronic health problems). The differences resulting from employing different sets of strata are greater, although neither set is consistently higher. In almost all cases, the difference between approaches is smaller than the bias resulting from not taking into account the sampling design. The major exception is the age parameter, where using the pseudostrata results in a design effect less than 1, compared to the design effect greater than 1 (1.11) with the true strata.

A different but related set of issues applies to the YHAP. It was a mixture of a near census and a probability sample of the community. This requires incorporating the selection design and sampling effects into the estimates and associated standard errors but recognizing that for the census there is no "pure sampling error." A model for this is discussed in Koch et al. (1975). A typical set of estimates is shown in Table 5-7, where the proportion of elderly living alone is shown by housing stratum and sex. As with the ECA data, since domain and subdomain estimates are to be compared, no finite population corrections have been applied (Cochran 1977:39, 142–146).

The first point is that within strata the unweighted estimates and the adjusted esti-

Table 5-5 ECA Sample Characteristics

	Unweighted (*n*)	Weighted (%)
Total	2569	100
Female	1570	60.4
Over 74 years of age	970	37.8
Chronic health problems	1529	59.6
Currently married	1125	53.5
Poor or fair mental health	592	23.3
Recent (6 mo) DIS disorder	178	6.7

Table 5-6 Design Effects in ECA Sample Logistic Regression Models Predicting Recent Psychiatric Disorder

	SRS[a]		Design effect[b]		
	Beta	Standard error	TS-Real	TS-Pseudo	BRR
Intercept	−3.12	0.247	1.23	1.44	1.54
Female	0.20	0.185	1.34	1.19	1.23
Age >74	−0.41	0.176	1.11	0.84	0.91
Chronic health problem	0.48	0.183	1.09	1.21	1.36
Married	−0.33	0.179	1.32	1.70	1.79
Poor/fair mental health	1.26	0.163	1.08	1.09	1.16

[a]SRS standard error normalized to actual sample size.
[b]Design effect = (design-based variance)/(SRS variance).

Table 5-7 Weighted and Unweighted Yale Health and Aging Project: Estimated Prevalence of Persons Living Alone by Sex and Housing Type (Standard Errors)

Estimator	Percent standard error (*N*: population, *n*: sample)	Housing type: Public (1)	Private (2)	Community (3)	Total (4)
		Males			
Weighted	%	68.8	45.6	18.7	25.3
	SE[a]	2.4	2.7	1.6	1.7
	N_h	436	563	4584	5583
Unweighted	%	67.8	45.3	18.3	36.1
	SE[b]	3.0	2.7	1.6	1.4
	n_h	240	333	594	1167
		Females			
Weighted	%	82.1	82.6	41.4	52.1
	SE[a]	2.1	2.3	2.3	2.4
	N_h	909	1646	7259	9814
Unweighted	%	81.4	81.6	41.2	66.3
	SE[b]	1.7	1.7	2.0	1.5
	n_h	488	535	622	1645

[a]Indirectly estimated using BRR (no fpc).
[b]Estimated using $\sqrt{p_h q_h / n_h}$ (no fpc) and $\sum_{h=1}^{6} N_h p_h q_h / N n_h$.

mates are extremely close. The adjustments reflect the sampling fractions, nonresponse rates, and undercoverage. However, when estimates for the entire city are of interest, the unweighted estimates are 9.8–14.2 percentage points too high for males and females, respectively.

The second important comparison is in terms of the standard errors. The weighted estimates were obtained using BRR and reflect not only the complexity of the weighting but also the clustering of selected households and subjects within households. These can be compared using the simple random-sampling formula shown at the bottom of Table 5-7. Surprisingly, the difference for males is quite small. However, for females there is a clear variance inflation because of the clustering. This design effect ranges from 32 percent in the community strata to 156 percent overall.

CONCLUSIONS

In conclusion, these two sample designs for surveys of the elderly involved differential sampling, response, and coverage rates. The latter two affect *all* population surveys whether they are probability samples or censuses. These differential rates affect not only estimates but also the associated standard errors. The use of probability samples, particularly in the community strata, permits inferences to much larger defined populations than would ordinarily be feasible. The limitations are in fact no different from those that apply to complete censuses of smaller populations, other than the limitations associated with sampling error; that is, nonresponse and coverage biases affect censuses and surveys equally.

These examples of stratified cluster samples with additional oversamples of elderly demonstrate the general principle that assuming a simple random sample may lead to spurious statistical significance when analyzing design-based data. Design-based procedures more appropriately specify the level of precision with which parameter estimates can be generalized to the study population. Moreover, the magnitude of design effects varies within a given data set by the specific parameter estimated, so that the effect of the sampling design cannot be estimated globally. It should be noted that the design effects reported here are not unusually high for these data or other data sets (Freeman et al, 1985; National Center for Health Statistics et al, 1987) and that design effects as high as 8.1 have been observed in the ECA data for some parameters (Leaf et al, 1985).

These observations lead to some general observations. For analytic purposes, where the defined population is of no special interest, we may choose to overlook the sampling structure and analyze the data as a "representative sample." That is, assume simple random sampling as is done in nonprobability samples. However, stratification variables should also be included as a "confounding variable." For inferences specific to a defined population, the design-based sampling weights and standard errors *must* be used.

The analyses presented indicate that different approaches to estimating design-based variances are roughly comparable and that the choice of which approach to employ is less important than the decision to use some design-based approach. However, it is useful to know the differences between the approaches when determining which approach or statistical package to employ for a specific problem—or which package to obtain for overall use.

In general, design-based variances estimation procedures consume more computer time than software that assumes simple random sampling. The increase is only moderate with the Taylor series models (and minimal for the RTILOGIT program for logistic regression), but it is very large for BRR models. In general, Taylor Series models are preferable over BRR when the software is available. When using Taylor Series modeling, indicators of the true sampling strata and psu's are preferable to the pseudoindicators. Pseudo-strata may be preferable when a project will be applying BRR to some of its analyses and Taylor series to other.

BRR has the advantage of being able to be run with smaller sample sizes than Taylor series models. This is especially useful when estimating variances in subgroups of the large study. Taylor series models tend to break down with subsamples of less than 500 observations. Another advantage of BRR is its widespread applicability. The procedures used in this chapter were written with SAS. Special software is not needed and the procedures can be adapted to any number of different analyses.

Today the choice of statistical techniques for use in calculating design-based variances is sizable, and there is a variety of statistical packages from which to chose. There is also choice in the way sampling error computing units are specified. Our results indicate that survey analysts have greater latitude in their choices about procedure, software, and calculating units than in deciding whether to take the sampling design into account when determining variances for inferences made to a larger population.

REFERENCES

American Psychiatric Association (1980). Diagnostic and Statistical Manual of Mental Disorders, 3rd ed. Washington DC, APA.

Bean JA (1975). Estimation and Sampling Variance in the Health Interview Survey. National Center for Health Statistics. Vital and Health Statistics, Series 2, No. 38, Public Health Services Pub. No. 1000, Washington DC.

Berkman LF, Berkman CS, Kasl S, Freeman DH, Leo L, Ostfeld A, Cornoni-Huntley J, Brody JA (1986). Depressive symptoms in relation to physical health and functioning in the elderly. Am J Epidemiol 124(3):372–388.

Bruce ML, Freeman DH, Leaf PJ (1987). Use of SAS Procedures for Estimating Design Based Logistic Regression Variances by Balanced Repeated Replication (BRR). Proceedings of the 12th Annual SAS Users Group International, pp. 1066–1070.

Cochran WG (1977). Sampling Techniques, 3rd ed. New York, Wiley.

Cohen SB (1983). Present limitations in the availability of statistical software for the analysis of complex survey data. Rev Public Use Data 11:338–344.

Cohen SB, Burt VL, Jones GK. (1986). Efficiencies in variance estimation for complex survey data. Am Stat 40:157–164.

Cohen SB, Kalsbeek WD (1981). NMCES Estimation and Sampling Variances in the Household Survey. National Center for Health Services Research, Department of Health and Human Services Pub. No. (PHS) 81-3281.

Eaton WW, Kessler LG (ed) (1985). Epidemiologic Field Methods in Psychiatry: The NIMH Epidemiologic Catchment Area Program. New York, Academic Press.

Fay RE (1985). A jackknifed chi-square test for complex samples. J Am Stat Assoc 80:148–157.

Francis I (1981). Statistical Software: A Comparative Review. New York, North-Holland.

Frankel MR (1971). Inference from Survey Samples: An Empirical Investigation. Ann Arbor, MI, Institute for Survey Research.

Freeman DH, Livingston MM, Leo L, Leaf PJ (1985). A comparison of indirect variance estimation procedures. ASA: Proc Survey Res Meth 313–316.

Hansen MH, Horwitz WN, Madow WG. (1953). Sample Survey Methods, Vol. 2. New York, Wiley.

Hauser RM, Koffel JN, Travis HP, Dickenson PJ (1975). Temporal change in occupational mobility: Evidence for men in the United States. Am Sociol Rev 40:279–297.

Holt MM (1977). SURRGER: Standard Errors of Regression Coefficients from Sample Survey Data. Technical report, Research Triangle Park, NC, Research Triangle Institute.

Holzer CE, Spitznagel E, Jordan KB, Timbers DM, Kessler LG, Anthony JC (1985). Sampling the household population. In Eaton WW, Kessler LG (ed), Epidemiologic Field Methods in Psychiatry: The NIMH Epidemiologic Catchment Area Program. New York, Academic Press.

Institute for Social Research (1981). OSIRIS IV User's Manual, 5th ed. Ann Arbor, MI, Institute for Social Research.

Kish L (1965). Survey Sampling. New York, Wiley.

Koch GG, Freeman DH, Freeman JL (1975). Strategies in the multivariate analysis of data from complex surveys. Int Stat Rev 43:59–78.

Leaf PJ, Livingston MM, Tischler GL, Weissman MM, Holzer CE, Myers JK (1985). Contact with health professionals for the treatment of psychiatric and emotional problems. Med Care, 23:1322–1337.

Leaf PJ, Myers JK (in press). Procedures used in the epidemiologic catchment area studies. In Robins LN, Regier DA (eds), Psychiatric Disorders in America. New York, The Free Press.

McCarthy PJ (1966). Replication: An approach to the analysis of data from complex surveys, in Vital and Health Statistics, Ser. 2, No. 14, National Center for Health Statistics, Public Health Service Pub. No. 1000, Washington, DC.

McCarthy PJ, Snowden CB (1985). The bootstrap and finite population sampling, in Vital and Health Statistics, DHHS Pub. No. 85-1369. Ser 2, No 95, Public Health Service, Washington DC.

National Center for Health Statistics (Fitti JE, Kovar MG) (1987). The supplement on aging to the 1984 National Health Interview Survey, Vital and Health Statistics. Ser. 1, No. 21, DHHS Pub. No. 87-1323, Public Health Service, Washington DC.

Rice DP (1987). Improvement of data resources for policy analysis for an aging population, ASA 1987 Proc Social Statistics Section, pp 22–26.

Robins LN, Helzer JE, Croughan J, Ratcliff KS (1981). National Institute of Mental Health Diagnostic Interview Schedule: Its history, characteristics, and validity. Arch Gen Psychiatr 38:381–389.

Robins LN, Orvaschel H, Anthony J, Blazer D, Burnam A, Burke J (1985). The diagnostic interview schedule. In Eaton WW, Kessler LG (eds), Epidemiologic Field Methods in Psychiatry: The NIMH Epidemiologic Catchment Area. New York, Academic Press.

SAS Institute (1985). SAS User's Guide: Statistics. SAS Institute, Cary, NC

Shah BV, Folsom RE, Harrell FE, Dillard CN (1987). RTILOGIT: Procedure for Logistic Regression on Survey Data. Research Triangle Park, NC, Research Triangle Institute.

Shah BV, LaVange LM (1981). Software for inference on linear models from survey data. Cary, NC, Research Triangle Institute.

Veroff J, Douvan E, Kulka R (1981) The Inner Americans: A Self Portrait from 1957–1976. New York, Basic Books.

Wallman K (1987). Coordination: A key to improving data about the aging population, ASA 1987 Proc Social Statistics Section, pp. 27–33.

Woodruff RS (1971). A simple method for approximating the variance of a complicated estimate. J Am Stat Assoc 66:411–414.

6

The Use of Survey Methods in Research on Older Americans

A. REGULA HERZOG AND WILLARD L. RODGERS

This chapter addresses the use of survey research methods for the collection of epidemiologic, behavioral, and social data on the older population. It takes the methods currently used in survey research as a given (for reference books on survey research methods see, for example, Babbie, 1989; Rossi et al, 1983) and emphasizes departures from them that may be necessitated by the age of the respondents. Although many older adults remain as alert and healthy as younger adults, they are more likely to be experiencing health and cognitive problems that may keep them from participating at all in surveys or that may introduce errors into their responses. These problems are particularly common among the very old or institutionalized. Thus, questions are often raised about the suitability of traditional survey techniques that rely primarily or exclusively on self-reports for collecting data about older persons and about ways to modify these techniques to accommodate them better.

In the major section of this chapter we shall review the available evidence to establish whether more frequent difficulties are encountered in collecting data from older persons by standard survey procedures, whether these difficulties produce greater error, and if so, which features of the standard survey seem to contribute to the difficulties. Throughout this section we will discuss possible modifications of standard survey procedures that may help in surveying the elderly. There follows a brief section about characteristics of advanced age that may be responsible for the observed effects. At the outset, we must point out that the literature bearing directly on potential errors in surveys with older adults is sparse, particularly with respect to needed modifications of standard procedures. Therefore, our chapter draws also on a much more broadly defined literature, sometimes forging rather speculative links to surveys with the elderly, and on informal observations by gerontological researchers, many of which still await systematic investigation.

ERRORS IN SURVEYS OF THE ELDERLY

We use a conceptualization of survey error proposed by Kish (1965) and elaborated more recently by Groves (1989). In general terms, error is defined as the deviation of a measure from the true value. More specifically, errors may be broken down into two broad components, usually labeled as "bias" and "variable error." *Variable error* is random, with an expected value of zero, and is due to random variation in irrelevant factors. Given sufficiently large sample sizes, the variable error in estimates of central tendency can be reduced to any desired level, because the positive and negative deviations balance out and the variance declines as a function of the number of respondents. *Bias*, on the other hand, is a systematic distortion introduced by survey procedures and personal characteristics and adds a constant factor to survey measures. It can sometimes be reduced by changing procedures but not, in general, by increasing the sample size. Two major types of bias and variable error are usually distinguished: sampling and nonsampling errors. Within nonsampling errors a further distinction can be made between those arising from nonresponse and those arising from responses.

Sampling

The most commonly used samples for epidemiologic studies of the population are household samples, because at any given time most people live within one particular household and each household has a specific location. By drawing a sample of households and of people within households with known probabilities, one can obtain a sample that is representative of the population living in a geographically defined area. The random error of the sample estimates can be reduced by drawing a larger sample.

There are several difficulties in using standard household sampling techniques to obtain samples of older adults. One problem is that such sample-based estimates may be biased by incomplete coverage of the target population (and may have variable error) because the household sampling frame includes only the population living in private households, whereas a substantial proportion of the older and the oldest old populations live in institutions (Havlik et al, 1987, Table 57; Rosenwaike, 1985, Table 7.6). Moreover, the institutionalized elderly are distinctly different from the noninstitutionalized elderly household population (cf. Rosenwaike, 1985): Among those age 85 and older, the institutionalized are much more likely to be female, to be white, to have hearing impairments (45 vs. 25 percent) and visual impairments (43 vs. 12 percent), and to require assistance in activities of daily living such as eating (36 vs. 5 percent) and walking (78 vs. 24 percent). It is clear, then, that surveys based on household samples may produce biased statistics about the entire population of older adults, particularly the oldest among them. In surveys of the elderly, every effort should therefore be made to sample older adults living in institutions as well as those living in the community.

Another problem with the standard household sampling technique for surveys of the elderly is the cost associated with screening by age. Although virtually every household contains at least one adult, only about every fourth household contains a person over 60 years of age (S. Heeringa, personal communication, 1989). Therefore, many sampled households will have to be approached repeatedly, only to discover eventually that nobody over 65 lives there. And the procedure becomes even more expensive when the target group is the oldest old. If this "screening" is conducted face to face, this can be a major component of the survey budget. Moreover, for some households, it will never be determined whether an older person lives there, because the household could not be screened at all. This fact makes it difficult to calculate the response rate because the exact number of eligible persons for the denominator is not known.

These problems have led to the use of lists that contain age information for sampling older adults. One widely used list is that of Medicare enrollees of the Health Care Financing Administration (HCFA). Although a large majority of the elderly U.S. population is enrolled in the Medicare program and thus is part of the list (Waldo and Lazenby, 1984), it remains unclear just how complete the coverage is (Rodgers and Herzog, 1982). In particular, poor people or illegal aliens may not be well represented by the Medicare files. Such files also become outdated rapidly because of deaths and moves. Finally, they are of limited usefulness for telephone surveys, because of the large proportion of unlisted telephone numbers.

Other sampling frames may be attractive with respect to certain subpopulations. A listing of all nursing home facilities is used as the sampling frame for the National Nursing Home Survey. This list is compiled from a variety of sources, many from states that keep a list because of licensing procedures. However, once the population of interest extends beyond residents of nursing homes to residents of *any* type of institution, a sampling frame may be more difficult to achieve, because there are many types of institutions, and the distinction between institutions and households is not always clear. If a person lives in a unit with its own bath and kitchen, but in a context where nursing care is provided by staff members, that person would be classified as living in a household according to the criteria applied in some current studies; other studies, however, would define the same person as institutionalized.

Other alternatives to the standard household sample are possible. One alternative—multiple frames—is used when no single frame with complete coverage exists, but it is possible to find several incomplete frames that, together, give a good overall coverage of the elderly. The list of Medicare enrollees, for example, may be supplemented by the Medicaid list to obtain coverage of a higher proportion of the elderly poor. It is not clear, however, how easy it is to use the Medicaid list. A promising system that is currently being developed is the MEDSTAT system, which incorporates Medicaid information.

Another alternative to the standard household sample is represented by the multiplicity sampling techniques originally proposed by Sirken (1970; Sudman and Kalton, 1986). This technique is based on the availability of a more general sample, the members of which are asked to list older family members who may then be contacted for an interview. For these procedures the referring person must report the age of the older person, but the accuracy rate for reports of the exact age of even a close relative is not known. Although the false positives can be eliminated at the point when the age is confirmed with the selected respondent, false negatives cannot be as easily detected. One procedure to minimize false negatives is to lower the age criterion for referral and to verify the exact age with the referred person directly at the point of contact. Such a procedure obviously broadens the screening operation and thereby reduces its efficiency.

This and other sampling techniques for rare populations that may be applicable to drawing samples of older adults are discussed in Kalton and Anderson (1989).

Nonresponse

Once households are sampled and respondents are selected from within households, respondents' participation in the survey has to be obtained. Even the best-designed sample may result in biased data if some of the selected respondents do not participate. The bias is a function both of the proportion and of the distinctive characteristics of nonrespondent (Moser and Kalton, 1972). Obtaining the participation of a high proportion of all selected respondents can be a real challenge, because participation is voluntary. In the following paragraphs the level of nonresponse is reviewed briefly, the likely bias is assessed, and reasons for nonresponse and possible suggestions for improving response rates are discussed.

Although survey researchers have focused primarily on overall response rates and their decline during the past few decades (Steeh, 1981), there is growing evidence that the nonresponse problem is more serious among older age groups than among the rest of the population (DeMaio, 1980; Hawkins, 1975; Herzog and Rodgers, 1988a; Mercer and Butler, 1967–1968; Weaver et al, 1975) and that it may be particularly low among those over 85 years of age (Herzog and Rodgers, 1988a; Wallace, 1987). In surveys that were designed to study just the elderly, reported response rates are generally high. For example, in the National Long Term Care Survey, conducted by the Bureau of the Census for the Health Care Financing Administration (HCFA), a response rate of 95 percent was obtained for persons in households and a rate of 97 percent was obtained for those in institutions, although a substantial proportion of the respondents were by proxy rather than by self-report. In the three initial Established Populations for Epidemiologic Studies of the Elderly (EPESE) sites, the response rates of adults 65 years of age and older ranged between 80 and 85 percent, although if partial, telephone, and proxy interviews are discounted the response rate for the oldest old (i.e., those 85 and over) is considerably lower (as low as 60 percent or less) (Cornoni-Huntley et al, 1986). Finally, in the Supplement on Aging to the 1984 National Health Interview Survey (SOA), a 93 percent response rate was obtained among adults 55 years of age and older when both proxy and self-reports were included (Fitti and Kovar, 1987). All the studies with relatively high response rates were specifically designed to survey an older population, and it is possible that they used procedures more appropriate for obtaining cooperation among the elderly than those used in general population surveys. However, methodological explanations must also be considered.

A difficulty in evaluating reported response rates is the fact that they can be calculated in many different ways, and published reports often do not include enough information to ascertain the method of calculation. For example, published reports often do not specify whether proxy respondents were included in the numerator or whether eligibles who died or were hospitalized before they could be interviewed were included in the denominator. Moreover, the specific procedures for obtaining participation are almost never documented. As a first step toward dealing with nonresponse in future research, it would be desirable to gather information about nonresponse rates (including those for screening interviews), uniformly defined, from several major surveys. This should include, whenever possible, tabulation of complete nonresponse, reluctant respondents, and proxy respondents, and the procedures used in each study (e.g., number of callbacks, criteria for going to proxies) should be documented in detail. A discussion of the calculation of response rates is presented in Herzog and Rodgers (1988a) and in Groves (1989).

The seemingly larger proportion of nonrespondents and panel drop-outs among the elderly carries a potential for larger bias, depending on whether a systematic difference exists between respondents and nonrespondents/drop-outs. Several studies have attempted to assess biases introduced by nonresponse. Most of these studies share the basic shortcoming of having less than perfect information available on nonrespondents. Information on nonrespondents is typically limited to relatively few characteristics and available only for a subset of all nonrespondents. Consequently, assessments of differences between respondents and nonrespondents are limited and potentially erroneous.

Several types of nonresponse investigations have been carried out. Some have simply examined the reasons given for nonresponse. There is some evidence that the proportion of outright refusals declines in older age to under half of all nonrespondents over the age of 75, whereas in other age groups refusals typically represent about two thirds to three quarters of all nonrespondents. Instead of simply refusing, older respondents (or members of their households) are more likely to cite health and mental health problems as reasons for nonresponse (Herzog, 1987; Herzog and Rodgers, 1988a). Similar findings have been reported with respect to reasons for attrition from panel surveys, where health problems are quite frequently given as reason for nonparticipation by older persons (Cooney et al, 1988).

Another type of nonresponse investigation involves comparisons between respondents and nonrespondents. In cross-sectional studies such information is generally limited to observations by interviewers or others, reports by respondents, or available records. Interestingly, this general literature has not yielded much evidence for consistent large-scale differences between respondents and nonrespondents. There is some, albeit inconsistent, evidence that social status, education, and race may be related to nonresponse (DeMaio, 1980; Goudy, 1976; Hawkins, 1975; Robins, 1963; Weaver et al, 1975). Limited evidence on characteristics beyond demographics suggests that nonrespondents are also less healthy, less happy, less active, and less socially involved than respondents (Herzog, 1987). Panel drop-outs (on whom information is available from previous waves of data collection) have been shown to be less educated and of lower socioeconomic status, but again, contradictory evidence has also been reported (Benney et al, 1956; Berelson et al, 1954; Reeder, 1960). Panel drop-outs are also less interested and involved in the topics of the interview (Baur, 1947; Belson, 1960; Berelson et al, 1954; Downes, 1952).

Some of the nonresponse studies have distinguished between different types of nonrespondents and have tended to show that nonrespondents who cite health reasons differ more clearly from respondents than do those who simply refuse (Cooney et al, 1988; Herzog, 1987; Norris, 1987; Riegel et al, 1967).

To summarize: Although the evidence regarding the level of nonresponse in surveys of the elderly is not entirely consistent and is difficult to evaluate because of variability in methodology, nonresponse among older adults appears to be more closely linked to health limitations than it is among younger age groups. This form of nonresponse introduces more substantial biases than nonresponse related to refusal. Because health-related biases are highly undesirable in surveys that are designed to assess health status and related characteristics, every effort must be made to keep nonresponse at a minimum. These efforts must target health-related nonresponse more aggressively than refusals, because of its greater potential for bias. Therefore, we turn now to a discussion of various procedural changes to increase response rates among older adults.

Sponsorship and Endorsement

The sponsorship of a survey is believed to be critical in attaining a high response rate, because it can confer legitimacy, credibility, and even authority on the survey. Yet there is little consensus on which sponsors are likely to be the most influential. It was felt that local sponsorship was more effective than federal sponsorship in the EPESE study in rural Iowa. Likewise, group discussions conducted in the Questionnaire Design Laboratory at NCHS suggested that the endorsement of a study by local seniors' groups would help in making the study credible to those asked to participate. On the other hand, the high response rate in the Supplement on Aging (SOA) was attributed to the fact that the Census Bureau—a national institution—conducted the interviews. Representatives from the Census Bureau felt that for the National Long Term Care Survey the sponsorship of another national institution, the NIH, would have been more effective in gaining access to institutions than was sponsorship by the bureau. Other researchers believe that endorsements elicited from well-known older personalities or senior advocate groups would be helpful. To our knowledge, no systematic data on the success of any such endorsements have been collected.

In some studies, such as the SOA and the New Haven EPESE, media coverage was sought at the beginning of the study. Copies of a resulting newspaper article were then provided to the interviewers, who could show it to respondents. The impression gained from this experience, which is typical of other studies, is that seeing the study mentioned in the newspaper lent it legitimacy. Media campaigns are suggested by many gerontological researchers as a general means of familiarizing the community with the ongoing survey, although some contend that such efforts may be lost on older persons with sensory impairments who do not read the newspaper or watch television programs.

More generally, some gerontological researchers are convinced that extended prior involvement in a community is necessary to obtain a high response rate. For example, in the New Haven EPESE, in which relatively high response and reinterview rates were obtained and in which only 20 out of 812 respondents have been lost in the six years of the study (A. Ostfeld, personal communication, 1989), the research staff attributes the high participation rate to the facts that they know the community well and that they enjoy the confidence of the residents. That experience suggests that anyone wanting to study an elderly population ought either to know well that population and its ways and problems or to get detailed information and assistance from those who do know it well. Local seniors' groups also can be very helpful in providing information and accessing seniors in a community, and so can local physicians and other health care providers.

Characteristics of Interviewers

Older interviewers may appear less threatening to older respondents, who are disproportionately worried about victimization (Clemente and Kleiman, 1976). There is at least anecdotal evidence to support such a notion. All the interviewers for the New Haven EPESE are women, because earlier experience had shown that older women are unlikely to open their doors to a strange man. In that study it was also observed that at least some of the respondents preferred older interviewers (that "gray hair" was welcome). This contention is based on a few call-backs to refusals, early in the initial data collection. Reasons given for the refusal included statements that the interviewer "was so young" or that the respondent "did not think she would understand" and an offer to provide a more mature interviewer was often welcomed. No instances of the reverse pattern were encountered. Based on this experience, older interviewers routinely called upon initial refusals and were able to increase the response rate by up to 7 percent. In the Iowa EPESE older interviewers were also preferred, partly because it was assumed that using interviewers of the same age group could reduce communication problems across generations. In summary, matched ages were believed to facilitate participation and to increase valid responding.

Older interviewers also might portray the image of an active and involved older person, and in turn might suggest a similar posture to the respondent. Because activity level and involvement are related to survey participation (Herzog and Rodgers, 1982; Schulz et al, 1988), the response rate might be increased. On the other hand, some respondents might compare themselves unfavorably with an active older interviewer, and consequently feel bad. Or again, younger interviewers might appear more novel and attractive to older individuals and thus facilitate participation. To summarize, speculations about the effect of the age of the interviewer abound. Moreover, it is well established that response rates vary considerably by interviewer. But it is less clear which interviewer characteristics account for the differences and whether the age of the interviewer has anything to do with the difference. In general, little rigorous research is available on this topic and we are unaware of any study examining the effect of interviewer age. Furthermore, the majority of work on interviewer effects concerns response effects only, rather than participation rates, and again, only minimal attention has been paid to age.

With respect to interviewer behavior, it has been suggested that it is particularly important to older respondents that the interviewer be on time and keep promises, however small. Interviewers in the New Haven EPESE wear white jackets and carry black bags, invoking a medical focus that is appropriate for that study, because a substantial number of the questions are health related.

Several investigators suggest that an advance letter introducing the survey and the interviewer should be sent. Several survey organizations include information about the interviewer in their advance letter and mention that the interviewer carries identification material to prove her legitimacy. This is generally believed to be useful and to alleviate fear of victimization and the unknown, although again no systematic tests seem to have been done.

Incentives

Incentives of a financial or other nature for survey participation have a long history in survey research. Most of the available research is on financial incentives, and it is inconclusive (Groves, 1989).

Current practice in gerontological research varies with respect to offering incentives to those who agree to participate in surveys. In surveys done by the Census

Bureau, incentives are not ordinarily offered, but if requests are made beyond a single interview, it is more common to offer some sort of gift or payment. A similar practice is observed by the Survey Research Center at the University of Michigan. Sometimes incentives are even offered for first-time contacts, when those are particularly onerous. NHANES offers monetary compensation for completion of the home interview and the health examination (which takes about 3.5 hours and requires the respondent to go to a mobile examination center), compensation of a lesser amount for the home interview and a shortened health examination given in the home (for those unable or unwilling to travel to the examination center), but no compensation for those who complete the home interview only.

Although sufficiently large incentives are likely to increase the response rate somewhat, they may also raise suspicion, thereby counteracting the positive effect. Furthermore, because of the cost, financial incentives are not feasible for many surveys. A further consideration with respect to a reward contingent on completion of an interview is the possibility that it introduces the idea of a business exchange into the interview context, and once this altered context is invoked, the size of the reward may be judged against a realistic hourly fee for services rendered, which may be quite high. In "communal" (as opposed to business) relationships, benefits are given in response to need or in order to please, rather than in return for favors received (Clark and Mills, 1979; Mills and Clark, 1982). In one instance, a benefit offered as a "sign of appreciation" was more effective than one offered as an "incentive" (Gould, 1984).

Anecdotal evidence from the Massachusetts Health Care Panel Study and from the Survey Research Center at the University of Michigan suggests that coffee mugs with the signet of the study, the sponsoring agency, or the like, and given before or at the outset of the interview are good incentives. Small gifts are also suggested by Carp (1989) as an incentive. Other nonfinancial incentives include a free medical exam or health-related information and feedback, but there appears to be little agreement among those involved in research on the elderly as to the effectiveness of such incentives. Some believe that a free health exam in itself is not of much value to elderly respondents because most of them receive medical care that is paid for by Medicare, and those who do not have such coverage may not want an examination. Others feel that a free examination, particularly for something not covered by standard health insurance, is often appreciated. The impression held by several gerontological researchers is that although incentives may have some marginal impact on some respondents, factors such as the perceived importance of the study, the sponsor of the research, the personality of the interviewer, and the burden (in terms of time and effort) placed on the respondents are much more important (e.g., Carp, 1989; Kaye et al, 1990). The incentive actually may be more important for the interviewer who feels that she can provide a reward for participation than for the respondent.

Mixed Modes of Data Collection

Surveys that use telephone and mail interviews in addition to face-to-face interviews in what is typically called a mixed mode may obtain higher response rates than surveys that rely on a single mode of data collection. Although all modes have their characteristic strengths and weaknesses in reaching respondents and obtaining their cooperation, combining them may overcome the limitations inherent in any one mode, adding up to an overall advantage for the response rate. For example, face-to-face interviews are unacceptable to those elderly who are concerned about victimization and unwilling to admit any strangers into their homes. A mixed-mode approach that combines telephone and face-to-face interviewing is particularly attractive, because in general the quality of the resulting responses does not differ in any substantial way across these two modes (Bradburn, 1983; Groves and Kahn, 1979), even for older respondents (Herzog and Rodgers, 1988b; Herzog et al, 1983).

Because the different modes reach and obtain interviews with somewhat different populations and vary in their relative costs but do not appear to produce data of vastly different quality, strategies that combine modes have proven useful in the general population, increasing response rates by 5–15 percent over those obtained with the original mode and sometimes reducing costs (Hochstim, 1967; Siemiatycki, 1979). The case for mixed-mode strategies for the elderly has recently been made by McKinlay and his colleagues (McKinlay, 1988; Tennstedt and McKinlay, 1987), who argue that mixed-mode surveys are cost effective in maximizing response rate, minimizing nonresponse bias, and ensuring high-quality data. Concerns remain, however, that there may be differences in the quality of data collected by different modes, or biases in data collected by one mode relative to data collected by another mode.

Telephone interviews have also been successfully used for follow-ups of face-to-face interviews, although mostly for reasons of cost efficiency rather than response rate (Herzog and Rodgers, 1988b; Kovar and Fitti, 1985). The modes of telephone and mail surveys of older persons are discussed and compared to face-to-face surveys in Herzog and Kulka (1989).

Finally, telephone and mail may be considered as modes for more efficient screening than the one that takes place on the doorstep (Hoinville, 1983).

Extended Field Period

Because health problems appear to represent an important reason for nonresponse among elderly persons, extended field periods that can accommodate respondents who are temporarily indisposed will eventually achieve a higher response rate than investigations that must be completed in a shorter time period. More generally, experience at the University of Michigan's Survey Research Center has shown that about a third of all initial nonrespondents agree to be interviewed when approached a few weeks or months after the initial request.

Proxy Reporters

Another way to reduce nonresponse is to seek information from another source about persons who are unwilling or unable to respond to an interviewer themselves. In existing surveys, a proxy reporter is generally someone who knows the sampled individual well. For those living in households, the proxy is almost always someone in the same household—preferably the spouse—whereas for those in institutions it is often a caregiver or a grown son or daughter.

Proxy reporters appear to be a much more important source of information about the oldest old than about younger adults, because of higher nonresponse rates among this age group and because of substantial proportions who, because of cognitive impairment or frail health, may be incapable of providing accurate responses to survey questions or even participating in the interview. For example, in the 1984 SOA of people 55 years of age and over, 8.5 percent of all the interviews were with proxies, but for those age 85 and older the rate was 26.6 percent (Fitti and Kovar, 1987). This increase in reliance on proxies for the oldest old parallels an increase of those having difficulty and/or receiving help with activities of daily living and those experiencing cognitive impairments (Fitti and Kovar, 1987, p. 22; Cornoni-Huntley et al, 1986). Indeed, in the longitudinal component of the SOA, those with proxy respondents were more likely to have died two years later than those who reported for themselves, confirming that they were sicker in 1984 (M. Kovar, personal communication, 1989). There appears to be a fair amount of consensus among gerontological investigators that proxy respondents must be used in research on the old and oldest old in order to avoid biasing the data in favor of healthy older persons.

Given that an interview with a proxy reporter may be the only way of obtaining information about frail older adults, how should the decision of choosing a proxy over the selected respondent be made? Some surveys, particularly those of the general population, do not accept proxy respondents at all. Many surveys of older adults permit a proxy if the sampled person is impaired but prefer to obtain the information directly from the sampled person. If the latter procedure is chosen, a set of decision rules has to be developed for determining whether the sampled older person is too impaired to answer for him- or herself. Several surveys leave the decision up to the interviewers, who have been trained in observing critical incidents of impairment. In some surveys (e.g., the New Haven EPESE), the interviewers review their assessment with the supervisor before inviting a proxy instead of the sampled older person. In other surveys, such as the NHANES and the Iowa EPESE, the interviewers decide on the spot but carefully document the reasons for their decision. Some surveys, such as the National Long Term Care Channeling Demonstration Project, permit switching to a proxy if the sampled respondent becomes confused or exhausted during the course of the interview. The specific decision rule involves a check point at the end of each section of the interview about the status of the respondent, with the possibility of skipping to the end of the interview for a few critical questions.

A formal test of cognitive impairment like the Mental Status Questionnaire is utilized in several surveys of the elderly. Although originally the instrument was included usually as a screening device, the unproven validity of such a test for establishing the ability of an older person to provide accurate information as requested in the survey is generally recognized. Another problem with the screening notion is that the interviewer has to score the respondent's answers on the spot and make a decision on how to proceed. This is considered by some investigators as too onerous a task to be completed reliably on the spot. As a consequence, the test results are often used ex post facto to supplement the interviewer's observation and assess the trustworthiness of the information obtained from the respondent, but are not used as a decision tool for choosing a proxy respondent to report in place of the selected respondent.

The issue of proxy reporters rests to a large extent on the trade-off between two sources of error: errors due to unit and item nonresponse may be reduced by seeking information from proxies, but errors due to inaccurate responding are often thought to be more frequent in proxy than in self-reports. To date, both of these assumptions remain unsubstantiated. We will discuss the quality of the proxy information later, when we discuss response error.

Cooperation From Institutions

Because of the high proportion of the old and particularly the oldest old who are institutionalized, consideration must be given to the cooperation of institutions in data collection efforts. Some level of cooperation is essential, whether the request involves gaining access to residents to ask for their participation, obtaining information about how to contact the resident's next of kin or other relatives, recording information from records on residents, or interviewing caretakers and other employees of the institutions.

Success in eliciting the cooperation of institutions apparently is related to a variety of factors that vary from state to state, including type of institution and regulations. Concerns about privacy laws seem to vary widely and to be reflected in rather idiosyncratic practices and requirements. In the follow-back study to the National Nursing Home Survey (NNHS), for example, in which telephone interviews were sought with the next of kin of those in the original institutionalized sample, it is estimated that names of next of kin were eventually obtained for about 80 percent of the selected persons. In some cases, the nursing homes sought permission from the next of kin before releasing their names to the study. A successful recruitment of long term-care institutions has been reported by Palumbo et al (1987). Factors affecting participation in nursing home studies have also been examined by Lipsitz et al (1987).

It is further suggested that an entire set of issues has to be negotiated with institutions, including confidentiality issues, informed consent issues, or access to information, and that the on-site manager is often the best person with whom to start such negotiations. If access to many different institutions is needed, this can become a costly enterprise.

Controlling Attrition in Panel Surveys

Sample maintenance in panel surveys must be a continuous effort and should not be relegated to the reinterview. Two critical aspects can often be addressed by essentially the same actions. First, the respondent's good will toward the study should be nurtured via reports about findings of the study, season's greetings, a small token of a gift, and the like. Second, the address and other pertinent information about the respondent should be kept current so that interviewing can start promptly whenever needed. Information about deaths, moves, and changes in address can be obtained from the post office in the process of a mailing to the original address. Useful discussions of relevant procedures are provided by Carp (1989) and by Freedman et al. (1980).

Item-Missing Data

Failure to answer a question can introduce further biases into statistics if those not answering the question systematically differ from those who do. Again, this source of bias appears to be potentially more serious for older people who give more frequent nonsubstantive responses consisting largely of "don't know" (DK) answers (Ferber, 1966; Francis and Busch, 1975; Gergen and Back, 1966). The age-related increase in number of DK answers appears to be larger for questions that deal with attitudes, feelings, and expectations than for those eliciting facts (Herzog and Rodgers, 1982). To gauge the bias resulting from item-missing data, one needs to know whether DK respondents are systematically different from those who give substantive answers. Research suggests that DK respondents tend to be less physically, cognitively, and psychologically healthy; less interested in survey content; less socially involved; less highly educated; and more likely to be female (Colsher and Wallace, 1989; Ferber, 1966; Francis and Busch, 1975; Glenn, 1969; Herzog and Rodgers, 1982).

Missing data can be distinguished according to whether the underlying reason is cognitive or motivational. Some DK and other nonsubstantive responses truly reflect lack of knowledge about the correct answer or difficulty in understanding the question. A prime example for this form of DK answer is missing data on intelligence measures or questions about medications. This form of missing response is likely to be related to age: Older adults are more likely to have difficulty understanding the question, organizing their thoughts, and framing their answers, and thus are more inclined to answer that they "do not know."

Other DK and nonsubstantive responses, however, reflect unwillingness to report or to try hard enough to retrieve the relevant information; these may also express themselves more directly as refusals. A prime example for this kind is missing data on questions about financial status. The correlates for the two forms of missing data are most likely different (Colsher and Wallace, 1989), and therefore biases resulting from different forms of missing data and procedures to reduce missing data must be different.

Missing data also depend on the nature of the question. Anecdotal evidence from the Survey Research Center at the University of Michigan suggests that questions referring to personal topics such as family and work yield lower proportions of missing data than questions on political and social topics; questions that are interesting to the respondent yield fewer missing data than those that are not; questions that are worded clearly and understandably yield fewer missing data than those that are not.

Response Errors

Finally, errors are often present in the responses of those who do participate in a survey and give a substantive answer. Investigations of the validity of answers to survey questions are mixed but have sometimes demonstrated rather large biases (Andersen et al, 1979; Cannell et al, 1965; Harlow and Linet, 1989; Sudman and Bradburn, 1974; U.S. Department of Justice, 1981). For example, between 20 and 35 percent of adults inaccurately reported whether they voted in various elections; and most of them erred in the direction of overreports, thereby creating bias in the estimates of voter participation (Rodgers and Herzog, 1987). The reasons for such errors in surveys are sometimes motivational, as when a respondent does not want to report the correct but unpleasant fact that he uses drugs or engages in other illegal behaviors. In other cases the reasons for errors are cognitive, as when a respondent misunderstands the survey question, cannot recall the requested information, or is otherwise misled by the survey process. It is possible that missing data and response errors are different symptoms of the same underlying problem. For example, a badly worded question that is difficult to understand may prompt one respondent to avoid an answer and another to guess, so that a respondent's behavior depends mostly on personal style. Based on this recognition, possible procedural modifications will be discussed together for both sources of error.

Response validity is usually assessed by one of the following methods: by comparing individual survey responses with independent information from records; by comparing average statistics based on survey responses with the same average statistics based on other data sources; and by comparing data resulting from different measures of the same concept, either in averaged form collected on split-ballot samples or in individual form on the same respondents on two different occasions. A fairly substantial body of research has addressed response validity of survey questions using one or the other form of design. Specific survey characteristics—such as the formulation of the survey questions and the response categories, the nature of the requested information, the context of the questions, and the mode of data collection—were also investigated. Good reviews are available in Andrews (1984), Bradburn (1983), Groves (1989), Schuman and Presser (1981), and Sudman and Bradburn (1974). Some very interesting work has been reported recently by cognitive psychologists examining the cognitive processes that underlie the answering of survey questions and affect the validity of the answers, but so far this work has not been tied to aging and surveys with the aged (e.g., Bradburn et al, 1987; Schwarz, 1989; Schwarz and Strack, 1989).

The survey process is often assumed to be particularly challenging for older adults because of some of the well-documented age differences in cognitive functioning. However, this assumption has not always been upheld. For example, Herzog and her colleagues found no increased error with age when examining factual survey questions that can be checked against external records (Herzog and Dielman, 1985; Rodgers and Herzog, 1987). Likewise, Bush et al (1989) found high agreement of self-reported medical conditions and medical records in a sample of persons over 65 years of age. There is a bit more evidence that the responses of older adults to attitudinal and other subjective items have more measurement error than those of younger adults, at least in part because the answers of older people are somewhat more influenced by question format and less by the substantive content of the question. However, the age differences are small and not entirely consistent (Andrews and Herzog, 1986; Kogan, 1961; Rodgers et al, 1988; Wallace, 1987). Colsher and Wallace (1989) observed less consistency in the responses of the oldest old than in the young-old adults, and they further documented that the inconsistencies were accounted for in part by relatively poor memory performance.

Three comments must be made about existing research on validity of responses among elderly adults. First, survey errors due to cognitive impairment are most likely to be found among the oldest old because cognitive impairments are relatively frequent in that age range. However, most of the investigations examining response error among the elderly do not include sufficient numbers of respondents over 80 or even over 70 for reliable estimates on these age groups. Therefore, the oldest old are usually combined with those over age 60 or 65, and because of their relatively small proportion they do not noticeably affect the findings for the broader age range. Two recent studies that directly contrast mildly cognitively impaired older adults with those not impaired are exceptions (Farrow and Samet, 1990; McHorney et al, 1990). Their findings indicate that with the possible exception of the level of missing data the two groups do not differ in data quality. Second, those older adults who are most likely to have difficulties in answering survey questions are also those least likely to participate in the survey. As noted in the preceding discussion on nonresponse, physical and mental health problems are a major reason for nonresponse. In other words, if all sampled older adults were to participate in the survey, most likely more difficulties with answering the survey questions would be observed. Third, age differences are not likely to be general across all types and formats of questions. Rather, we would expect interactions, with older adults displaying particular problems with specific question formats. For example, it has often been argued that questions about information that has to be retrieved from long-term memory are more difficult for the elderly.

In the following paragraphs we review the evidence for response errors among the elderly with regard to specific aspects of the interview process and discuss suggestions for improvements to facilitate higher-quality data.

Characteristics of the Survey Questions

Differences in the meaning of questions for different age groups have been pointed out by gerontological researchers. For example, today's elderly seem to be less willing than younger age groups to draw comparisons between themselves and others, as is often requested by survey questions ("Compared to others your age . . ."), because admitting that one is better than others would seem presumptuous. Moreover, older adults seem less comfortable with the kinds of psychological self-descriptions that are the mainstay of personality and mental health scales. In particular, it has been suggested that questions assessing satisfactions with various domains of life and similar evaluative questions may yield biased answers among older adults because of the desire among the elderly to maintain a positive view about themselves and associated defensive mechanisms (Carp and Carp, 1981; Herzog and Rodgers, 1986). More generally, older adults dislike the highly standardized format of the typical survey questions and response categories, and they often attempt to avoid direct responses by digressing from the question and by rewording answers without using the provided categories (Jobe and Mingay, 1990; Kane and Kane, 1981).

Anecdotal evidence reported by several gerontological researchers suggests that survey questions developed on younger adults can be too complex for older adults. A prime example of this is provided by the items from the Rotter Internal-External Control Scale (Rotter, 1966) that require respondents to hold in mind two highly abstract and lengthy sentences in order to decide which one applies to them. Typically, interviewers must repeat the Rotter items frequently and nevertheless are often left with the impression that the response was chosen haphazardly. Using simpler wording and offering a statement of just one of two alternatives to be judged as right or wrong would improve the questions. Double-negative questions provide another example of a survey question that is too complex for many older adults. Although double-negative questions are often deliberately worded that way and included in batteries of items in order to control response set, they appear to be very taxing to the cognitive flexibility of older adults. Because of their difficulty, question formats like these will often lead to missing answers or to invalid responses. Gerontological researchers must be very careful about the wording of established and well-validated scales, if the validation was conducted on younger respondents alone.

Similar questions have been raised about surveys that require a great deal of detailed information on a fairly specific topic such as food consumption or performance of activities (Jobe and Mingay, 1990; Kelsey et al, 1989). In these types of surveys, information about the frequency of many different food or activity categories is requested, and for each category the size of the portion or the intensity of the activity is also desired. Research on the use of these types of questions among older respondents is needed.

One aspect of the question wording that has received a good deal of confirmation through actual research is the number of response categories. Seven to nine categories result in responses of higher validity than do two to four (Bollen and Barb, 1981; Cochran, 1968; Cox, 1980). Although concerns had been raised in the past that fewer response categories may be easier for older respondents and therefore produce more valid responses (Lawton, 1977), recent largely unpublished work (Rodgers et al, 1988) demonstrates that seven to nine categories are probably optimal for those over as well as those under 60 years of age.

Seven to nine response categories might indeed seem like a large number to present to an older respondent. A particular format that appears to aid in the presentation of a relatively large number of categories is that of unfolding. According to this format, the response categories are presented in a step-wise fashion, with major distinctions (e.g., "Do you agree or disagree?") asked first and minor distinctions probed thereafter (e.g., if the respondent agrees, "Do you agree very much or just somewhat?"). Some of our preliminary data support such a format.

Length of Interview

The opinion is often expressed that interviews may be tiring for elderly respondents, resulting in relatively high nonresponse rates and in poor data quality. Quantitative substantiation of this assertion is less easy to come by. Moles (1987) reports that the length of the interview and the proportion of respondents who feel tired at the end of their interviews increases with their age. Herzog et al (1983) report similar and pronounced age differences for telephone interviews. Gibson and Aitkenhead (1983) corroborate the basic age effect in a sample of Australians within the restricted age range of 60 years of age and older.

By keeping the interviews as short as possible, tiredness and its effects may be minimized. Another way of dealing with a lengthy and tiring interview is proposed by Gibson and Aitkenhead (1983), who used an abbreviated interview that could be administered to an impaired respondent or to a proxy respondent. In the Iowa EPESE and in a study on hip fractures (Kelsey et al, 1989), visits were sometimes split into two sessions. Carp (1989) also suggests dividing the interview into two halves and conducting the parts on different days. All methods have their shortcomings. If abbreviated interviews are administered, information on many variables will be missing. If the interviews are split into two or more sessions, the break between sessions allows respondents to refuse the completion of the interview. Nevertheless, all procedures attempt to deal with a real problem: how to obtain information from those who may not be able to sustain a lengthy interview because of physical or cognitive problems.

A slightly different interpretation holds that it is the complexity of many of the standard survey questions, the tedious sequencing of many surveys, and the respondents' lack of interest in the topic of the survey, rather than the sheer length, that accounts for its tiring effect. Procedures that have been suggested to deal with these problems include (1) structuring the sequence in which the questions are asked, so as to put exhausting and less important questions toward the end, and (2) breaking up long sequences of questions by changes in topic areas or interspersing physical activities.

Interviewer Training

Interviewers in studies of older adults are generally given at least some special training to acquaint them with the problems often encountered with such respondents. Such procedures include, for example, the use of video tapes and role-playing exercises. In some studies—most notably, the evaluation of the National Long Term Care Channeling Demonstration Project conducted by Mathematica Policy Research (MPR)—considerable effort went into sensitizing interviewers who are not elderly to physical problems often faced by old and frail people. For example, a tape, the "Unfair Hearing Test," simulates what it is like to be hearing impaired. Impaired vision was simulated by having the interviewers wear glasses smeared with Vaseline. Popcorn in the interviewers' shoes simulated the discomfort of walking for someone with problems such as arthritis. The interviewers also read a lot of material about the elderly, and poems by the elderly about what it is like to live in a body that is not working well. The results of this sensitization program have been promising, but we are not aware of any systematic evaluations, and the apparent effects of sensitization may be confounded with existing characteristics of the interviewers. MPR has also developed a video tape on interviewing the elderly that is available and has been used elsewhere. Actors were hired to play the role of elderly respondents.

Another problem that needs addressing during interviewer training is that of the burden that interviews with the elderly put on the interviewer. Interviews with the elderly take longer (an observation corroborated by every survey with which we are familiar; see also Moles, 1987). Older adults are more likely to digress from the topic of the question (Kelsey et al, 1989) and less willing or able to use the standardized response categories (Jobe and Mingay, 1990). For these reasons, interviewing the elderly is in some respects more strenuous than interviewing younger adults (Gibson and Aitkenhead, 1983). The interviewer must be more attentive to catch possible deviations from appropriate response behavior and must be more tactful in drawing respondents back to the original questions. More frequent interviewer assistance in interviews with elderly respondents has been documented (Herzog and Rodgers, 1988b; Moles 1987).

Given the increased assistance that is required from interviewers, it is particularly important to instruct interviewers to avoid influencing respondents' answers. Indeed, slightly higher interviewer effects have been observed for older adults (Collins, as reported in Hoinville, 1983; Herzog and Rodgers, 1982).

Interviewers may further experience a disproportionate amount of distress when faced with the many problems expressed by and observed in older people. As in any interview that brings difficult issues to the surface, interviews that deal with issues of aging can raise awareness and empathy among the interviewers for problems faced by the aged. Discussion of such a burden and its origin during interviewer training and suggestions on how to deal with it helps to minimize problems and burnout during field work. Referral information with respect to services for specific problems that might be discussed during the interview can also be carried by the interviewer and provided to respondents when appropriate. Another suggestion is that the standard number of completed interviews per time unit and the expected length per interview as they are specified by some survey organizations should be relaxed explicitly in a survey of older adults to acknowledge the increased burden. At the same time (and this is worth pointing out during training), many interviewers express delight at the rich reports, the vitality, and the wisdom displayed by many older adults and experience a shattering of their stereotypes of older age (Gibson and Aitkenhead, 1983).

Respondent Training

Training and intervention procedures have been used in survey research and in gerontological research on cognitive functioning. In survey research, one set of procedures (Cannell et al, 1981) is based on the recognition that those who are selected for an interview are often unclear about what is expected of them in the role of respondent, and that instructing them in this role improves their reporting. The procedures, which include three dimensions—commitment, instructions, and feedback—have been shown to improve reporting in face-to-face and telephone interview surveys on health and mass media use (Cannell et al, 1977; Cannell et al, 1981; National Center for Health Statistics, 1987b).

In research on intellectual processes among older persons, considerable evidence exists to show that with proper training older adults can improve their performance in intelligence tests and other problem-solving tasks (Baltes and Willis, 1982). Characteristics of training procedures that appear to be successful include modeling, direct instructions, and possibly feedback (for review see Denney, 1979). Although most training procedures for cognitive functioning consist of extensive efforts, there are some indications that even a minor exposure can have a beneficial effect. For example, Baltes and Willis (1982) note an improvement from pre- to posttest of cognitive functioning, as assessed, conducted on an older control group. They suggest that this reflects a facilitative effect of the first experience with the test. Likewise, Colsher and Wallace (1989) observed a decline in missing data from an earlier to a later interview among older adults (using a similar interview schedule). One of the interpretations that they suggest for the decline is the effect of the experience with the first interview.

Because today's older adults have had less experience with standardized testing and interviewing than younger cohorts, they might benefit from some guidance on how to view and relate to a survey interview. Procedures such as those developed by Cannell and his colleagues should be investigated.

Proxy Reporters

Although a body of research evaluates the relative quality of responses provided by proxy reporters, most of this research is flawed by a critical design feature: Sampled persons for whom a proxy is sought are different in their physical and mental health from sampled persons who can respond for themselves. Consequently, in most studies it is impossible to separate the effects of proxy reporting on response quality from the effect of self-selection: Either proxy information is collected on a subset of respondents who are not healthy enough to answer for themselves and the quality of this information is contrasted with the quality of self-reports by those healthy enough to do so, or proxy and self-reports are collected on the same persons, but only those who are healthy enough to report for themselves are eligible. Both designs are flawed because of confounding and likely bias. Furthermore, external validation criteria are rarely available to establish which of two discrepant reports is more accurate. These and other methodological problems affecting most existing investigations of the quality of proxy responses are discussed in a recent literature review by Moore (1988).

With these caveats in mind, the existing literature on proxy information in epidemiologic studies suggests that its validity varies considerably, depending on the relationship of the proxy to the respondent, the type of information sought, and the time period over which information is being sought. Regarding the relationship of the proxy, household surveys typically ask a close relative, such as the spouse or an adult son or daughter, to serve as proxy; in institutional settings the immediate caretaker is often sought. However, some surveys retain the original proxy even if the sampled person moves into an institution. One aspect of the proxy that might be critical is how often the proxy interacts with the sampled person; a number of well-designed studies are relevant here. For example, proxies who live with the respondent provide more highly corresponding, but also more biased information, than proxies who do not live with the respondent (Magaziner et al, 1988). Bassett and Magaziner (1988) have recently reported that the frequency of contact is positively related to the response quality of the proxy, if the proxy does not live with the sampled person. Results reported by Epstein et al (1989) indicate that proxy reporters who helped the older person more frequently were more discrepant in their assessment of the respondent's health from the respondent's own assessment than were proxies who helped less frequently. Because the frequency of helping is related to health status, interpretation of this finding is difficult, but one possible explanation is that proxies who provided a lot of care were justifying that level of care by describing the respondent as in particularly bad health.

It seems logical that the choice of proxy should be determined by the nature of the information sought. For example, caretakers may be more knowledgeable than family members about the physical health and functional symptoms of institutionalized respondents, whereas family members might be more knowledgeable about personal and family history, economic situation, and the like. Among family members, wives have been shown to be particularly reliable proxy reporters for dietary information (Kolonel et al, 1977) and siblings for events of childhood years (Pickle et al, 1983). More generally, spouses appear to provide less missing and more consistent survey answers than children or friends (Farrow and Samet, 1990).

Regarding the type of information, the assumption is widely shared that proxies can be asked to report about factual information but not about feelings, such as satisfactions or depression, or about cognitive performance. Recent findings (Bassett and Magaziner, 1988; Epstein et al, 1989; Rodgers and Herzog, 1989) suggest that reports by properly chosen proxies can provide information that is about as valid as self-reports. However, biases may be present; for example, proxies tend to judge the respondent as less satisfied than does the respondent himself. It is also suggested that subjectively experienced symptoms may indeed be less accurately reported by proxies than specific conditions or observable functions (Magaziner et al, 1987; Magaziner et al, 1988).

One final issue concerns the setting in which the proxy interview occurs. Although in many surveys the proxy respondent is interviewed alone, and sometimes over the telephone, in the New Haven EPESE the proxy answers the survey questions in the presence of the sampled person. This provides an opportunity for the two to assist each other in retrieving the requested information. We shall return to this issue in a more systematic fashion in the next section.

To summarize, responses by proxy are unavoidable in surveys of the elderly to represent those who are truly unable to report for themselves and who cannot be reached because of institutional regulations or protective families. Although some reassuring evidence documents the quality of proxy responses, more systematic research on this topic is needed. We suspect that the final verdict will depend on who the proxy respondent is, what information must be obtained, and the interaction between the two. In the meantime, it is certainly wise to pay attention to the proportion of proxy respondents as a potential confounding variable in subgroup comparisons (e.g., comparisons of the oldest-old with younger groups of older Americans; Kelsey et al, 1989).

Assistors

By standard practice, survey interviews are sought in private, and participation by other family members is actively discouraged on the assumption that the presence, and especially the participation, of another person may influence the respondent and thereby decrease response accuracy. This may be true for younger respondents, but one can speculate that family members or caregivers could actually play a beneficial role for older adults, because some older adults may find it difficult to deal with a rather formal interview conducted by an interviewer they do not know. The presence of a familiar and trusted adult might make the older respondent more comfortable with the interview situation. More important, the familiar adult might assist the older respondent to recall some information, or could even conduct the interview under the interviewer's guidance, thereby alleviating fears about the interview situation and facilitating communication during the interview. An interesting example is reported by Fischer et al (1989), who showed that caregivers could reliably administer a modified version of a cognitive examination themselves if careful instructions were given. At the most extreme, the familiar adult would answer the questions instead of the older respondent, effectively acting as a proxy, as discussed earlier.

Obtaining Information from Administrative Sources

A promising means of upgrading the quality of data on older adults is to supplement self-reports with administrative records, especially if the source of such records is different from the respondent. The National Death Index (NDI) is rapidly gaining popularity as a means of following up respondents who are lost from a panel and may have died and as a means of confirming reports by others that the panel member has died. The NDI was created for nationwide tracking of deaths that have ocurred in research populations (Rogot et al, 1983; Wentworth et al, 1983). Upon approval by the NDI, the NDI will match submitted names and identify the states in which the deaths occurred, the dates of the deaths, and the corresponding death certificate numbers. Various pieces of personal information and ideally the Social Security number are needed for successful matching. Copies of the actual death certificates including the cause of death can then be obtained from the appropriate state offices for a fee. The matches have to be done carefully because neither research nor administrative files are perfect; generally, the more identifying information available for each person, the more successful the matching procedure.

The Medicare file compiled from data collected by HCFA, disscussed earlier as a possible sampling frame, also represents a source of information on dates of hospitalizations and diagnoses. It can also be matched with research data to supplement self-report information.

The MEDSTAT files that are currently being developed will contain information on Medicaid enrollees that can be linked to research data files. The information is compiled and managed by HCFA and includes information on eligibility history, health service utilization, expenditures, and personal information.

Interviewer Observations and Systematic Tests

Another form of bolstering self-report information with information from the interview context proper is to conduct standardized tests and systematic interview observations. Although tests have often been considered off-limits to the personal survey, several recent examples document the feasibility of including tests of verbal intelligence and memory into a personal interview. For example, a free recall test was included in the Iowa EPESE study (O'Hara et al, 1986), a free recall test in the East Boston EPESE (Scherr et al, 1988), a free recall and a recognition test in the Study of Michigan Generations (Herzog and Rodgers, 1989), a sentence completion test to assess a form of crystalized verbal intelligence from the Lorge-Thorndike Intelligence Test in the Americans' Changing Lives Survey conducted by the Survey Research Center at the University of Michigan, and a test of cognitive flexibility from Schaie's Test of Behavioral Rigidity in the Study of Michigan Generations (Herzog and Rodgers, 1989). Tests of cognitive impairment in the form of the Mental Status Questionnaire (Pfeiffer, 1975) and the Mini-Mental Status Questionnaire (Folstein et al, 1975) were included in many surveys of the aged, among them the EPESE studies conducted by NIA, the many studies using the OARS methodology, the MESA Study conducted at the University of Michigan, and the Americans' Changing Lives Survey conducted by the Survey Research Center at the University of Michigan.

Tests of physical performance have also been developed and used in surveys of older adults. For example, a test of a range of motion was used by Branch and Jette in the Masssachusetts Health Care Panel Study. More recently, the MacArthur Program on Successful Aging has developed a number of balance and gait measures that are currently being used in several sites.

Systematic observations by interviewers are usually collected upon the completion of an interview but are mostly aimed at some very global assessment of the respondent's willingness and ability to participate and of the physical environment. These observations could be expanded to include critical incidents of cognitive and physical impairment. In most instances such observations could also be improved by more specific and particularly behavioral description of the characteristics to be rated and by more careful development of the rating scales.

Mode and Form of Survey Administration

Mode of survey administration—by telephone, by mail, or face to face—was discussed at an earlier point in this chapter as a tool in reaching different groups of eligible respondents and thereby reducing nonresponse. Mode is also related to item nonresponse and to response error and thus must be considered when attempting to reduce these forms of error. Compared to surveys conducted face to face, telephone surveys result in higher proportions of item-missing responses but yield similar response distributions (Groves and Kahn, 1979). These findings do not differ if only older respondents are examined, but the interview is experienced as more burdonsome by the elderly when it takes place on the phone than face to face (Herzog and Rodgers, 1988b;

Herzog et al, 1983). The findings suggest that telephone surveys can be conducted with older adults, but that special attention and interviewer training may have to be devoted to reduce item-missing responses and that the length of the interview has to be controlled rigorously.

Telephone surveys may also be considered as a means of conducting follow-up surveys or for completing an interview that had to be cut short because of frailty and tiredness of the respondent.

Much less is known about mail surveys with elderly adults. Although there are examples of mail surveys conducted with older adults, the mail mode has not been systematically evaluated for use with this age group. Pertinent information is summarized by Herzog and Kulka (1989) and led to the conclusion that mail surveys should not necessarily be discounted as a means of data collection by gerontological researchers but that more systematic research is needed.

A related issue refers to self-administered questions and measures that are presented as part of a face-to-face interview. This mode of administration is often chosen in order to accommodate a larger number of questions. Anecdotal evidence from surveys conducted at the Survey Research Center suggests, however, that this rationale may not work for all older respondents, because many do not see well enough or do not trust their competence and thus request that the interviewer read the questions. (See also Toner et al, 1988, for similar observations.) And if questions or response categories are presented in written form, the presentation must be very carefully designed. For example, to assure legibility, letters must be large enough and the figure–ground contrast must be strong enough.

In the following paragraphs we summarize some characteristics of older adults that may explain the difficulties experienced in survey interviews.

POSSIBLE FACTORS AFFECTING SURVEY DATA OF THE ELDERLY

Health and Functional Impairments

Perhaps the most obvious characteristic associated with old age is deteriorating health. Most health problems reported by the oldest old are chronic rather than acute (Havlik et al, 1987), and these often limit daily activities (cf. Rosenwaike, 1985). Moreover, vision and hearing impairments become increasingly frequent and severe with age (Corso, 1977; Havlik, 1986), as do severe cognitive impairments (Gurland et al, 1980; Myers et al, 1984; Pfeffer et al, 1987). Memory performance and certain dimensions of intelligence decline (Craik, 1977; Perlmutter, 1978, 1986; Poon, 1985; Schaie, 1979). Many of these conditions are particularly prevalent among the oldest old (Cornoni-Huntley et al, 1986; Havlik, 1986; Havlik et al, 1987).

Indeed, the problems associated with interviewing the old and oldest old are often conceived as those arising from the minority who can be classified as "the frail elderly" who are "not institutionalized, but . . . cannot function independently" and who "tend to be neglected . . . because they are more difficult to locate and to interview" (Streib, 1983, p. 40; see also Shanas, 1962). They or their caretakers may judge that their cognitive impairments would make it too difficult for them to follow interview questions and to provide accurate information. Or they may judge that physical and functional health problems would interfere with sustained effort and a pleasant exchange. Based on such considerations, they may decline the request to be interviewed. Of course, in such decisions the respondent or caretaker is prejudging not only the respondent's own functioning but also the requirements of the interview situation. We are unable to assess how realistic the latter judgments may be or how amenable they are to modification, because very little information is available about the preceptions that the public, and in particular the elderly, hold about the typical interview.

Once participation has been secured, sensory, cognitive, and physical health problems may affect performance in a standard interview. The respondent has to understand the question properly and retrieve the relevant information from memory. Many distortions may occur during retrieval. If the information cannot be retrieved, rules of inference may be applied to reconstruct the information (Bradburn et al, 1987; Loftus et al, 1985; Turner and Martin, 1984). Older adults are more likely than younger adults to disregard the standardized scale format and respond in terms that do not easily translate into the given format (Jobe and Mingay, 1990). They also tend to sidestep questions and converse "on the side" (Moles, 1987). As a consequence, older adults generate more missing data problems (Colsher and Wallace, 1989; Gergen and Back, 1966; Glenn, 1969) and need more frequent assistance from the interviewer in the form of repeating questions and response categories (Herzog and Rodgers, 1988b). Moles (1987) reports a systematic assessment of interviewer assistance in the form of repeating question stems and response categories, each of which is a permissible interviewer action even in a highly standardized interview. The proportion of respondents who received such assistance is higher for older and particularly for the oldest respondents.

Personality and Motivational Factors

Other potential explanations for the possibility that survey data from older adults might contain more errors refer to personality and social characteristics rather than physical and cognitive health. First, with respect to nonresponse, the older adult has less frequent contact with unfamiliar persons because of the termination of work and family roles that involve regular contact with strangers. Fear of crime, often cited to explain the recent drop of response rates in cities (House and Wolf, 1978), is disproportionately high among older adults (Clemente and Kleiman, 1976) and may make them hesitant to admit a stranger into their homes. Several gerontological investigators believe that fear of crime and concern for safety are critical factors in nonresponse among the elderly. It is also conceivable that older persons who are unable to keep their homes and themselves presentable because of physical impairments and a lack of help may be too embarrassed over their condition and that of their homes to admit a stranger.

Increased introspection with age (cf. Botwinick, 1978; Neugarten, 1968) may reduce interest in political and social developments and the eagerness to talk about them. Loss of interest, in turn, may contribute to nonresponse (Goyder, 1985; Heberlein and Baumgartner, 1978; Hoinville, 1983; Yu and Cooper, 1983), to more frequent DK answers (Herzog and Rodgers, 1982), and possibly to less accurate reporting.

The great adaptability of the human organism contributes further to response error or at least confounds age comparisons. As people grow older and experience fewer societal opportunities and more personal limitations, they continuously adapt by behavioral compensations and cognitive restructuring in order to maintain a positive view of the self (Atchley, 1982). As a consequence, older adults will still answer that they can drive an automobile, although they may have curtailed their driving at night and in bad weather (Transportation Research Board, 1988). Or they will answer that they are satisfied with their housing although they may have modified their housing standards (Campbell et al, 1976).

Cohort Differences

Although many of the characteristics of older adults discussed so far are probably related to chronological age, a few cohort-related differences should also be mentioned. Those persons who make up today's population of older adults received, on average, fewer years of formal education and during their schooling and work life encountered fewer tests and standardized interviews than today's younger adults. Thus, today's older adults may differ from older adults of the future in their understanding of the necessity of these procedures, as well as in their familiarity and comfort with them. Such differences in experience may explain why today's older adults are more likely than today's younger adults to resist the standardized question and response format, to formulate responses in their own words, and to digress from the task of answering into a discussion of the question or the general topic of the interview. Also, the meaning of certain topics and the ease with which people think and talk about them differ by age or cohort. For example, as we mentioned earlier, many gerontological researchers have observed that today's older adults appear less comfortable than younger generations in talking about psychological phenomena.

Nature of Information

Chronological age and its correlates impact on the survey process in yet another way. The information that is requested in a survey interview may be inherently different for different age groups or cohorts. For example, because older persons have lived for many more years, the information of interest in many social and epidemiologic surveys is more complex than that for younger persons. Telling examples are nutritional histories in research on cancer and heart disease etiology; employment and earnings histories in economic research; and life event histories in stress and coping research.

CONCLUDING COMMENT

In this chapter we have reviewed currently available survey research methods with respect to surveying the elderly and have evaluated the use of these methods with older populations in light of the existing evidence. Although much systematic research remains to be carried out, we are willing to venture some suggestions. In our own work and that of others we have not been able to identify disproportionate response errors among surveys of older Americans. To be sure, data collected with survey techniques potentially contain many forms of errors, but this is true for the entire adult population and does not appear to be more serious among those over 60 years of age. Also, we do not deny that the structure and meaning of specific measures may differ for different age groups and that careful evaluation of measurement equivalence is always necessary for age comparisons. But in this review we have focused more narrowly on the quality of survey data collected from older adults, addressing a concern that is often voiced in the context of discussions on data needs on older Americans.

However, we do believe that such a concern may be justified with respect to the oldest old, and particularly the impaired and unhealthy among them. These persons are less likely to participate in the survey, and by their absence they may produce a nonresponse bias. If they do participate, they are less likely to provide a usable answer; and they are more likely to provide an answer of questionable quality. Methodological research efforts need to focus on this particular group.

It has been suggested that the highly structured and standardized interview format typical for most surveys may have to be relaxed for interviews with some of these elderly. Standardized interview questions and procedures are the rule in established survey research organizations because variations in survey and interview procedures can introduce variable error and bias into resulting data. But the inflexibility of these methods may introduce errors of their own into surveys of older and particularly the oldest old: Information is lost when respondents refuse to participate in what they judge to be an onerous interview or decline to answer an unintelligible question; and information is erroneous when respondents guess answers or misunderstand questions. Critics have pointed out that standardized interviews violate norms of ordinary discourse, thereby introducing error; and they point out that interviews should more closely follow the conventions of normal discourse, which has several characteristics that distinguish it from the course of the typical survey interview (Briggs, 1986; Jordan and Suchman, 1987; Mishler, 1986). This criticism may be particularly relevant to interviews with specific subgroups such as older respondents (as noted in the collaborations between cognitive psychologists and survey methodologists; cf. Jabine et al, 1984), among whom resistance to the standardized interview format has been noted by many researchers. Efforts to design more flexible interview procedures that can be adjusted to the specific respondent are therefore needed.

Another way in which data from older adults may be improved is to augment self-report data with data from other sources such as systematic observations, information from proxies, tests, and administrative records. We have discussed several of these suggestions.

A good understanding of the limitations and potentials of the various types of survey methods is critical for an informed interpretation of the resulting data and certainly for the mounting of actual data collection efforts. We hope that we have been able to raise the appreciation among our readers for the types of the errors that can be introduced into the data by the choice of methods. We even hope that some of our readers may consider undertaking further methodological investigations of their own, thereby contributing to a solid and much needed foundation of survey research methods with the elderly.

ACKNOWLEDGMENTS

The preparation of this chapter was supported by NIA Grant R01-AG02038. The authors are grateful to their colleague Robert Groves for many discussions on possible improvements of survey methods for older adults, to many gerontological researchers for sharing their experiences in investigating the elderly, and to Jennifer Kelsey, L O'Brien, and Richard Schulz for useful comments on an earlier version.

REFERENCES

Andersen R, Kasper J, Frankel MR, et al (1979). Total Survey Error. San Francisco, Jossey-Bass.
Andrews FM (1984). Construct validity and error components of survey measures: A structural modeling approach. Public Opinion Quart 48:409–442.
Andrews FM, Herzog AR (1986). The quality of survey data as related to age of respondent. J Am Statist Assoc 81:403–410.
Atchley RC (1982). The aging self. Psychother Theor Res Pract 19:388–396.
Babbie ER (1989). The Practice of Social Research, 5th ed. Belmont, CA, Wadsworth.
Baltes PB, Willis SL (1982). Plasticity and enhancement of intellectual functioning in old age: Penn State's Adult Development and Enrichment Project (ADEPT). In Craik FIM, Trehub S (eds), Aging and Cognitive Processes, Vol. 8. New York, Plenum, pp 353–389.
Bassett SS, Magaziner J (1988). The use of proxy responses on mental health measures for aged, community-dwelling women. Presented at the 41st Annual Scientific Meeting of The Gerontological Society of America, San Francisco.
Baur EJ (1947). Response bias in a mail survey. Public Opin Quart 11:594–600.
Belson WA (1960). Volunteer bias in test-room groups. Public Opin Quart 24:115–126.
Benney M, Gray AP, Pear RH (1956). How people vote. New York, Grove Press.
Berelson BR, Lazarsfeld PF, McPhee WN (1954). Voting. Chicago, University of Chicago Press.
Bollen KA, Barb KH (1981). Pearson's R and coarsely categorized measures. Am Sociol Rev 46:232–239.
Botwinick J (1978). Aging and Behavior, 2nd ed. New York, Springer.
Bradburn NM (1983). Response effects. In Rossi PH, Wright JD, Anderson AB (eds), Handbook of Survey Research. New York, Academic Press.
Bradburn NM, Rips LJ, Shevell SK (1987). Answering autobiographical questions: The impact of memory and inference on surveys. Science 236:157–161.
Briggs CL (1986). Learning How to Ask. Cambridge, Cambridge University Press.
Bush TL, Miller SR, Golden AL, Hale WE (1989). Self-report and medical record report agreement of selected medical conditions in the elderly. Am J Public Health 79:1554–1556.
Campbell A, Converse PE, Rodgers WL (1976). The Quality of American Life: Perceptions, Evaluations, and Satisfactions. New York, Russell Sage Foundation.
Cannell C, Fisher G, Bakker T (1965). Reporting of hospitalization in the Health Interview Survey. Vital and Health Statistics, Ser. 2, No. 6. Washington, DC, U.S. Government Printing Office.
Cannell CF, Miller PV, Oksenberg L (1981). Research on interviewing techniques. In Leinhardt S (ed), Sociological Methodology 1981. San Francisco, Jossey-Bass.
Cannell CF, Oksenberg L, Converse JM (1977). Striving for response accuracy: Experiments in new interviewing techniques. J Mark Res 14:306–315.
Carp FM (1989). Maximizing data quality in community studies of older people. In Lawton MP,

Herzog AR (eds), Special Research Methods for Gerontology. Amityville, NY, Baywood, pp 93–122.
Carp FM, Carp A (1981). It may not be the answer, it may be the question. Res Aging 3:85–100.
Clark MS, Mills J (1979). Interpersonal attraction in exchange and communal relationships. J Pers Soc Psychol 37:12–24.
Clemente F, Kleiman MB (1976). Fear of crime among the aged. Gerontologist 16:207–210.
Cochran WG (1968). The effectiveness of adjustment by subclassifications in removing bias in observational studies. Biometrics 24:295–313.
Colsher PL, Wallace RB (1989). Data quality and age: Health and psychobehavioral correlates of item nonresponse and inconsistent responses. J Gerontol Psychol Sci 44:P45–P52.
Cooney TM, Schaie KW, Willis SL (1988). The relationship between prior functioning on cognitive and personality dimensions and subject attrition in longitudinal research. J Gerontol (Psychol Sci) 43:P12–P17.
Cornoni-Huntley JC, Brock DB, Ostfeld AM, Taylor JO, Wallace RB (eds) (1986). Established populations for epidemiologic studies of the elderly. National Institute on Aging. NIH Pub. No. 86-2443.
Corso JF (1977). Auditory perception and communication. In Birren JE, Schaie KW (eds), Handbook of the Psychology of Aging. New York, Van Nostrand Reinhold.
Cox EP, III (1980). The optimal number of response alternatives for a scale: A review. J Mark Res 17:407–422.
Craik FIM (1977). Age differences in human memory. In Birren JE, Schaie KW (eds), Handbook of the Psychology of Aging. New York, Van Nostrand Reinhold, pp. 384–420.
DeMaio TJ (1980). Refusals: Who, where and why. Public Opinion Quart 44:223–233.
Denney NW (1979). Problem solving in later adulthood: Intervention research. In Baltes PB, Brim OG, Jr. (eds), Life-span Development and Behavior, Vol. 2. New York, Academic Press.
Downes J (1952). The longitudinal study of familes as a method of research. Milbank Memorial Fed Quart Bull 30:101–118.
Epstein AM, Hall JA, Tognetti J, Son LH, Conant L, Jr. (1989). Using proxies to evaluate quality of life. Medi Care 27:S91–S98.
Farrow DC, Samet JM (1990). Comparability of information provided by elderly cancer patients and surrogates regarding health and functional status, social network, and life events. Epidemiology 1:370–376.
Ferber R (1966). Item nonresponse in a consumer survey. Public Opinion Quart 30:399–415.
Fischer L, Visintainer PF, Schulz R (1989). Reliable assessment of cognitive impairment in dementia patients by family caregivers. Gerontol Soc Am 29:333–335.
Fitti JE, Kovar MG (1987). The supplement on aging to the 1984 National Health Interview Survey. Vital and Health Statistics, Ser. 1, No. 21. DHHS Pub. No. (PHS) 87-1323. Public Health Service, Washington, DC.
Folstein MF, Folstein SE, McHugh PR (1975). "Mini-mental state": A practical method for grading the cognitive state of patients for the clinican. J Psychiatr Res 12:189–198.
Francis JD, Busch L (1975). What we know about "I don't know." Public Opinion Quart 39:207–218.
Freedman DS, Thornton A, Camburn D (1980). Maintaining response rates in longitudinal studies. Sociol Meth Res 9:87–98.
Gergen KJ, Back KW (1966). Communication in the interview and the disengaged respondent. Public Opinion Quart 30:385–398.
Gibson DM, Aitkenhead W (1983). The elderly respondent: Experiences from a large-scale survey of the aged. Res Aging 5:283–296.

Glenn ND (1969). Aging, disengagement, and opinionation. Public Opinion Quart 33:17–33.

Goudy WJ (1976). Nonresponse effects on relationships between variables. Public Opinion Quart 40:360–369.

Gould R (1984). Fundraising as a communal exhange: Donor response and the availability heuristic. Proceedings of the American Psychological Association, Consumer Psychology Division, August.

Goyder J (1985). Face-to-face interviews and mailed questionnaires: The net difference in response rate. Public Opinion Quart 49:234–252.

Groves RM (1989). Survey Errors and Survey Costs. New York, Wiley.

Groves RM, Kahn RL (1979). Surveys by Telephone: A National Comparison with Personal Interviews. New York, Academic Press.

Gurland B, Dean L, Cross P, Golden R (1980). The epidemiology of depression and dementia in the elderly: The use of multiple indicators of these conditions. In Barret JE, Cole JO (eds), Psychopathology in the Aged. New York, Raven.

Harlow SD, Linet MS (1989). Agreement between questionnaire and medical records: The evidence for accuracy of recall. Am J Epidemiol 129:233–248.

Havlik RJ (1986). Aging in the eighties: Impaired senses for sound and light in persons age 65 years and over. Advance data from Vital and Health Statistics, No. 125. DHHS Pub. No. (PHS) 86-1250. Hyattsville, MD, Public Health Service.

Havlik RJ, Liu BM, Kovar MG, et al (1987). Health statistics on older persons, United States, 1986. Vital and Health Statistics, Ser. 3, No. 25. DHHS Pub. No. (PHS) 87-1409. Washington, DC, Public Health Service.

Hawkins DF (1975). Estimation of nonresponse bias. Sociolog Meth Res 3:461–488.

Heberlein TA, Baumgartner R (1978). Factors affecting response rates to mailed questionnaires: A quantitative analysis of the published literature. Am Sociol Rev 43:447–462.

Herzog AR (1987). Nonresponse in Sample Surveys of Older Adults. Presented at the 40th Annual Scientific Meeting of the Gerontological Society of America, Washington, DC, November.

Herzog AR, Dielman L (1985). Age differences in response accuracy for factual survey questions. J Gerontol 40:350–357.

Herzog AR, Kulka RA (1989). Telephone and mail surveys with older populations: A methodological overview. In Lawton MP, Herzog AR (eds), Special Research Methods for Gerontology. Amityville, NY, Baywood, pp. 63–89.

Herzog AR, Rodgers WL (1982). Surveys of older Americans: Some methodological investigations. Final Report to the National Institute on Aging. Ann Arbor, MI, Institute for Social Research.

Herzog AR, Rodgers WL (1986). Satisfaction among older adults. In Andrews FM (ed), Research on the Quality of Life. Ann Arbor, MI, Institute for Social Research, The University of Michigan, pp. 235–251.

Herzog AR, Rodgers WL (1988a). Age and response rates to interview sample surveys. J Gerontol (Soc Sci) 43:S200–S205.

Herzog AR, Rodgers WL (1988b). Interviewing older adults: Mode comparison using data from a face-to-face survey and a telephone resurvey. Public Opinion Quart 52:84–99.

Herzog AR, Rodgers WL (1989). Age differences in memory performance and memory ratings as measured in a sample survey. Psychol Aging 4:173–182.

Herzog AR, Rodgers WL, Kulka RA (1983). Interviewing older adults: A comparison of telephone and face-to-face modalities. Public Opinion Quart 47:405–418.

Hochstim JR (1967). A critical comparison of three strategies of collecting data from households. J Am Stat Assoc 62:976–989.

Hoinville G (1983). Carrying out surveys among the elderly: Some problems of sampling and interviewing. J Mark Res Soc 25:223–237.

House JS, Wolf S (1978). Effects of urban residence and interpersonal trust and helping behavior. J Pers Soc Behav 36:1029–1043.

Jabine TB, Straf ML, Tanur JM, Tourangeau R (eds) (1984). Cognitive Aspects of Survey Methodology: Building a Bridge Between Disciplines. Washington, DC, National Academy Press.

Jobe JB, Mingay DJ (1990). Cognitive laboratory approach to designing questionnaires for surveys of the elderly. Public Health Rep 105:518–523.

Jordan B, Suchman L (1987). Interactional troubles in survey interviews. Proceedings of the Section on Survey Research Methods, American Statistical Association.

Kalton G, Anderson DW (1989). Sampling rare populations. In Lawton MP, Herzog AR (eds), Special Research Methods for Gerontology. Amityville, NY, Baywood, pp. 7–30.

Kane RA, Kane RL (1981). Assessing the Elderly: A Practical Guide to Measurement. Lexington, MA, Rand Corporation.

Kaye JM, Lawton P, Kaye D (1990). Attitudes of elderly people about clinical research on aging. Gerontologist 30:100–106.

Kelsey JL, O'Brien LA, Grisso JA, Hoffman S (1989). Issues in carrying out epidemiologic research in elderly. Am J Epidemiol 130:857–866.

Kish L (1965). Survey Sampling. New York, Wiley.

Kogan N (1961). Attitudes toward old people in an older sample. J Abnorm Soc Psychol 62:616–622.

Kolonel LN, Hirohata T, Nomura AMY (1977). Adequacy of survey data collected from substitute respondents. Am J Epidemiol 106:476–484.

Kovar MG, Fitti JE (1985). A linked follow-up study of older people. 1985 Proceedings of the Section of Survey Research Methods of the American Statistical Association. Washington, DC, American Statistical Association, pp. 179–184.

Lawton MP (1977). Morale: What are we measuring? In Nydegger CN (ed), Measuring Morale. Washington, DC, Gerontological Society.

Lipsitz LA, Pluchino FC, Wright SM (1987). Biomedical research in the nursing home: Methodological issues and subject recruitment results. J Am Geriatr Soc 35:629–634.

Loftus EF, Fienberg SE, Tanur JM (1985). Cognitive psychology meets the national survey. Am Psychol 40:175–180.

Magaziner J, Hebel JR, Warren JW (1987). The use of proxy responses for aged patients in long-term care settings. Compr Gerontol Bull 1:118–121.

Magaziner J, Simonsick EM, Kashner TM, Hebel JR (1988). Patient–proxy response comparability on measures of patient health and functional status. J Clin Epidemiol 41:1065–1074.

McHorney C, Teno J, Lu JF, Sherbourne C, Ware J (1990). The use of standardized measures of functional status and well-being among cognitively impaired and intact elders: Results from the Medical Outcomes Study. Presented at the 43rd Annual Scientific Meeting of the Gerontological Society of America, Boston, MA.

McKinlay J (1988). Optimal methods for studying health related behaviors of the elderly in household surveys. Presented at the International Symposium on Data on Aging: Developing Research on Measuring Health and Health Care. Bethesda, MD, National Center for Health Statistics.

Mercer JR, Butler EW (1967–68). Disengagement of the aged population and response differentials in survey research. Soc Forces 46:89–96.

Mills J, Clark MS (1982). Exchange and communal relationships. In Wheeler J (ed), Review of Personality and Social Psychology, Vol. 3. Beverly Hills, CA, Sage, pp. 121–144.

Mishler EG (1986). Research Interviewing. Cambridge, MA, Harvard University Press.
Moles EL (1987). Perceptions of the Interview Process. Presented at the 40th Annual Scientific Meeting of the Gerontological Society of America, Washington, DC, November.
Moore JC (1988). Self/proxy response status and survey response quality: A review of the literature. J Off Stat 4:155–172.
Moser CA, Kalton G (1972). Survey Methods in Social Investigations, 2nd ed. New York, Basic Books.
Myers JK, Weissman MM, Tischler GL, et al (1984). Six-month prevalence of psychiatric disorders in three communities: 1980 to 1982. Arch Gen Psychiatr 41:959–967.
National Center for Health Statistics (1987a). Proceedings of the 1987 Public Health Conference on Records and Statistics, DHHS Pub. No. (PHS) 88-1214. Hyattsville, MD.
National Center for Health Statistics (1987b). An experimental comparison of telephone and personal health surveys, Vital and Health Statistics, Ser. 2, No. 106. Washington, DC.
Neugarten BL (1968). The awareness of middle age. In Neugarten BL (ed), Middle age and aging. Chicago, University of Chicago Press.
Norris FH (1987). Effects of attrition on relationships between variables in surveys of older adults. J Gerontol 42:597–605.
O'Hara MW, Hinrichs JV, Kohout FJ, Wallace RB, Lemke JH (1986). Memory complaint and memory performance in the depressed elderly. Psychol Aging 1:208–214.
Palumbo FB, Magaziner JS, Tenney JH, Goren LM, Warren JW (1987). Recruitment of long-term care facilities for research. J Am Geriatr Soc 35:154–158.
Perlmutter M (1978). What is memory aging the aging of? Dev Psychol 14:330–345.
Perlmutter M (1986). A life span view of memory. In Baltes P, Featherman D, Brim P (eds), Advances in Life Span Development and Behavior, Vol. 6. Hillsdale, NJ, Erlbaum.
Pfeiffer E (1975). A short portable mental status questionnaire for the assessment of organic brain deficit in elderly patients. J Am Geriatr Soc 23:433–441.
Pfeffer RI, Afifi AA, Chance JM (1987). Prevalence of Alzheimer's disease in a retirement community. Am J Epidemiol 125:420–436.
Pickle LW, Brown LM, Blot WJ (1983). Information available from surrogate respondents in case-control interview studies. Am J Epidemiol 118:99–108.
Poon LW (1985). Differences in human memory with aging: Nature, causes, and clinical implications. In Birren JE, Schaie KW (eds), Handbook of the psychology of Aging, 2nd ed. New York, Van Nostrand Reinhold, pp. 427–462.
Reeder LG (1960). Mailed questionnaires in longitudinal health studies: The problem of maintaining and maximizing responses. J Health Hum Beh 1:123–129.
Riegel KF, Riegel RM, Meyer G (1967). A study of the drop-out rates in longitudinal research on aging and the prediction of death. J Pers Soc Psychol 5:342–348.
Robins L (1963). The reluctant respondent. Public Opinion Quart 27:276–286.
Rodgers WL, Herzog AR (1987). Interviewing older adults: The accuracy of factual information. J Gerontol 42:387–394.
Rodgers WL, Herzog AR (1989). The consequences of accepting proxy respondents on total survey error for elderly population. In Fowler FJ (ed), Health Survey Research Methods. National Center for Health Services Research and Health Care Technology Assessment, Public Health Service, U.S. Department of Health and Human Services, DHHS Pub. No. (PHS) 89-3447, pp. 139–146.
Rodgers WL, Herzog AR (1991). Collecting data about the oldest old: Problems and procedures. In Suzman RM, Willis DP, Manton KG (eds), The Oldest Old. New York, Oxford University Press.
Rodgers WL, Herzog AR, Andrews FM (1988). Interviewing older adults: Validity of self-reports of satisfaction. Psychol Aging 3:264–272.
Rogot E, Feinleib M, Ockay KA, Schwartz SH, Bilgrad R, Patterson JE (1983). On the feasibility

of linking census samples to the National Death Index for epidemiologic studies: A progress report. Am J Public Health 73:1265–1269.
Rossi PH, Wright JD, Anderson AB (1983). Handbook of Survey Research. Orlando, FL, Academic Press.
Rosenwaike I (1985). The Extreme Aged in America: A Portrait of an Expanding Population. Westport, CT, Greenwood Press.
Rotter J (1966). Generalized expectancies for internal vs. external control of reinforcement. Psychol Monogr 609.
Schaie KW (1979). The primary mental abilities in adulthood: An exploration in the development of psychometric intelligence. In Baltes PB, Brim, OG, Jr. (eds), Life-span Development and Behavior, Vol. 2. New York, Academic Press.
Scherr, PA, Albert MS, Funkenstein HH, Cook NR, Hennekens CH, Branch LG, White LR, Taylor JO, Evans DA (1988). Correlates of cognitive function in an elderly community population. Am J Epidemiol 128:1084–1101.
Schulz R, Tompkins CA, Rau MT (1988). A longitudinal study of the psychosocial impact of stroke on primary support persons. Psychol Aging 3:131–141.
Schuman H, Presser S (1981). Questions and answers in attitude surveys: Experiments on question form, wording, and context. New York, Academic Press.
Schwarz N (1989). Assessing frequency reports of mundane behaviors: Contributions of cognitive psychology to questionnaire construction. In Hendricks C, Clark M (eds), Research Methodology, Vol 11. Beverly Hills, CA, Sage.
Schwarz N, Strack F (1989). Evaluating one's life: A judgement model of subjective well-being. In Strack F, Argyle M, Schwarz N (eds), The Social Psychology of Well-being. London, Pergamon.
Shanas E (1962). The Health of Older People. Cambridge, MA, Harvard University Press.
Siemiatycki J (1979). A comparison of mail, telephone, and home interview strategies for household health surveys. Am J Public Health 69:238–245.
Sirken MG (1970). Household surveys with multiplicity. J Am Stat Assoc 65:257–266.
Steeh, CG (1981). Trends in nonresponse rates, 1952–1979. Public Opinion Quart 45:40–57.
Streib GF (1983). The frail elderly: Research dilemmas and research opportunities. Gerontologist 23:40–44.
Sudman S, Bradburn NM (1974). Response effects in surveys: A review and synthesis. Chicago, Aldine.
Sudman S, Kalton G (1986). New developments in the sampling of special populations. Ann Rev Sociol 12:401–429.
Tennstedt SL, McKinlay JB (1987). Choosing the most appropriate field approach for older populations: The case for mixed-mode surveys. In Proceedings of the 1987 Public Health Conference on Records and Statistics, Pub. No. (PHS) 88-1214. Hyattsville, MD, U.S. Department of Health and Human Services, pp. 427–432.
Toner J, Gurland B, Teresi J (1988). Comparison of self-administered and rater-administered methods of assessing levels of severity of depression in elderly patients. J Gerontol (Psychol Sci) 43:P136–P140.
Transportation Research Board (1988). Transportation in an aging society: Improving mobility and safety for older persons. In Committee Report and Recommendations, Vol 1. Special Report 218. Washington, DC, National Research Council.
Turner CF, Martin E (eds) (1984). Surveying Subjective Phenomena. New York, Russell Sage.
U.S. Department of Justice (1981). Issues in the measurement of victimization. Bureau of Justice Statistics, NCJ-74682, Washington, DC.
Waldo DR, Lazenby HC (1984). Demographic characteristics and health care use and expenditures by the aged in the United States: 1977–1984. Health Care Financ Rev 6:1–29.
Wallace RB (1987). The relationship of cognitive function, health status and mood to missing

data and inconsistent responses in an interview survey of the elderly. In Proceedings of the 1987 Public Health Conference on Records and Statistics. Pub. No. (PHS) 88-1214. Hyattsville, MD, U.S. Department of Health and Human Services, pp. 423–426.

Weaver CN, Holmes SL, Glenn ND (1975). Some characteristics of inaccessible respondents in a telephone survey. J Appl Psychol 60:260–262.

Wentworth DN, Neaton JD, Rasmussen WL (1983). An evaluation of the Social Security Administration master beneficiary record file and the National Death Index in the ascertainment of vital status. Am J Public Health 73:1270–1274.

Yu J, Cooper H (1983). A quantitative review of research design: Effects on response rates to questionnaires. J Mark Res 20:36–44.

7

The Pragmatics of Survey Field Work Among the Elderly

FRANK J. KOHOUT

Published reports of survey results rarely pause to describe the many problems and unforeseen events that occurred during data collection. Likewise, most textbooks on survey methods leave the novice with little appreciation for the obdurate reality of field work. Despite the hygienic precision and objectivity that such publications depict, survey field work never runs as smoothly as we would wish.

This chapter offers practical suggestions for imposing order on this inherently disorderly process. The suggestions are based largely on personal experience and anecdotal evidence reported by others, because definitive experimental evidence is lacking for much of what is covered. The chapter is intended as a complement to that of Herzog and Rodgers, which focuses on the literature of survey research methods.

The problems and issues addressed were selected mainly because they tend to be glossed over in methods textbooks and are the most likely to catch the novice researcher unprepared. The focus is on population-based surveys, which draw respondents from naturally occurring and geographically defined populations and which usually involve interviewing in respondents' homes or other remote sites. Much of this chapter applies to any type of community survey, but special attention is given to problems that arise in studying older people. Examples are drawn mainly from the multisite EPESE project (Cornoni-Huntley et al, 1986), and more particularly from the Iowa Established Populations for Epidemiologic Study of the Elderly (EPESE) site, an epidemiologic study in which the 65-and-older population of two rural counties was followed through eight annual surveys.

To dispel the notion that the practical work of survey research is merely a mechanical process, the opening section deals with some "theoretical" notions that must guide each step in designing and implementing surveys of the elderly.

THE FIRST STEP IN SURVEY DESIGN: GAINING AN APPRECIATION OF THE "ELDERLY"

For economy of expression, we commonly refer to the "elderly" or "older people" when we wish to distinguish a subpopulation. However, these labels can mislead us into assuming we are dealing with a homogeneous group. If applied to people 65 and older, for example, the term *elderly* refers to an age range of perhaps 35 years, and within this range there is as much diversity as there is in earlier years. This range is equivalent to that from the ages of 15 through 50. We would not fail to recognize the diversity in this range in designing surveys or in analyzing data.

Speaking of "the elderly" can lead to ecological fallacies: Because a higher proportion of people over 65 suffer from chronic diseases, cognitive decline, and limitations in physical function, we are apt to ascribe these characteristics to any individual in the "elderly" group. Such ecological fallacies can have subtle but serious effects on the design of questionnaires and interview protocols, the training of interviewers, and nearly every other aspect of data collection. For example, we may neglect to ask about current occupation and occupational exposures, under the assumption that "the elderly" are retired. Or we may neglect to ask detailed questions about exercise, travel, sexual behavior, or intellectual pursuits, assuming these activities have been curtailed. Then, because of our failure to include sufficiently discriminating measures, we are likely to find nothing but the homogeneity we assumed in the first place.

Within the "elderly" group, there are not only large age differences but cohort differences, which we must attend to in the design of interview content and format. We must be aware that both age and cohort differences could make the comparability of questions between the age strata of the "elderly" population problematic. That is, because of age and cohort differences, a given questionnaire may not be perceived in the same way by the various strata of the "elderly" population, so that they are, in effect, responding to different instruments.

For example, when we ask about childbearing experiences, a woman of 65 is reporting about events that occurred about 30–45 years ago, whereas a woman of 85 is reporting events 50–65 years ago. In addition to "real" differences between these women, the demands on their recall are quite different. If we fail to recognize this difference, we may attribute the older woman's lack of recall to cognitive decline. Similarly, questions about menopause may lack comparability across the "elderly" age range. If, for example, we ask a woman of 85 whether she used estrogen, she may reply in the affirmative, although she took some other drug, whose name she has forgotten.

When we ask about occupational exposures, a man of 85 will be hard-pressed to recall the names of chemicals he handled on a factory job he held for five years during the 1930s or earlier. A farmer of the same age may be able to recall using certain types of fertilizer, herbicides, and pesticides but may be unable to recall how long and in what years he used them.

Although chronological age can produce strong response effects, cohort differences may have an even greater impact. Cohort effects arise from environmental factors that change over time and that produce marked cultural, social, and psychological differences that survey designers must take into account.

For example, a man born in 1905 would have entered the labor force in the early 1920s and would have retired around 1970 to 1975. People in this cohort are likely to have been born at home, perhaps with a midwife or family member attending, and their mothers probably had no prenatal physician care. Until late in adulthood, when the health care system was more fully developed, they were unlikely to have seen a physician except when they were seriously ill. Many were foreign born or were born to recent immigrants. They were exposed to a number of epidemics during childhood and as teenagers were exposed to a worldwide influenza epidemic. A large proportion terminated their education with the eighth grade and few went on to college. Those who became factory workers probably worked long hours under sweatshop conditions.

By contrast, people born in 1925 are more likely to have been born in a hospital, and a physician is likely to have attended those born at home. A much higher proportion finished high school before entering the labor force, which was during World War II. The men are likely to have served in the armed forces, and more of the women entered the labor force than had done so previously. Those who worked in factories during and after the war were exposed to a new array of toxic substances, which resulted from advances in chemical technology.

Although cohort differences are important for assessing past exposures, they may have an even greater impact on basic attitudes, which are formed relatively early in life and are influenced by the prevailing norms of the time. Thus, a person who entered the labor force during the depression of the 1930s is likely to have markedly different attitudes on economic and political issues from one who reached adulthood in the boom years of the 1920s. Those who came of age during World War II are likely to have yet another world view.

It is interesting to speculate how future cohorts of the elderly will differ, because of the effects of mass media exposure, more prolonged education, innovations in health care, and the like. However, until these cohorts reach old age, we must attune survey methods to their seniors. We cannot assume that today's "elderly" are merely chronologically older than cohorts to follow.

The distinction between age and cohort effects is familiar in epidemiology, and these effects are recognized for the theoretical and analytical problems they entail. However, one must also appreciate age and cohort effects in terms of their implications for survey design and, more particularly, for the design of questionnaires and interviewing procedures. One must be aware that age and cohort effects have implications not only for the content of interviews, but also for their format and structure.

For a variety of reasons it is desirable to use closed-end questions in interviews: This format reduces administration time, facilitates data entry and analysis, and reduces the effects of interviewer's subjective judgment. However, we cannot assume that elderly respondents, like today's college students, are familiar with the closed-end format from multiple-choice exams and their professors' questionnaires. On average, the elderly have had less formal education, and if they were ever exposed to multiple-choice exams, these experiences occurred in the remote past. Moreover, they have not been trained to think in terms of a Likert scale, from "strongly agree" to "strongly disagree," much less in terms of "1-to-10" rating scales, so they may be uncomfortable and unfamiliar with such formats. Thus, we should not be surprised that many elderly respondents are unprepared to deal with closed-end items in a face-to-face interview.

Respondents interviewed for first time may be unfamiliar with answering questions by choosing from set categories. This may be frustrating for respondents who wish to explain their answers and expect the interviewer to listen and record them, prolix as they may be. In longitudinal studies, it is common to find that "don't know" responses and item refusals decrease at each successive follow-up. Although this may be due in part to increasing interviewer expertise, it is also likely that respondents are learning the role expected of them in the interview situation and have adapted to the closed-end format. Because "trained" respondents are more tractable, interviewers can more easily keep them focused and can reduce interviewing time while seemingly maintining better rapport.

Respondents who previously answered "don't know" to attitude items that they had never considered may now acquiesce to an "agree" or "disagree" response option. Those who gave "don't know" responses to factual items may now be willing to offer a guess, even if they really do not know the requested facts. Further, when respondents acquiesce, they are likely to select the most socially desirable response option from those they are given (Backstrom and Hursch-Cesar, 1981).

At first glance, it might appear that the tendency to acquiesce, to give socially desirable responses, and to play the role of a "good subject" will have marked effects only on questions dealing with facts and opinions and that this tendency will have minimal effects on performance tests, such as tests of physical or cognitive function. However, these biases may also enhance the respondents' motivation (to cooperate and show the interviewer how well they can do), which in turn can improve their performance on tests of physical and cognitive function.

SAMPLING AND SUBJECT SELECTION

The obvious goal of sampling is to obtain a subset of cases that is representative of the population from which it is drawn. However, although sampling is often viewed as a purely statistical matter, at least two nonstatistical considerations take precedence: An appropriate sample depends first on one's research questions and second on what is feasible.

To estimate prevalence or incidence rates for a certain well-defined population, we would want to draw a probability sample from that population. However, to identify risk factors or correlates of a disease it may be more appropriate to use a convenience sample of persons known to be free of the disease at the outset of the study. Likewise, if we are studying a relatively rare disease, it may be more appropriate to sample cases that have already been identified by the health care system (e.g., by sampling hospital records). Moreover, if we wish to generalize to some population beyond that which we sample, a convenience sample may be just as good as a probability sample. Despite common misconceptions, the statistics that support inferences from a probability sample to a population do not support generalizations to any broader population.

The advantages of population-based surveys must also be weighed against their cost, which is usually greater than those based on convenience samples of equal size. Costs of population-based surveys can be reduced by using mailed questionnaires or telephone interviews, perhaps with random-digit dialing. However, such methods preclude the use of physical measurements and may still be more expensive than in-person interviews done with a smaller, but well-chosen, convenience sample.

Adding to the cost of population-based surveys of older people is the cost of generating the sample in the first place. Only rarely is a list of, say, the 65-and-older population available. Thus, one must first develop such a list, a sampling frame, or employ area probability sampling. The former usually involves taking a census by door-to-door canvass or other means; the latter involves doing a brief screening interview at randomly selected residences to locate age-eligible respondents.

Three different approaches were used to generate population lists in the various EPESE sites (Cornoni-Huntley et al., 1986). The East Boston EPESE project used the canvassing approach to build a list, which was partially checked for completeness against patient records at the East Boston Neighborhood Health Center, where most older residents of their survey area go for primary care. The Iowa EPESE project, before interviewing in small towns and rural areas, used local informants to build an initial list, which was checked against state driver's license records and a mailing list obtained from the local Area on Aging Office. Interview appointments were then made by telephone, at which time age eligibility was verified with respondents. The New Haven EPESE project represents one of the rare instances where lists of older people were already available. A large proportion of the New Haven elderly live in retirement housing projects, which maintain lists of their residents. For those living elsewhere in the community a list was available from the utility company, which registers 65-and-older persons, because they are entitled to reduced rates.

Notably, all the EPESE projects involved large-scale surveys with rather lengthy interviews, so the costs of developing sampling frames were a relatively small percentage of the budget even in Iowa and East Boston. Had sample sizes been under 1000 or so, the cost of complete enumerations would have been prohibitive.

Assuming that it is a complete enumeration, a sampling frame not only facilitates probability sampling but enables one to assess biases in the sample that is ultimately obtained. Unfortunately, it is often not feasible, even at great expense, to generate a complete sampling frame for natural populations, so biases are inherent in the frame itself and impossible to assess, except through approximate comparisons with U.S. Census tabulations.

Curiously, we often overlook the deficiencies of a bad sampling frame or a poorly executed probability sample, presumably under the assumption that any attempt at probability sampling is superior to resorting to samples of convenience. The obverse also seems to hold: Convenience samples are suspect, no matter how well constructed. This is not to say that our faith in probability sampling is not misplaced; the problem is that we too often excuse departures from it.

The adequacy of a sampling frame must be closely scrutinized, particularly for population segments that might be underrepresented or left out entirely. Whether or not a sampling frame is used, the sampling design may systematically underrepresent or exclude certain segments, such as the oldest, the sickest, or those who can afford protracted vacations for the period in which a survey is done. Finally, because of selection biases that result from refusals, not-at-homes, and unlocatable respondents, the sample of completed interviews may depart markedly from those that were randomly drawn.

Assuming we recognize and can accurately characterize disproportionate representation in our sample, we can correct for it by appropriate weighting when analyses are performed. However, we can make no such correction for segments that are completely excluded, and if we do not have an accurate estimate of disproportionate representation, weighting is sure to produce erroneous results.

Although funding restrictions may constrain one to work with a convenience sample, one need make no excuses for doing so as long as the inherent design limitations are observed. One such limitation, which often goes unrecognized, is due to disproportionate representation on variables whose distribution in a population is completely unknown. Representativeness of a sample is usually checked by comparing the sample with a population on a limited number of demographic variables that have known distributions, perhaps using U.S. Census data. However, representativeness with regard to the main variables of interest in a given study may never be checked and may indeed be impossible to check. Unlike random sampling, which ensures reasonable representation on all variables, convenience samples cannot be trusted to be representative with regard to variables with unknown distributions.

The problem of representativeness becomes more complicated when we consider combinations of variables as they are manifest in individual members of a natural population. If, for example, a sample does not represent the population distribution of comorbid conditions and associated constellations of correlates, no statistical procedures will allow us to isolate risk factors for the population. This underscores the value of probability sampling from natural populations and the corresponding limitations of convenience samples. The latter can certainly be useful in suggesting possible relationships and in providing leads for further inquiry, but they should never be viewed as a substitute for probability sampling, even if they appear to "represent" a natural population with regard to univariate distributions on known demographic variables.

Sampling from Subpopulations

Population-based surveys, with probability sampling, can be done economically if one is willing to focus on a relatively small population or subpopulation, such as small communities or neighborhoods in larger cities. Such populations may be particularly appropriate for studying older people: In and around most cities it is usually possible to locate relatively self-contained communities or neighborhoods with large concentrations of older people. Further, despite additional limitations on representativeness, retirement communities and vaction areas that attract older people may also be strategic sites for exploring some epidemiologic questions.

These subpopulations will tend to be homogeneous with regard to such factors as race, ethnicity, socioeconomic status, and the sources of health care. However, the economies inherent in surveying small, condensed groupings may make it possible to select two or more subpopulations for comparative studies. Developing a sampling frame is also likely to be less costly, since it may be possible to identify respondents through local informants (as was done in the Iowa EPESE project) or from existing lists, such as church or club records.

Sampling from small populations that have a high concentration of people in the 65-and-older range may make it easier to locate respondents in the oldest-old range of 75 or 80 and older, but this is not always the case. For example, some retirement communities and vacation areas will be populated mainly by people under 80. Finding frail elderly respondents may also be difficult, because many relocate to be closer to their adult children or enter nursing homes outside the area. The lesson here is not to assume that the desired type of respondent will be available but to do a thorough check before selecting a subpopulation for study.

Availability of Respondents

The preceding admonition applies universally, not just to the special case of small subpopulations. Countless projects have been stymied by the lack of research subjects that investigators have assumed would be available. Further, the problem may not be that too few eligible subjects are present but that too few can be located and contacted or that too few are willing and able to cooperate with the research. In sampling patients, for example, an investigator may rely on a clinician's guess of the number of patients seen in a given time period. Instead of trusting to chance, a prudent investigator will ask for clinic records or other documentation of subject eligibility. He or she will also get the clinician and other involved staff to sign a letter specifying what they will do to assist in subject recruitment. Investigators working in other settings should likewise obtain letters of cooperation from anyone who is to assist in recruiting subjects.

One must also be assured that identified subjects will be willing to cooperate. No matter how thorough and precise the sampling plan, the resulting sample may be utterly useless if the response rate is below about 70 percent. The loss of nearly a third of the sample to self-selected refusals and other causes makes it difficult to argue that the remainder constitutes a probability sample or an otherwise representative sample of the target population. To make matters worse, it is usually impossible to assess adequately the characteristics of the lost cases, so no amount of statistical adjustment will enable one to correct for resulting biases.

Obtaining an adequate response rate involves a multitude of factors, including early public relations efforts, questionnaire design, and interviewer training and competence, to name just a few. To ensure that all these factors are working in favor of the response rate, there is no substitute for pretesting. In psychology, there is an old aphorism that says, "Never run an experiment until you're sure it will work." The message here is that extensive pretesting of instruments and methods is a necessary prelude to running an experiment. It applies equally well to surveys.

Although pretesting can be time-consuming and seemingly cause delays, it is time well spent. Each aspect of the survey should be pretested, from sampling prodecures to data processing. In addition to pretesting these aspects in isolation, it is advisable to do a formal pilot study, in which the entire survey is performed on a miniature sample (Babbie, 1973; Babbie, 1989). More will be said later about pretesting and pilot studies.

PLANNING AND ORGANIZING FIELD WORK

Field work is never as ordered and predictable as we would wish, and certainly not as tractable as our research proposal may suggest. Even if we make an appointment, the respondent may not be at home. The respondent may be surrounded by family and there may be no place to conduct a private interview. A respondent may be occupied with other activities, such as baking, repair projects, or a TV show, and may insist on continuing them throughout the interview. The respondent may be sick, intoxicated, distraught over a recent tragedy, or in the midst of an argument with a spouse, who refuses to leave.

All these are seemingly improbable situations, but over the course of a study they may constitute a sizable proportion of interviews. Further, they all entail at least minor deviations from the standard protocol and require the interviewer to decide what alternative course to take. Assuming that interviewers are well trained, they will be able to cope with many anomalous situations and, with experience, will become proficient in completing interviews under adverse conditions. However, the danger is that they may need to make ad hoc decisions about modifying the interview, and if they are allowed to deviate from the protocol as they deem appropriate, standardization is jeopardized.

Although it is impossible to plan for every contingency, it is certainly feasible to draw up a general contingency plan to cover broader categories of problem situations. This plan should provide interviewers with definite rules that specify when they may use their own judgment and when they may not, when they may terminate an interview, when they may truncate an interview and schedule a time for completing it, when they may seek medical attention for the respondent, and when and how they may seek out a proxy respondent.

Contingency plans should specify which personnel are authorized to make ad hoc decisions when certain problems are encountered, but even supervisors and investigators must be limited in the sort of ad hoc modifications they may make once field work begins. A thorough contingency plan, in writing, should specify procedures they too must follow in problematic situations. Using the "war game" approach in planning sessions, attempting to imagine worst-case scenarios and appropriate responses, is a useful strategy in constructing contingency plans.

Even with a thorough contingency plan, unforeseen situations will arise and call for ad hoc decisions. All such decisions, no matter who makes them, should be documented as they are made, entered in a logbook, and promptly disseminated to other members of the field staff. Prompt and regular reporting to investigators should also be built into the system, so that they can assess the implications of ad hoc decisions for subsequent analysis and interpretation of results.

Decisions about when to use a proxy are best left to the supervisory staff, although interviewers may be authorized to locate the most appropriate proxy once it is decided to use one. Ideally, a physician should be designated to decide what to do for respondents needing immediate medical attention, and the contingency plan should specify the conditions under which a family member or the respondent's physician should be called, transportation should be offered, and referral to a physician or hospital should be made. The contingency plan should also specify procedures for referrals to social service agencies.

Investigators who lack field work experience, particularly in surveys of the elderly, will probably need assistance in contemplating the sort of problems that will arise and in formulating contingency plans. Textbooks on survey methods (Babbie, 1973; Backstrom and Hursh-Cesar, 1981; Hoinville et al., 1977) and interviewing (Mishler, 1986; Richardson et al, 1965) are useful at the start. Perhaps better than formal textbooks is a book by Converse and Schuman (1974), which presents a collection of interviewer experiences, many described in the interviewer's own words. As a next step, consultations should be sought with experienced investigators, especially those who get involved with field work. Just as valuable, if not more so, would be consultations with interviewers and filed supervisors who have worked with older respondents. Finally, investigators and staff involved in planning field work should be sure to do at least a few interviews during the pretesting or piloting phases of the project.

Managing Field Work

No matter how experienced and trustworthy interviewers may be, supervision is essential. Smaller projects can be done with a single field supervisor, but larger studies usually require a staff with clear lines of authority. The field supervisor should be in daily contact with interviewers and should be accessible whenever interviewing is in progress. This person acts not only as a straw boss but as a counselor and resource person for the interviewers. The required number of field supervisors depends on many factors, but if interviewers report to the field supervisor daily, there should be one supervisor for every 10 interviewers.

On smaller projects, field supervisors may be responsible for scheduling the interviewers' work, but on larger projects they usually assign work as scheduled by a higher-level coordinator. Preferably, field supervisors are themselves experienced interviewers; besides directing the work of interviewers, they must be able to provide technical advice and emotional support. Field work suffers if interviewers get the impression that they know more about interviewing than their supervisor or if they believe that the supervisor lacks authority to direct their work. The field supervisor generally works long hours and is busy throughout the day with a myriad of details and unforeseen problems. It is not a job for someone who flusters easily.

In the Iowa EPESE project, field supervisors were stationed at local headquarters as interviewing proceeded from one town to another, with a crew of about 10 interviewers assigned to each supervisor. Interviewers reported to the headquarters each morning to receive their day's assignments and returned at the end of the day to submit their completed questionnaires. Field supervisors immediately reviewed their crew's questionnaires and noted any missing data, improperly scored items, or illegible comments. If an interviewer did not have an adequate explanation for such items, the field supervisor directed her to revisit or telephone the respondent to get whatever additional information was needed. During the middle of the day the field supervisors again reviewed the previous day's questionnaires in search of errors. They also exchanged and field-edited the questionnaires from one anothers' crews, so each questionnaire was reviewed three times before it reached the central office for final editing.

As noted earlier, the interviewer's authority to make ad hoc decisions must be clearly circumscribed, in the interests of standardization. However, field supervisors are typically given more leeway to decide on deviations from the protocol, but they must also be instructed to document any such ad hoc decisions and to inform the investigators promptly when they occur. Should major problems arise, the field supervisor should contact the investigator before allowing field work to proceed.

For example, during the baseline survey for the Iowa EPESE project, refusal rates in one town were running inexplicably high for about three days until one refuser commented that "Mrs. X told everyone not to talk to you." Mrs. X, it turned out, was the widow of the town's sole physician and had become their unofficial primary care provider when he died. None of the project's local informants had hinted about her influence in the community, so she was not contacted for an endorsement. When her role was discovered, however, field work was suspended until the investigators could inform her about the study. When interviewing resumed a few days later, several respondents noted that Mrs. X had called to recommend participation and nearly all who refused previously granted interviews.

Commonly, field supervisors are also responsible for conducting validation interviews (also called verification interviews), which usually entail a brief phone call to a random sample of respondents to verify that interviews were actually done. Validation interviews often involve reasking a small number of questions dispersed throughout the questionnaire in order to check that complete interviews were done. In studies using a relatively brief protocol, a sample of respondents may be given a complete interview for validation purposes. However, even in the latter cause, validation interviews serve mainly as a deterrent against slipshod and "curbside" interviews; only rarely will they detect cheating interviewers.

With all the technical responsibilities assigned to the field supervisor, it is sometimes difficult to attend sufficiently to interviewer morale. However, this is another critical function that the supervisor must perform, and time must be allowed for it (Converse and Schuman, 1974). An interviewer's morale is dealt a severe blow when she returns from a particularly trying day only to have the supervisor edit the questionnaires and point out errors. Conversely, if the interviewer has had a particularly good day, the last thing she needs is an immediate lecture on writing more legibly. The supervisor must take time to chat about the interviewers' experiences, reassuring them on bad days, sharing their joy on good days, and always expressing appreciation for their efforts. Higher-level staff, particularly investigators, should also participate in morale-boosting activities, perhaps relieving the supervisor in this function on days when the workload is particularly heavy. In the process, investigators will glean valuable insights into the problems encountered in the field.

DEVELOPING QUESTIONNAIRES FOR ELDERLY RESPONDENTS

It should be noted that the term *questionnaire* has both broad and narrow usages. In its broad sense it refers to any form on which questions are printed and responses are recorded. When differences between modes of administration are at issue, it is customary to restrict the term *questionnaire* to self-administered forms and refer to an interviewer-administered form as an "interview schedule." However, since this chapter deals only with interviews, *questionnaire* is used in its broad sense, which includes interview schedules. It should also be noted that *interview protocol,* which is sometimes used as a synonym for *interview schedule,* is used in this chapter to refer to the set of rules and procedures that interviewers are supposed to follow in gaining access to respondents, conducting interviews, recording responses, and reporting to their supervisors.

Research Questions vs. Questionnaire Items

It should be obvious that one must define one's research questions before one can write questions to ask respondents. All too often, however, investigators forge ahead to questionnaire development before their research questions are clearly formulated in detail and in writing. A short list of hypotheses or general questions will not do. What is needed is a longer list of questions and subquestions that serves to justify the inclusion of each item as well as the exclusion of any tangential items. As Sudman and Bradburn (1982) have admonished, items whose only justification is that they would be "interesting to know" or "nice to know" should be excluded. There is rarely sufficient time and funding available for tangential items.

In addition to, or in place of, a list of research questions, it is helpful to draw a diagram that clearly illustrates how variables relate to one another (de Vaus, 1986).

Even if no cause–effect relationships are involved, the sort of diagram used to represent causal models, as in a path analysis, is quite useful at this stage. In this diagram, each theoretical variable should be enclosed in a box and linked to others with arrows that indicate a hypothesized direction of influence. Then, as the questionnaire is developed, each item should be placed in one of the boxes along with the variable it will index. At this stage, it is desirable to use more than one item or scale to index each variable, but items that do not fit logically in any box (either as dependent, independent, or control variables) are good candidates for deletion. Subsequent pretesting will likely indicate that the questionnaire is too long, and it will be necessary to delete or shorten some items. The diagram will again be helpful at this point, since it will clearly show which variables are indexed by multiple measures, which variables would be dropped from the design if certain items are deleted, and so forth. This may not make dropping one's favorite items any more palatable, but it will help to make such decisions more logical.

Types of Questionnaire Items

A number of writers have made the important distinction between factual items and attitudinal items in interviews (Babbie, 1989; Backstrom and Hursh-Cesar, 1981; Sudman and Bradburn, 1982). Factual items ask for information that can be verified, at least in principle, by sources other than the respondent. Attitudinal items ask for opinions, judgments, and self-perceptions, which only the respondent can provide. Each of these two types confronts the questionnaire designer with a somewhat different set of problems. In writing factual items we must first be able to assume that respondents possess the facts we are interested in, so we can design questions that assist them in recalling the facts and reporting them truthfully. With attitudinal items we must first be able to assume that respondents have thought about, and formed attitudes toward, objects that concern us, so we can design questions that assist them in expressing attitudes openly.

Investigators tend to be so deeply involved with the knowledge of their discipline that they can easily fall prey to false assumptions about the knowledge and attitudes of respondents (Backstrom and Hursh-Cesar, 1981). Thus, they may assume that all but a few respondents will know the factual information they seek and that all but a few will have opinions about all the issues relevant to the study. Of course, allowances are usually made for "don't know" responses, but these may be erroneously attributed to faulty recall (for factual items) or indecision (for attitudinal items). These deviant respondents are often lumped into the residual "don't know" category and treated as missing data in subsequent statistical analyses.

In fact, a substantial proportion of respondents will simply not know certain facts that they "ought" to know, such as their annual income, the number of times they saw a physician in the past year, or the particulars of their Medicare coverage. Likewise, many respondents will have no opinions about, and may have never thought about, issues that "should" concern them. If we are fortunate, these unwarranted assumptions will be disclosed during interview pretesting, through an obviously large number of "don't know" responses and refusals on certain items. However, some items may encourage acquiescence and may not yield an obviously poor distribution of responses. Thus, it is good practice to instruct pretest interviewers to record all instances where respondents say they are guessing, say they have no opinion, or otherwise indicate that the respondent is acquiescing to a given response option. Also, early pretests should provide for debriefing respondents, at which time they may be asked which items they found difficult to answer.

For factual items, "Refuse," "Don't Know," and "Not Sure" have considerably different meanings and should not be relegated to a common residual category. For attitudinal items, "Refuse," "No Opinion," "Neutral," and "Undecided" are all legitimate response categories, not to be treated as missing data or replaced with imputed values without due consideration. Improved question clarity and interviewer probing will serve to minimize such "deviant" responses, but it is unlikely that they can be eliminated entirely. If possible, therefore, one should include categories on the questionnaire for all these residual responses, to allow for subsequent analyses.

In most epidemiologic studies of the elderly, interviews include multiple-item indices or scales, which do not fit neatly into the foregoing factual–attitudinal categories. Here it is more appropriate to distinguish two other types: assessment devices and performance tests. The former include scales designed to measure depression, morale, or mental illness; the latter include memory tests, dementia tests, and tests of strength, mobility, vision, and hearing. Because the development of multiple-item indices requires substantial time and effort, as well as expertise in measurement, investigators commonly borrow indices that have appeared in the literature. In principle, such borrowing is desirable, since it presumably ensures that results of the borrower's study are comparable to those of others. However, as argued in the next subsection, borrowing is not without its pitfalls.

Validity and Reliability of Borrowed Indices

It is a common misconception that a measurement instrument has inherent degrees of validity and reliability that are established by its developer and that carry over to other settings, so long as the instrument is not modified in any way. Thus, when researchers adopt a previously used instrument, they often cite validity and reliability statistics from previous studies and neglect to calculate such statistics for their own samples.

This misconception is especially troublesome when a presumably "standard" scale, developed on samples of clinical patients or college students, is adopted for use with community-dwelling older people. It discourages modifications that would make the scale more appropriate for old people and, at the same time, encourages false confidence in its validity and reliability.

When a scale is modified, comparisons with previous studies are indeed problematic. On the other hand, if we use an unmodified "standard scale," we could be deceived into assuming that comparisons are legitimate when indeed they are not. Without explicit evidence, there is no assurance that the scale measures the same thing in older people as it did in the people on which it was developed. For example, a depression index developed for clinical patients and normally administered by a physician is likely to be received much differently when a lay interviewer administers it in an older person's home. Respondents may be more reluctant to tell a lay interviewer that they have contemplated suicide or have suffered crying spells and instead will present a more optimistic front. On the other hand, many somatic symptoms associated with depression in younger people and featured prominently in clinical depression scales may be more indicative of the chronic diseases and physical disabilities common in the elderly.

The situation is further complicated by the more common use of proxies in studies of the elderly. Although it is unlikely that a proxy would be asked to respond to performance tests or such things as a depression scale, it is common to ask them to respond to seemingly more factual scales, such as those that index physical function or activities of daily living.

To summarize, the message of this subsection is twofold. First, the validity and reliability of even a so-called standard scale cannot be assumed, but must be assessed for each subgroup in each study. Second, the comparability of "standard scales" across studies cannot be assumed. Investigators who lack expertise in reliability and validity assessment are well advised to seek assistance from a measurement specialist.

Writing Questionnaire Items

Questionnaires are rarely developed from scratch, but instead are built by combining a researcher's own items with others gleaned from the literature. Typically, the researcher's own contribution consists of individual questions that are needed for the current project, whereas components borrowed from prior research consist mainly of multiple-item instruments that measure more complex variables, such as functional or cognitive status. This section deals with writing single items, a task that nearly all investigators must undertake when designing a survey.

To emphasize the importance of proper item wording, Payne (1980) demonstrated that seemingly minor changes in wording can result in differences of 20 percent or more in an item's response distribution, which is a considerably stronger effect than such things as sampling bias typically produce. Despite its importance, however, item-writing technique has received so little attention in the literature that it remains an art form (Backstrom & Hursh-Cesar, 1981; Sudman and Bradburn, 1982; Payne, 1980). There are no formal principles for writing good items, only countless rules of thumb. Following is a list of only 10 rules of thumb, adapted largely from Payne (1980), which are particularly relevant to items written for the elderly.

1. Keep questions brief; twenty or fewer words should suffice. Consider breaking longer questions into two sentences, but beware of the effect of pauses described under Rule 4.
2. Use simple, familiar words and minimize the use of polysyllabic words. Keep in mind that a large proportion of the elderly have no more than an eighth-grade education.
3. Use the active voice and avoid the passive voice. The active voice usually yields clearer, shorter questions. For example, use "Has a doctor ever told you that . . . ?" but not, "Have you ever been told by a doctor that . . . ?"
4. Avoid compound sentences; they often confuse respondents and cause them to respond prematurely. Consider, for example, "Do you go to a dentist regularly, that is, at least once a year, or do you go only when you have a dental problem?" If an interviewer recites this at a comfortable pace for the elderly,

many would answer "yes" or "no" by the third comma pause and never hear her recite the final clause.

5. Avoid technical terms; health science nomenclature is jargon to elderly respondents. Many will misunderstand even terms that are in general use, such as hypertension, malignancy, or cholesterol. Many cannot distinguish Medicare, Medicaid, Social Security, and health insurance. If technical terms are unavoidable, they must be defined.
6. Use good grammar, but use an informal style, so that questions do not sound stilted or pretentious. For example, ending sentences with prepositions is usually preferable to using such formal constructions as *with which, to which,* and the like. Indeed, because *which* often sounds pompous, consider replacing *which* with *that* wherever respondents would do so in everyday speech.
7. Avoid slang and folksy colloquialisms. Some respondents may not understand the intended meaning; others may interpret such usage as patronization. Slang or folksy wording also precludes the use of an item in other times and places: How will it sound 10 years hence or in another city?
8. Avoid words with more than one meaning. Most respondents will give an appropriate answer to a question such as, "When was the last time you saw a doctor?" but we may never know how many were caught by, or mischievously seized upon, the double entendre.
9. Never use double negatives, such as "Do you disagree that doctors should not make house calls?"
10. Avoid hypothetical questions. These are confusing and are rarely useful anyway. Note that any question could become hypothetical if its asks about something that the respondent is able to do (e.g., asking someone who cannot walk whether they get chest pains when walking). Interviewers should be instructed to skip questions that do not apply to the respondent.

Large surveys use few open-ended questions, because answers must be recorded verbatim and subsequently coded. Almost all items will instead be closed-ended, a format similar to a multiple-choice test. Thus, along with writing the main body of a question, one must also write appropriate response categories. Following are 10 rules of thumb for writing response categories:

1. Make all responses short, preferably a single word.
2. Avoid using responses of markedly different length.
3. Response options should be mutually exclusive and exhaustive, unless the respondent is allowed to choose more than one option. Use an "Other (specify)" to obtain an exhaustive list, but be aware that such responses may require coding later on or may never be usable.
4. Use as few options as necessary. The respondent could be confused by too many options, and the interviewer spends at least as much time reading response options as she does asking questions. In some cases, five or more options must be used to obtain a good "spread" of responses, but fewer options, even a yes–no dichotomy, usually will suffice.
5. Present options in a logical order. Number lists should be in ascending or descending order. Attitude options should be arranged from most positive to most negative, or vice versa. However, note that even on factual items respon-

dents tend to select an option near the middle of a list when they are unsure or guessing.

6. If many items use the same set of response options, consider placing them in sequence.
7. Avoid enumerating response options in the question itself. Instead, read the question, then introduce the response options with, "Would you say . . .?" Then read the response options.
8. Provide a complete set of residual response options to every item. On factual items, respondents may be classified as "Refused to answer," "Don't know," and so forth. On attitude items they may be classified as "Refused to answer," "Don't know," "Undecided," and so forth. As noted earlier, differences between these residual categories could be important analytically, so they should be coded separately on the questionnaire.
9. Never read residual options to the respondent. They should be told at the outset of their right to refuse and should be aware that they can answer, "Don't know." However, reading these options will encourage respondents to use them more frequently than they would otherwise.
10. Use prompt cards, but use them sparingly. Handing the respondent a printed list of response options is most useful when (a) the options are numerous, (b) the options are lengthy, and (c) a series of items uses the same options. Prompt cards save time and help to clarify the response options. However, they cannot be used for vision-impaired people and they may cause embarrassment for those who are illiterate.

Obviously, no list of rules can guarantee good items. They can only assist in producing initial drafts, which must be tested empirically before they are judged acceptable. As a first test, each item should be read aloud at a pace that interviewers will use. Is it as clear when it is recited as it was when it was written? Does it sound stilted? Does it contain tongue-twisting phrases, alliteration, or easily mispronounced words that will sound odd or cause the interviewer to stumble? This recitation test should be done by several people, including some who are unfamiliar with the project.

When all items are judged satisfactory, they can be combined into a complete draft of a questionnaire. At this point, the dependencies among items should become apparent. For example, some items presuppose that others have been asked earlier, and some items become inappropriate for respondents who gave certain answers to previous items. Thus, the questionnaire should tell the interviewer which items to skip and under what conditions she should skip them. Often, with the addition of a screening question, it becomes possible to skip large blocks of questions for many respondents, thus reducing average interviewing time.

Question Order

Interviews should begin with items that have low emotional impact. This puts respondents at ease and enables the interviewer to set an initial tone and pace for the interview. If screening questions must be asked to determine respondent eligibility, these must of course be asked first. Besides these, demographic items are good candidates for the opening section, but those that may elicit a large proportion of refusals (e.g., income) are better postponed until the end of the interview. Moreover, the "innocuous" opening section should not be prolonged, because the respondent's interest and attentiveness may be sacrificed. This section should be limited to five minutes or less, and if more demographic information is needed, the remaining items may be used to close the interview.

Immediately after the opening section, the questionnaire should ask some interesting, nonthreatening questions that, from the respondent's viewpoint, are germane to the purpose of the interview. In health interviews, for example, some questions about health should be asked as soon as possible, but to avoid establishing a pattern of refusals or "don't know" responses they should be easy to answer. In some cases it may be necessary to add items to the interview solely to provide a transition to difficult, threatening, or embarrassing items. For example, asking respondents to rate their own health is a good prelude to more specific health history questions, even if self-rated health will not be used in subsequent statistical analyses.

The main body of the questionnaire should be divided into discrete sections that contain, from the respondent's viewpoint, logically related items. For each section the interviewer should recite a brief, standard introduction to orient the respondent and, if needed, to provide a rationale for asking certain questions. In a health interview, respondents can be oriented quickly to a section devoted to such matters as chronic diseases, and the interviewer may simply say, "Now, I have some questions about medical problems that many older people have." On the other hand, respondents may not see the relevance of sections dealing with certain exposures, stress, cognitive status, or social support, and must be given a rationale for their inclusion. However, the rationale should be stated briefly and matter-of-factly. It should not emphasize how embarrassing or sensitive the questions will be and should not provoke debate over the section's relevance, nor should it divulge the researcher's hypotheses, because doing so is likely to color the respondent's answers. It is often sufficient to tell respondents that certain questions will be asked "because doctors need to know if these things are related to a person's health," or "because we're trying to find out if these things either cause or prevent health problems for older people."

The various questionnaire sections should be ordered logically, with those of similar content juxtaposed, to minimize abrupt transitions. However, a respite should be provided between sections that are particularly stressful or fatiguing, perhaps by separating them with more agreeable sections or by providing time for the respondent to stand and stretch.

Ideally, interviews should end on a positive note, so it is good practice to close with a few items that enable respondents to express optimism or report something desirable about themselves. This "decompression" is especially important for respondents who had to report many health problems and functional deficits and who did poorly on performance tests. In such cases, the interviewer should also take a little extra time following the interview for pleasant conversation about something other than the interview. It should go without saying that the interviewer should always express sincere appreciation for what the respondent has contributed to the research.

Pretesting Questionnaires

Pretesting is not merely a luxury enjoyed by well-financed projects; it is a necessary prelude to any study. If anything, pretesting is even more critical in surveys of older people, not only because they present special problems to interviewers, but because we can so easily make erroneous assumptions about similarities and differences between old and young respondents.

No questionnaire and no single item within it should ever be used until it is pretested with respondents of every type to be included in the survey. It should be obvious that pretests cannot be limited to younger and healthier volunteers if the survey will ultimately draw upon very old, sick, or frail respondents. Less obvious and often overlooked is the need to include proxy respondents in a pretest if the latter will be employed in the survey. A thorough pretest will also include any type of respondent who will present special problems during the survey, such as those with dementia, those with hearing or vision impairments, and those who speak little English. Moreover, pretests should be done with "real" respondents of each type rather than with someone who is merely role playing.

Pretesting is not a one-time task. Ideally, one does a series of pretests as a questionnaire is refined, culminating with a full-scale pilot study in which interviews are done under the same conditions that will be encountered in the actual survey. For example, if interviews will be done in respondents' homes, the pilot study should be done there also.

As noted later, the questionnaire should be pretested extensively before the training of novice interviewers begins, which means that the investigators, project director, field supervisors, or others with interviewing experience must do the pretesting. On the other hand, the pilot study should be done after interviewers are trained, so that real interviewers as well as real respondents will be involved. During and immediately after the pilot, debriefing sessions with interviewers should be held and statistical analyses should be done promptly. Because interviewers have been hired at this point, final questionnaire revisions and procedural changes must be done as quickly as possible, to minimize interviewer retraining and associated costs. Another detail, questionnaire printing, could delay the field work, so it is common to use photocopies during the first week or two of a survey.

Pretesting will expose items that are grossly confusing, unclear, or overly sensitive. These will probably be identified through respondents' reactions as well as through the bunching of responses into a single category or an unusually large number of item refusals or "don't know" responses. For example, a large proportion of "don't know" responses may indicate that an item is worded vaguely, that more response options are needed, that more probing is needed, or that a better introduction to the item is needed. However, the item may suffer from the more basic problem noted earlier: It may ask for information that many respondents cannot provide or may ask about attitudes they have not formulated.

Unfortunately, items that do not yield the obvious response anomalies noted earlier may still have serious biases. The wording of a question or its response options may subtly encourage over- or underreporting, and such a problem may be overlooked if the pretest does not yield a markedly skewed distribution. For example, if we ask older people to rate their overall health, they will tend to rate themselves somewhere near the middle of the categories they are given. So if we ask them to rate their health as Excellent, Good, Fair, or Poor, a smaller proportion will rate themselves as Poor than would do so if we added a lower category, Very Poor.

Perhaps the only effective way to detect such biases is through a quasi-experimental pretest, in which alternatively worded items and response options are randomly administered to subsamples (Babbie, 1973; Bradburn et al, 1979; Payne, 1980). If alternate forms of an item yield similar response distributions, it is probably safe to use either form, assuming that they are not biased in the same direction. On the other hand, if they yield markedly different distributions, it may not be clear which form should be used, and it may be necessary to pretest even more forms of the item until a preferred form is found.

INTERVIEWER SELECTION

In most respects, selecting interviewers for the elderly is done according to the same criteria that apply in surveys of younger people. Interviewers should have sufficient education to cope intelligently with the questionnaire and other demands of the role, which usually implies a high school degree. They should have reasonably good grammar, an amiable interpersonal style, and sufficient social skills to manage the stressful and awkward situations that are bound to occur. Interviewers must be nonthreatening yet sufficiently assertive. Prior experience with interviewing is usually desirable, but this does not necessarily reduce the time required for training. Unfortunately, it is not usually feasible to observe potential interviewers interacting with older people, to see how they relate.

Although little research has been done to determine who makes the best interviewers, most experts would agree that, all other things being equal, middle-aged women are the best choice for interviews with the elderly (Backstrom and Hursh-Cesar, 1981). This preference is based not on demographic characteristics, but on the grounds that middle-aged women are most likely to possess all the personal qualities that interviewers should have, including maturity, empathy, reliability, and social skills. There is, of course, no guarantee that any given middle-aged woman will have these and other requisite qualifications for interviewing, but such women are so commonly employed in surveys of the elderly that it is appropriate to use the pronoun *she* when referring to an interviewer.

Because interviewers are usually employed for the duration of a project, they must be willing to accept temporary employment. They must also be willing to work irregular hours: part-time in some periods and overtime in others. Ordinarily, interviewers are paid hourly or by the interview, so their pay will vary from one week to the next. These conditions again favor middle-aged women, in the sense that they are the most likely to apply for interviewing jobs and the most likely to stay on the job until a project is completed. This self-selection process will doubtless change as it becomes more common for women in this age group to be permanent members of the labor force.

Conventional wisdom also dictates that interviewers should be as similar as possible to respondents, presumably because respondents will be more likely to consent to interviews with someone who has similar cultural and personal characteristics and will feel most comfortable in discussing personal matters with such a person (Babbie, 1973; Backstrom and Hursh-Cesar, 1981). Thus, although it may be impossible to find elderly interviewers to match elderly respondents, this "similarity principle" tells us that an interviewer in the 40 to 60 age range is preferable to a college student under

20. Further, because women outnumber men in most elderly populations, it tells us that women are preferable to men as interviewers.

Actually, the "similarity principle" is most cogent with respect to cultural and personal characteristics that do not depend entirely on age and sex. Here it tells us to match, or avoid extreme mismatches between, interviewers and respondents on such factors as education, speech patterns, dress, and demeanor. It points to the folly of sending a city-bred interviewer into rural areas, sending someone with a New Jersey accent to interview in Appalachia, or sending an overdressed interviewer into a working-class neighborhood. Although a skilled interviewer may be able to establish rapport with a markedly dissimilar respondent, such respondents are likely to remain somewhat inhibited, especially with regard to items for which the interviewer's visible characteristics are most salient (Bradburn, et al, 1979; Sudman and Bradburn, 1974).

In the Iowa EPESE project, which was done in two rural counties, interviewers were recruited from the small towns in the survey area. They worked in their own counties, but to maintain confidentiality, they never interviewed in their home towns and never interviewed anyone who was not a complete stranger. Many of them were former nurses and most had more education than their respondents, yet they were similar in most other respects to the respondents' friends and relatives. It is generally a good idea to recruit indigenous interviewers, and this may even be a necessity when special subpopulations, such as ethnic neighborhoods, are to be surveyed.

INTERVIEWER TRAINING

The time required for interviewer training depends mainly on two factors: (1) the prior experience of the interviewers and (2) the length and complexity of the interview. The average training course takes about two 40-hour weeks, but a longer course may be needed if novice interviewers will be employed to do interviews averaging one or more hours duration (Babbie, 1973).

The course should provide ample practicum experience as well as didactic sessions. Most of the first week is typically devoted to teaching basic interviewing techniques, familiarizing interviewers with the questionnaire, and conducting mock interviews. The second week is usually spent doing practice interviews under field conditions. Ideally, the questionnaire has been extensively pretested and is in near final form when training begins, because novices are easily confused when required to adapt to frequent changes at the same they they are learning basic techniques.

If a pilot study is to be done, it should follow the training period. Otherwise, interviewers will be too inexperienced to provide a realistic pilot, and many problems that derive from their inexperience could be mistaken for problems with the questionnaire or management procedures.

The course should be planned and scheduled as thoroughly as possible, down to such details as preparing manuals and study materials, scheduling practice interviews, and scheduling lunch and refreshment breaks. In most cases, interviewers are paid during their training, and an ill-designed course can add substantially to a project's cost. Notably, the cost of interviewer training is often either underestimated or neglected entirely when investigators develop a project budget, although it is wise to budget a little extra in case the additional training proves necessary. Often overlooked in the budget are incentive payments to volunteer respondents for practice interviews, and costs of training extra and replacement interviewers needed to compensate for those who are discharged or quit, payment of guest lecturers and extra training staff, and costs of periodic continuing-education sessions that are often needed.

Although the training course will necessarily have a didactic component, lengthy, abstract lectures are out of place. Lectures and presentations should be brief, concrete, and confined to that material that cannot be taught by any other mode. Practical demonstrations should be emphasized, and sessions should be scheduled in manageable chunks to avoid information overload. There is relatively little benefit in a lecture about such abstractions as "rapport," but interviewers can learn how to establish and maintain it through concrete examples and practical advice in dealing with factors that affect rapport, such as how to dress, what to say, and what not to say in an interview. Demonstrations showing how to and how not to apply various techniques, such as probing, keeping the respondent focused, and maintaining neutrality, are much more effective than lectures.

The course should provide trainees with ample opportunities to practice interviewing and to get feedback on their performance. Within the first few days they should receive the questionnaire, and after its content has been reviewed by an instructor, they should be told to familiarize themselves with it as a homework assignment. They should be told to read all questions verbatim, but to practice reading them aloud until their delivery is so smooth and natural that a listener would be unable to tell they are reading. By the third or fourth day of training they should be prepared to begin practice interviews.

Initially, they should practice on one another, which is less intimidating than working with "real" respondents. For the first few trials, their performance should not be critiqued, but they should be encouraged to discuss any problems they may have had in conducting their interviews. After three or four such sessions, they should be comfortable with tape recording a few interviews with their fellow trainees and discussing their performance with a trainer. By the beginning of the second week they should do at least two tape-recorded practice interviews on real elderly respondents. As before, a trainer should offer feedback on the interviewer's performance. By the end of the second week, interviewers should have done at least five more interviews with elderly respondents, which need not be recorded but which should be followed by debriefings with the trainer. The latter should be done in the same settings as those that will be encountered in the field. Ideally, they should be done with volunteer respondents who vary in age, functional ability, hearing and vision, and so forth, to expose trainees to at least a few difficult cases.

It is good strategy to incorporate a continuing education program for interviewers, especially if the survey will span several months. This will help to ensure that all interviewers are adhering to the standard protocol and have been informed about any modifications that have been decided upon since field work began. Even when a continuing education program has not been built into the study design, investigators may find that interim training sessions are needed, as ad hoc protocol modifications accumulate.

This section was not intended to give exhaustive coverage to all the topics that are covered in a typical interviewer training course, nor would space allow it. However, a few words about these other topics are in order before closing this section. Obviously, interviewers should learn about such things as the purposes of the study, its funding source and sponsorship, its investigators, and the rationale for various items in the questionnaire (Backstrom and Hursh-Cesar, 1981). Here again, however, training should be restricted to the practical. In other words, interviewers should be taught what to tell respondents about these matters, but not to understand them as the investigators do. For very good scientific reasons, they should not be told the hypotheses, how the data will be analyzed, nor what every index is intended to measure. This admonition is based on research in experimental settings (Rosenthal and Rosow, 1975), where it has been demonstrated that observations are biased in favor of the experimenter's hypotheses and expectations. These results suggest that in survey research a dutiful interviewer who knows the hypotheses will be biased toward confirming them, consciously or not, by the manner in which she reads questions, probes, and records responses. It is a good idea to tell interviewers when information is being withheld. Indeed, most will accept the explanation that having certain information will make it difficult for them to remain neutral toward their respondents.

INTERVIEWING ELDERLY RESPONDENTS

Although an interview is generally viewed as a unitary social encounter, it is useful to break it into smaller phases and to examine the special problems that must be solved during each phase. Three discrete phases are discussed in the subsections to follow, beginning with the problem of gaining access to elderly respondents, which usually involves a good deal of preparatory work before the interviewers take to the field.

Gaining Access to Elderly Respondents

Prior to beginning survey field work, potential respondents should be made aware of the project and, ideally, informed that they have been selected for participation. For large projects it is usually appropriate to launch an extensive public relations campaign, consisting of press releases or advertisements in newspapers, investigator appearances on local radio and TV talk shows, and presentations at service clubs, church groups, congregate meal sites, and senior citizen centers. Even for smaller studies contact should be made with political authorities, the police, the local medical association, and such relevant service agencies as the Area Agency on Aging and the Visiting Nurse Association. It is also wise to identify and contact influential individuals, whose endorsement could be valuable in convincing potential respondents to participate.

If respondents' names and addresses are known in advance, letters should be sent to potential respondents informing them that they have been selected for interviews, explaining what their participation will entail, and describing in general terms the purpose and significance of the project. Letters should be brief, written in plain English, and printed in easily readable type. It is important to note that the initial letter merely serves to announce the study: It should not ask for a reply or an interview appointment, which would give respondents an opportunity to refuse an interview before someone could explain the study more fully and counter respondents' objections.

In the announcement letters and other public relations, sponsorship and auspices must be explained with caution, lest respondents mistake a scientific study for, say, a government fact-finding activity. In the Iowa EPESE project, for example, it was found that many respondents confused the sponsoring National Institute on Aging with the Social Security Administration or Medicare and were concerned that results of the study would affect their benefits. Additional effort was thus required to counter such beliefs and to ensure respondents that the study was being done by University of Iowa researchers for scientific purposes.

When interviews are to be done in respondents' homes, interviews are most commonly obtained by what may be called the drop-in approach, in which interviewers have the task of gaining access to respondents: The interviewer merely appears at the door of a potential respondent and requests an interview. If the respondent is willing, the interview is done on the spot; otherwise, the interviewer attempts to schedule a later appointment. If the respondent resists, the interviewer politely withdraws (preferably before the respondent becomes adamant) and reports an "initial refusal" to the supervisor, along with a report on the respondent's reasons for refusing. The supervisor assigns the case to a troubleshooter, usually the most skilled and experienced interviewer on staff, who recontacts the respondent by telephone or in person and again attempts to get an interview. If the troubleshooter fails to convert the refusal, the case may be reported to the investigator, who decides whether further conversion attempts should be made. In the East Boston EPESE project, the Principal Investigator, a physician who is well known in the community, telephoned the most recalcitrant refusers and was able to convert many (Cornoni-Huntley, 1986).

It is important to realize that the interaction that occurs in recruiting a respondent sets the tone for the subsequent interview. Although skillful interviewers can usually establish rapport with reluctant respondents, they will fail to do so in a significant minority of cases. Further, respondents who are pressured to relent may be more adamant the next time they are approached: This is particularly troublesome in longitudinal studies, where refusals at follow-up are just as undesirable as those at baseline.

The alternative to the drop-in is the scheduled-appointment approach, in which respondents are contacted by phone and asked to schedule an interview appointment at a convenient time. A troubleshooter makes another call to initial refusers and is careful not to invoke an adamant refusal. If the respondent continues to decline, a troubleshooter is sent to make an in-person contact. The scheduled-appointment approach is more consistent with the norms of polite interaction and places less pressure on respondents to comply. Those who participate understand more clearly that they are doing so by choice and are more likely to grant subsequent interviews. This approach was used during the baseline survey of the Iowa EPESE project, which has succeeded in retaining 96 percent of its respondents through seven annual follow-ups. It should be noted that this project switched to the drop-in approach for subsequent in-home follow-ups in order to reduce costs, but it appears that the salutary effect of scheduled appointments at baseline carried over to the follow-ups.

Notably, in both the drop-in and scheduled-appointment approaches, a large proportion of refusals may be made by someone other than the respondent, particularly when respondents are very old, sick, or frail. In such cases, the caretakers, spouses, or adult children may decide whether an interviewer is allowed to see the respondent, and when the caretaker refuses an interview, the respondent may never be consulted. Of course, even for younger and healthier respondents a spouse or family member may deny access. For example, in the Iowa EPESE project many refusals were made by wives, who always answered the phone or appeared at the front door and said they were "sure" that their husbands would not want to participate. Yet when the interviewer succeeded in talking directly to the husbands, they usually consented. Thus, interviewers must be as adept at dealing with and getting past gatekeepers as they are in interviewing elderly respondents.

When interviewing is to be done in nursing homes, investigators or other higher-level staff must usually arrange for access to respondents. The first obstacle to surmount is getting the nursing home's permission to interview on the premises, which may involve lengthy negotiations, assuming that the administration agrees to negotiate at all. Further, the head of nursing services must be brought into the negotiations, since administrators may withhold permission until she is convinced that interviews will cause no disruption of established procedures. In most cases, the administrator will also require written permission for the interview from the respondent's next of kin, legal guardian, and physician. All the latter must thus be contacted and convinced that the research is important and that the interview will cause the respondent no physical or emotional discomfort.

Once all the gatekeepers have granted access to a patient, most interviews will proceed fairly smoothly. Ordinarily, nursing home patients welcome the diversion that an interview offers and present few special problems, so long as they are capable of responding to the questionnaire. However, since a large proportion of nursing home patients is too sick or cognitively impaired to handle an interview, it will often be necessary to use proxies. Depending on the content of the interview, a nursing home staff member, rather than a spouse or family member, may be the most appropriate proxy, in which case it may be necessary to pay the proxy respondent for his or her time.

Interviewers should be well informed about the arrangements that have been made with each nursing home and should be careful to comply with any limitations that the nursing home requires. They must, of course, avoid inconveniencing the nursing home staff, placing demands on their time, or interfering with their schedule.

Meeting and Greeting

Like the interaction that occurs during respondent recruitment, the first few minutes after the interviewer enters a respondent's home are critical in setting the tone of the interview. So the interviewer must be able to appraise the situation she has entered as quickly as a quarterback reads a defense. Other family members may be present and there may be no place for a private interview. The respondent may be occupied with such activities as baking, repair projects, a TV show, or a chat with neighbors and may insist on continuing them throughout the interview. The interviewer may have awakened the respondent from an afternoon nap or arrived at the respondent's usual nap time. The respondent may be sick, intoxicated, distraught over a recent tragedy, or in the midst of an argument with a spouse. The point is that something was going on before the interviewer arrived and she must assist the respondent in making the transition to the interview situation.

The interviewer must be aware that she may be the first visitor that an elderly respondent has had in many days. To those who treasure their solitude she may be an intruder; to others she may be a rescuer from loneliness. To those surrounded by younger family members she may offer a rare chance to talk about things that concern older people; to others her questions will be impertinent. The interviewer must quickly adjust her demeanor to become the kind of person with whom the respondent would share confidences (Babbie, 1973).

Upon entering the house, the interviewer must also balance the need to observe social amenities with the need to get on with the business of interviewing. Some respondents will brusquely insist on beginning immediately and getting it over as quickly as possible, so the interviewer must slow the pace and digress occasionally to establish rapport without appearing to waste time. Other respondents will be exceedingly hospitable, offer food or beverages, and treat the interviewer as an honored guest. Here the interviewer might cause offense if she proceeds too quickly and acts too impersonally.

In the Iowa EPESE project, where interviews were scheduled in advance, elderly respondents commonly baked pastry or made a special trip to the store in anticipation of the interviewer's visit. Because refusing offers of food could cause offense, the interviewer simply asked to postpone eating until after the interview. If offered coffee, tea, or a soft drink, she usually accepted, because this gave her an opportunity to acknowledge the respondent's hospitality without delaying or interfering with the interview. However, interviewers were instructed to decline any alcoholic beverage and to do so without appearing judgmental, since the interview contained questions about alcohol consumption. They merely said, "Thank you very much for the offer, but I still have more interviews today," or, "It would make me too sleepy to finish all the work my boss assigned me today."

Setting the Stage

The interviewer should select a site that offers comfortable seats, adequate light, and freedom from distractions. The interviewer should sit close enough to be heard without shouting and to hand the respondent prompt cards, consent forms, and so forth, but should avoid sitting too close. Kitchen or dining room tables are usually good sites, because they provide the interviewer with a work surface, but these may not be desirable if they are located where other household members will be intruding frequently. For long interviews, a comfortable living room chair is best for the respondent.

When two respondents, usually married couples, are to be interviewed, it is usually best to send two interviewers to interview them simultaneously in separate rooms, so that both will have privacy. The interviewer who finishes first must, of course, keep her respondent occupied while the other completes the interview. If respondents can overhear one another's interviews, they may be distracted from their own and may begin commenting on, offering corrections to, or even bickering about one another's responses. Such events can usually be prevented if, at the outset, an interviewer simply closes a door between the two rooms.

Conducting the Interview and Maintaining Rapport

Although an interview is a unique form of social interaction, it is governed by society's norms, which tell us that seniority entitles older respondents to deference. When interviews are done in their homes, ownership of the "turf" also entitles them to deference. These norms apply whether the interviewer is a lay person or a health professional.

This is not to say that an interview requires anything more than common courtesy. Indeed, exaggerating or feigning deference, in the manner of the stereotypical used car salesman, is just as inappropriate as blatant disrespect. Part of the interviewer's social skills is her ability to comply with the society's norms in such a way that they are transparent.

One of the obvious ways to express deference is through modes of address. Thus, although older respondents may address the interviewer by her first name, she should always use the more formal *Mr., Mrs.,* or *Miss,* unless specifically asked to use a first name. An occasional *Yes sir* or *Yes ma'am* is also fitting, but overuse of these phrases could make the interviewer appear patronizing or obsequious.

Some older people, especially the very old or functionally impaired, may respond slowly and, as a result, may give the impression that they are either hard of hearing or that they failed to understand what was said. Novice interviewers are commonly prone to such misperceptions and begin shouting at the respondent or speaking almost in baby talk. This is sure to threaten rapport, and even if the respondent completes the interview without complaint, he or she will think twice about consenting to a follow-up.

With experience, interviewers learn that they just cannot rush a slow respondent and that interviewing time must be cut by improving their own efficiency and minimizing their own digressions. If an interview drags on so long that the respondent shows signs of fatigue, it may be strategic to truncate the interview and schedule an appointment to complete it on another day. Of course, this avenue is not open to the interviewer unless investigators have authorized her to use it.

Many older people will respond fairly quickly, but will also elaborate on each response with a lengthy explanation. This mode of responding, as noted elsewhere, probably indicates that the respondent has not been trained to deal with fixed-choice interview items and is trying to give a logical or socially acceptable answer. By pausing to record these elaborations in detail or by asking for even more clarification, the interviewer encourages the respondent to provide more of them. Thus, unless the respondent insists or provides a truly relevant qualification, the interviewer should refrain from writing long notes on the questionnaire and move to the next item as quickly as courtesy allows. If this ploy is unsuccessful, the interviewer may gently hint that there are many more questions to follow and that a later question may allow the respondent to elaborate further on the present topic.

If the interviewer is adequately trained, she should be able to read questions without stammering or hesitation. She should read all questions verbatim, but her tone, pace, and inflection should sound so natural that she gives the impression that she, rather than the questionnaire, is doing the asking. Of course, if the respondent finds any question offensive, she must point out that she was instructed to read it exactly as written. She risks losing rapport if she accepts blame for offending items.

Interviewing with Others Present

It is generally believed that the presence of a third party inhibits a respondent, threatens the validity of responses, and violates interview standardization. Yet in virtually all in-home surveys, some interviews are done with a third party present, and such interviews may be more numerous in surveys of the elderly, where a large proportion of respondents are living under the protection of caretakers, because of illness, frailty, or cognitive impairment. Interviewers are usually instructed to do their best to clear the room of third parties or, failing this, to attempt to reschedule the interview for a time when the respondent will be alone. However, the physical setting may not allow for complete privacy, or the respondent or a third party may insist that the latter remain. So the only alternative to accepting the presence of another person may be no interview at all. Bradburn et al (1979) have suggested that it is better to accept biases caused by the presence of others than to force a refusal, because the former can be assessed and corrected for, whereas the latter can never be adequately assessed. These authors review data from a number of surveys, which indicate that biases due to the presence of others may not be as pronounced as we might expect, although they may account for 25 percent or more of all interviews. Moreover, as noted later, a third party may be helpful in many cases.

If third-party biases (harmful or helpful) are to be assessed, we must collect sufficient information about them. Unfortunately, such information is rarely collected, much less reported in the literature. All questionnaires should at least provide a place for the interviewer to record whether another person was present and, if so, whether that person helped or hindered the interview. To do a more thorough analysis of response effects, the interviewer should record the third party's sex, age, relationship to the respondent, and, if the third party eventually left, what parts of the interview were done in private. Although it is rare to have more than one other person present, the questionnaire should provide space for documenting these occurrences as well.

Interviewers must also be trained to handle third parties, not by ignoring them but by using them constructively. If they begin answering for the respondent, the interviewer should re-ask questions and specifically request that the respondent give his or her own thoughts. Or each time the third party offers an answer, the interviewer may ask the respondent, "Is that right, Mr. X? Do you agree with that?" Usually, a third party who is hindering the flow of an interview will eventually get the message and leave. If the ordering of items is not critical, it may be wise to allow interviewers to postpone some sections of the interview until she either gets the other person to leave or determines that the person will never leave.

In most cases, the third party is indeed helpful in providing answers to factual questions and in interpreting the respondent's answers. Still, the interviewer should postpone recording a response until she confirms it with, "Do you agree with that, Mr. X?" If Mr. X does not agree, she should record his response and, if appropriate, note the other person's response in the margin of the questionnaire for later review by the supervisor. She must not allow the in-person interview to turn into a proxy. Instead, she must subtly manipulate the third party to playing the role of "helper." Once she has done so, she can usually get that person to withdraw for particularly sensitive parts of the interview or those that demand concentration, such as psychological assessments and performance tests.

SAMPLE MAINTENANCE AND SURVEILLANCE IN LONGITUDINAL STUDIES

Attrition in longitudinal studies has essentially the same effect as refusals at the time of the baseline survey, although we have more information about lost cases for use in assessing resulting biases. As noted earlier, obtaining commitment at baseline is crucial in maintaining respondent participation, but perhaps even more important is the baseline interview itself. If the interviewer was unable to maintain rapport, or if the interview was too lengthy or stressful, a respondent is likely to refuse a follow-up.

Of course, many other factors lead to refusals at follow-up, some of which are beyond the researcher's control. For example, illness will render some respondents incapable, cognitive decline may make some fearful of an interview, and deteriorating housing conditions may make others reluctant to admit interviewers into their homes. Some respondents will have come under the watchful eye of a caretaker or moved to a nursing home, so that new gatekeepers now control access to them. In most of these instances, it may be possible to conduct follow-up interviews with proxies, but where a suitable proxy cannot be found, the respondent becomes a refusal.

Refusals usually account for most attrition in longitudinal studies, but other types of attrition are also troublesome. Although older people are not as mobile as younger groups, many move to warmer climates soon after retirement and many move closer to adult children when their health declines. If one maintains a good tracking system, it should be possible to find respondents who relocate and to interview them by phone or perhaps by a mail-out questionnaire that captures at least part of the information that an in-person interview would yield.

In the EPESE projects, baseline respondents were asked to provide the names, addresses, and telephone numbers of two or three persons not living with them who would always know where they were living. These contact persons have proved invaluable in locating respondents who moved from the target areas: In the Iowa EPESE project, which has a somewhat lower mobility rate than the other sites, not a single case was lost to follow-up in seven years.

If the time between baseline and follow-up will be several years, annual contacts of some other form should be provided for in the study design. One such contact is a periodic newsletter, which not only serves to maintain respondents' interest in the project but provides an unobtrusive method of tracking their whereabouts, through the services of the postal system. The phrase ADDRESS CORRECTION REQUESTED should be printed in large block letters on the front of the envelope or folded newsletter. Seeing this message, a postal worker will not forward the newsletter to a new address but will instead return it to the sender with an address correction, assuming the Post Office has a new address. (The Post Office charges a small fee, perhaps a dollar, for each address correction they process.) Because there may be local variations in handling address corrections, one should of course check with the Post Office for instructions on handling these mailings.

A somewhat more limited means of tracking respondents is through lists or computer files maintained by hospitals, nursing homes, Area Agencies on Aging, and government agencies, including Medicare, Medicaid, and state drivers' license databases. All these sources are limited, in that they are unlikely to cover all the relevant cases and may not be current. However, if access to such data sources is feasible, it is a relatively simple matter to check one's respondent list against them.

In most epidemiologic studies, mortality is an important end point or outcome variable, not merely another source of respondent attrition. In any event, a mortality surveillance system that detects deaths in a timely manner is essential for field work. To appreciate this need, one need only imagine how embarrassing it might be if an interviewer were to request an interview with someone who died nearly a year earlier or if she were to be greeted by a presumed-dead husband when on arrival to interview his widow about the circumstances of his death. Although it may be impossible to eliminate all such occurrences, they can be minimized if thorough mortality surveillance procedures are in place. Because mortality surveillance is covered elsewhere in this book, details about designing a surveillance system will not be given here.

CONCLUSION

This chapter began by exhorting the reader to gain an appreciation of "the elderly" before undertaking the design of survey research, and it is fitting to return to that theme at the close.

There is good reason to believe that research in older populations will continue to increase in the coming decades. This means that older people will be asked to shoulder an increasing burden of research participation. Although the number of surveys may increase, the burden on any given respondent should not. Thus, we must be just as concerned with respondent burden as we are with the efficiency and technical quality of our survey instruments. We must recognize that every item we add to a questionnaire adds to the respondents' fatigue, and every item has the potential to aggravate the stress we impose on them. And as noted earlier, we must recognize that the greatest burden will be placed on those who are probably least able to cope—the oldest, sickest, and frailest, who will usually be forced to endure the longest interviews and to report the most problems.

Fortunately, the goals of efficiency and technical quality are, for the most part, consistent with that of minimizing respondent burden. For all these goals, brevity and stress reduction are paramount.

REFERENCES

Babbie ER (1973). Survey Research Methods. Belmont, CA, Wadsworth.
Babbie ER (1989). The Practice of Social Research, 5th ed. Belmont, CA, Wadsworth.
Backstrom CH, Hursh-Cesar G (1981). Survey Research, 2nd ed. New York, Wiley.
Bradburn NM, Sudman S, et al (1979). Improving Interview Method and Questionnaire Design. San Francisco, Jossey-Bass, 1979.
Converse JM, Schuman H (1974). Conversations at Random: Survey Research as Interviewers See It. New York, Wiley.
Cornoni-Huntley JC, Brock DB, Ostfeld AM, Taylor JO, Wallace RB (eds) (1986). Established Populations for Epidemiological Studies of the Elderly. Washington, DC, National Institute on Aging, NIH Pub. No. 86-2443.
de Vaus DA (1986). Surveys in Social Research. London, George Allen & Unwin.

Hoinville G, Jowell R, et al (1977). Survey Research Practice. London, Heinemann.
Mishler EG (1986). Research Interviewing. Cambridge, MA, Harvard University Press.
Payne SL (1980). The Art of Asking Questions. Princeton, NJ, Princeton University Press.
Richardson SA, Dohrenwend BS, Klein D (1965). Interviewing: Its Forms and Functions. New York, Basic Books.
Rosenthal R, Rosow RL (1975). The Volunteer Subject. New York, Wiley.
Sudman S, Bradburn NM (1974). Response Effects in Surveys: A Review and Synthesis. Chicago, Aldine.
Sudman S, Bradburn NM (1982). Asking Questions: A Practical Guide to Questionnaire Design. San Francisco, Jossey-Bass.

8

The Use of Proxy Respondents in Health Studies of the Aged

JAY MAGAZINER

The standard procedure in most health surveys of young and old alike is to attempt to interview a sampled respondent, and if that person is unable to provide information for himself, to interview a surrogate or proxy respondent instead. Proxy responses are then substituted for those of the missing subject, and analyses proceed using data from both sources. This practice of substituting proxy responses for those of the missing subject is used widely in health surveys of the aged, where it is not uncommon for more than 20 percent of community dwellers and 50 percent of nursing home residents to be unable or unwilling to participate themselves (Cornoni-Huntley et al, 1986; Hing et al, 1989). The proportion of subjects unavailable for health surveys increases with advancing age among those 65 and older (Fitti and Kovar, 1987; Herzog and Rogers, 1988), as does the proportion of "don't knows" and refusals to answer specific items (Colsher and Wallace, 1989), making it most difficult to obtain information directly from the oldest and frailest, who are often those of greatest interest in health surveys.

The impact of excluding information on those subjects unable to provide it for themselves is not well studied. If those excluded are not representative of the population of interest, error may be introduced into surveys of this group. This problem may be compounded in longitudinal surveys, where drop-out is not random and where some evidence suggests that those not responding and dropping out are the frailest among the elderly (Norris, 1985; Herzog and Rogers, 1988; Rogers and Herzog, 1989). Missing data on survey items may also be problematic, as those who do not answer specific questions appear to differ from those who do (Colsher and Wallace, 1989; Rogers and Herzog, in press).

The approach of using proxies to substitute for missing subject-derived information has its advantages. This strategy has been shown to increase the number of available subjects substantially (Cornoni-Huntley et al, 1986; Fitti and Kovar, 1987; Heyman et al, 1984; Magaziner et al, 1988) in studies of the elderly. Further, proxies can generally be identified and are willing to participate (Burnam et al, 1985; Cornoni-Huntley et al, 1986; Magaziner et al, 1987, 1988). The practice of using proxies has potential drawbacks as well. Although the old adage that some data are better than none has prevailed in survey research circles, a critical appraisal of the potential limitations of using proxy reports is warranted. The remainder of this chapter provides an overview of some problems that may be encountered when using proxy-derived data, reviews existing research on the use of proxies in older populations, and provides a series of practical strategies that those confronted with the problem of using proxy respondents might follow.

THE ISSUES

Two issues are of primary concern when evaluating the use of proxy reports: response precision and response bias. These issues of reliability are no different from the general concerns about error in all scientific measurement. Both precision and bias contribute to agreement (i.e., the degree to which the proxy's response agrees with that which would have been obtained from the subject had that subject been interviewed directly). One way to deal with poor agreement attributable to low precision is to increase the sample size and thereby reduce standard errors of estimates. This strategy is appropriate when the variability relating to subject–proxy response agreement is random (i.e., when proxies do not systematically over- or underreport in relation to subject reports).

The second concern, that of bias, may be more important and more difficult to address. Bias in this context is defined as the systematic under- or overreporting of responses by proxies in comparison to those that would have been obtained from the subject had that subject been interviewed directly. The effect of biased proxy reports is that estimates derived from proxies or the combination of proxies and subjects will be misleading. Bias cannot be remedied simply by increasing the sample size. Depending on the research issue under study, bias need not always be viewed as detrimental, however. For deriving population estimates, where unbiased estimates are needed, it is always problematic. Under some circumstances, however, as when testing specific hypotheses, the bias introduced by using proxy reports may provide a more conservative test of that hypothesis. For example, if we hypothesize that patient functioning will improve as a result of a given treatment and if proxies are known to report lower levels of functioning than patients report for themselves, then a finding that functioning improves following treatment (based all or in part on proxy-derived data) provides a conservative test of the hypothesis. On the other hand, had proxies been known to report better functioning than patients, then the bias attributable to proxy reports that now has the same direction as the hypothesis prevents us from using these data to test the hypothesis. In this case, we cannot be certain whether the treatment or reporting bias is responsible for the result.

This example serves to demonstrate that although not all bias is bad, it is essential to know whether the bias exists and, at the very least, its direction. Although simple in concept, the practical realities of estimating the bias introduced by proxies are relatively complex, since the usual reason for relying on proxies in most health studies is that subjects are not available for evaluation and hence are not likely to be available for comparisons needed to estimate bias. The problems of response bias may be compounded when attempting to evaluate change over time in longitudinal studies. When subjects drop out because of mental or physical health problems, the simple substitution of a proxy at time 2 may introduce additional bias. As with cross-sectional comparisons, this need not be fatal but must be evaluated in the context of the research hypotheses and the direction of bias.

PREVIOUS STUDIES OF PROXY REPORTS IN THE AGED

Few studies of proxy responses have been conducted in the aged. The problems inherent in using proxy-derived data in younger subjects (<65 years) have been a concern of epidemiologists for many years (Enterline and Capt, 1959; Gordis, 1982; Herrmann, 1985; Humble et al, 1984; Kolonel et al, 1977; Lerchen et al, 1986; Marshall et al, 1984; Maclean and Genn, 1979; Rocca et al, 1986) and are the subject of a recent review (Moore, 1988). These studies of younger persons have addressed such topics as dietary habits, smoking history, occupational exposures, and health symptoms. For the most part, the reliability of proxies has been evaluated for recalling behaviors in the distant past: Few have evaluated the use of proxies for the subject's current health status, a primary focus of epidemiologic studies in the aged.

Response Agreement

Response agreement incorporates elements of both precision and bias. Efforts to evaluate the systematic variations attributable to proxies (i.e., bias) have been made and are discussed in the next section. No efforts have been made to assess precision directly; instead, efforts have been directed to understanding response agreement. Although few studies exist and reproducibility across studies and settings is limited, available data on the aged in community, hospital, and long-term care setting suggest that agreement is a function of the type of information sought, characteristics of the proxy, and characteristics of the older subject. In studies to date (Bassett et al, 1990; Clipp and Elder, 1987; Epstein et al, 1989; Magaziner et al, 1987, 1988), agreement appears better for question areas that are relatively objective and observable, such as age, gender, the presence of medical diagnoses and conditions, observable symptoms (e.g., blackouts), and clearly defined functional characteristics (e.g., ability to walk or feed oneself). Agreement is poorer for more private conditions and those that are less observable, relying more on opinion than on observation, such as perceived health status, whether or not a urinary catheter is used, and ability to hear and see. Response comparability also tends to be poorer for more complex tasks of daily living, such as the ability to handle money, shop, or do housekeeping (Magaziner et al, 1988). Interestingly, agreement for tests of cognitive ability are relatively good, as are ratings of depression and emotional status (Epstein et al, 1989; Bassett et al, 1990). Studies involving evaluation of general psychological well-being and satisfaction, both based on experiential and nonobservable symptom complexes, yield conflicting results, with some (Bassett et al, 1990; Epstein et al, 1989) reporting poor agreement and others (Clipp and Elder, 1987; Rogers, 1988) reporting relatively good agreement.

Studies providing information on characteristics of proxy informants indicate that some proxies are better than others in providing information for subjects who cannot be interviewed themselves (Bassett et al, 1990; Clipp and Elder, 1987; Epstein et al, 1989; Magaziner et al, 1987, 1988; Rubenstein et al, 1984). Such proxy characteristics as age, relationship to subject, living arrangement in relation to subject, and amount of time spent with the subject have all been considered. To add to the complexity of this problem, it appears that agreement of proxy reports is also a function of the specific question being asked of particular proxies. In one study, for example, where proxy characteristics were evaluated in relation to response agreement, proxy characteristics did not influence subject–proxy agreement on measures of social activity, emotional status, overall health, or functional status; but proxies who lived with subjects or who had more frequent contact with them provided answers with higher agreement for a measure of satisfaction (Epstein et al, 1989). In another study (Magaziner et al, 1988), older proxies and those who were first-order relatives provided answers that agreed more with those of subjects for both physical and instrumental activities of daily living. Those living with respondents provided more comparable answers for physical activities of daily living, though no differences were seen with regard to living arrangement and instrumental activities of daily living. In contrast, those providing assistance to subjects gave more comparable answers on instrumental tasks of daily living with no differences seen for physical tasks of daily living. In another study (Bassett et al, 1990), neither the proxy characteristics of gender, age, education, relationship to subject, living arrangement, nor amount of visiting for those not living with subjects influenced agreement on measures of general well-being. With the exception of less comparability among those proxies who visit with subjects frequently, none of these proxy characteristics were associated with ratings of depressive symptomatology either. For cognitive status evaluation, better agreement was observed for those living with subjects and those visiting with them more frequently (Bassett et al, 1990). In yet another study (Clipp and Elder, 1987), functional ratings by friends were more comparable with self-reports of functioning than were spousal reports.

Although scant, there is some evidence to suggest that subject characteristics also influence response agreement. For the few studies addressing this issue, it appears that if subjects are in better health, agreement is better on measures of satisfaction (Epstein et al, 1989) and instrumental tasks of daily living (Magaziner et al, 1988) but that for physical tasks of daily living, better agreement is observed when the subject is more impaired. When subjects are depressed, subject–proxy agreement tends to be poorer for both measures of physical and instrumental tasks of daily living (Magaziner et al, 1988).

Response Bias

As with response agreement, studies of bias also indicate that characteristics of the question, proxy, and subject are associated with systematic over- or underreporting of responses. In the few studies of the elderly conducted to date (Bassettt et al, 1990; Clipp and Elder, 1987; Epstein et al, 1989; Magaziner et al, 1987, 1988; Rogers and Herzog, 1989; Rubenstein et al, 1984), proxies generally rated more impairment and disability than subjects. Variations on this general theme were seen across studies, however. For example, whereas three studies (Clipp and Elder, 1987; Magaziner et al, 1988; Rubenstein et al, 1984) found ratings of greater disability by nonprofessional proxies for measures of physical and instrumental activities of daily living, another study (Epstein et al, 1989) reported no bias for a measure of general functional status. In a study of cognitive status and affect (Bassett et al, 1990), it was found that proxies underrated affect and overrated cognitive status compared to subject-derived ratings on these measures. This is similar to the results in a study asking subjects and proxies about memory ability (cognitive) and depression (affect) (Rogers and Herzog, 1989).

The relationship of the proxy to the subject is a factor in estimating bias, although consistent results across studies are not evident. In one study (Rubenstein et al, 1984), nurses ratings of functional status yielded less disability than ratings by family proxies but more disability than ratings by patients themselves. In another study (Magaziner et al, 1988), first-order relatives provided less-biased reports than other relatives on measures of functioning, although on these same measures, more bias was observed for female proxies, proxies living with subjects, and proxies providing assistance to subjects in performing their activities of daily living. In another study (Rogers and Herzog, 1989), it was found that husbands rate their wives as having less difficulty remembering things than wives self-ratings. This was not the case for wives' ratings of husbands, however, where no differences were observed.

Subject characteristics also appear to be associated with the bias observed between proxies and subjects. In one study (Magaziner et al, 1988), proxies reported more disability than patients for measures of physical activities of daily living among subjects who were unimpaired on measures of physical health and depression. For measures of instrumental tasks of daily living, however, proxies reported more disability than patients when patients were impaired on measures of physical health and depression. In another study (Clipp and Elder, 1987), subjects with lower feelings of personal efficacy and self-esteem and those feeling less competent or in control of their own aging reported their own health to be better than did proxies compared to subjects without such feelings.

Overall, the limited evidence available indicates that both agreement and bias are functions of the question being asked, proxy characteristics, and subject characteristics. Because of the limited number of studies and their variety with respect to populations, settings, and questions, it is difficult to draw detailed conclusions about the manner in which agreement and bias are affected by the question, proxy, and subject characteristics. Aside from the general statements that proxies seem to provide more agreeable responses on objective items and that family proxies tend to report more disability on measures of functional status than subjects themselves, little else is consistent across studies. Suffice it to say, these are important issues that must be considered when using proxies, though the specific impact of using a proxy in any given study may not be predicted confidently, a priori, given data presently available.

PRACTICAL CONSIDERATIONS FOR RESEARCH

Until definitive directives on the use of proxies can be provided, several practical strategies might be followed.

Question Design

Given that there is better proxy–subject agreement for more objective questions, where possible, researchers should design questions that are clear and objective and that minimize respondent interpretation, judgment, and opinion. Although this seems obvious, this strategy is frequently not followed. Many standard activities of daily living scales, for example, require respondents to evaluate degrees of subject dependence for a variety of functions. Depending on task complexity and the degree of generality captured by the question, such questions may lead to varying interpretations by different reporters. To minimize this, consideration should be given to rewording standard questions to refer to discrete, observable aspects of more global activities. Rather than asking if subjects are able to perform housework independently, respondent interpretation might be minimized by asking whether respondents are able to dust, vacuum, wash floors, and so on. Likewise, rather than asking if subjects are able to dress themselves, it might be more appropriate to ask whether they are able to put on a shirt, button it, put on trousers, buckle a belt, put on a dress, put on socks, tie shoes, and so on. Taking this step one further, instead of calling for evaluation of one's ability to perform tasks, better agreement and less bias might result from questions pertaining to actual performance of discrete activities (e.g., "Do you put on your shirt?" versus "Can you put on your shirt?") Of course, the decision of whether or not to ask questions in this way must rest on whether the interest is in capacity (ability) to perform tasks or actual performance of activities in daily life.

Use of Proxies Only

Consideration should be given to relying solely on proxies rather than on mixing data derived from proxies and subjects. This may be especially important in longitudinal studies of change in health and functioning, since subjects are likely to drop out because of disability and health problems and proxies are known to rate greater degrees of disability for many functional domains than subjects report for themselves. Changing to a proxy for follow-up data may result in more decline than is actually present. Of course, in attempting to obtain information only from proxies, it might be necessary to seek subjects when proxies are not available, or to change proxies, both of which may introduce additional complications.

Pilot Studies

Given that agreement and bias are functions of questions asked, proxy characteristics, and patient characteristics, careful pilot studies are needed in which the specific question areas to be used and the proxies to be encountered in the population under study are evaluated. These pilot efforts should consider both proxy–subject agreement and bias. Regarding agreement, attention should be given to random variability in response and the sample size required for deriving parameter estimates. Bias should be evaluated for both direction and magnitude.

One difficulty with this strategy of comparing subject and proxy responses for a sample of subjects and proxies that typify the study sample is that those subjects for whom many proxies are needed (i.e., the cognitively and physically impaired) cannot be interviewed for comparative purposes. Thus, in making comparisons of proxies with subjects who can be evaluated, one must make the assumption that for the characteristic in question, subject–proxy agreement and bias will not vary as a function of subject status. In light of what we know about the effect of subject characteristics on response agreement and bias, this may not be a justifiable assumption. The use of other data sources (e.g., medical charts, laboratory tests, utilization records, or patient examinations by health professionals) may be helpful in estimating the agreement and bias of proxies for impaired subjects. Of course, care must be taken to assure that source documents themselves do not derive from the same proxy's reports (e.g., history information in hospital admitting notes frequently comes from proxy reports).

Several techniques for evaluating proxy–subject agreement and bias have been used. To compare the agreement of proxy and subject scores on continuous measures, a Pearson correlation coefficient has been employed; for categorical measures, Cohen's Kappa statistic has been used (Bassett et al, 1990; Epstein et al, 1989; Magaziner et al, 1987, 1988). Although the proportion agreement is easily expressed and widely used as a measure of interrater agreement, unlike Kappa, it does not take into account agreement by chance. The values of both Kappa and correlation coefficients range from 0 to 1. Kappa values greater than .75 may be interpreted as an indication of excellent agreement, whereas values below .40 may be viewed as indicating poor agreement (Fleiss, 1973). Similar values have been used for interpreting correlation coefficients (Bassett et al, 1990; Magaziner et al, 1988). To test for beyond-chance agreement (i.e., statistical significance), for Kappa, a Z score based on kappa and its standard error may be computed; for correlation coefficients, t-tests may be used.

Techniques for estimating whether proxies over- or undervalue responses compared to subjects (i.e., bias) have also been described (Bassett et al, 1990; Epstein et al, 1989; Magaziner et al, 1987, 1988). For continuous measures, bias has been expressed as a mean difference score, using a paired comparison t-test to evaluate statistical significance (Epstein et al, 1989; Magaziner et al, 1988). To evaluate bias and compare continuous measures with different value ranges and metrics, subject–proxy differences have been computed and expressed relative to the subjects' standard deviation in order to obtain a standardized difference (Bassett et al, 1990). By this technique, bias = (D/SD_s), where D is the difference between proxy- and subject-derived score, and SD_s is the subject standard deviation. Bias expressed in this way will range from 0 to 1, where .2 may be considered small and .8 large (Cohen, 1977). To evaluate proxy bias with categorical measures, the percentage bias has been compared (Magaziner et al, 1987), and its statistical significance evaluated using McNemar's chi square test (Fleiss, 1973). Percent bias was calculated as the ratio of the difference between the proportion of affirmative responses of proxies and patients expressed as a percentage of the proportion of patients responding affirmatively.

Accounting for Proxies in Data Analysis

Although not a solution to the problem of using proxy responses, it is important to account for the use of proxies in data analyses. Several techniques for estimating the effect of using proxy-derived data have been suggested (Heyman et al, 1984; McLaughlin et al, 1984; Mosley and Wolinsky, 1986; Walker et al, 1988). Although none of these techniques can evaluate the bias attributable to using proxies, since the effect of the information source may be attributable to the proxy or to the reason for using a proxy (i.e., some systematic difference attributable to subjects not available for evaluation themselves), use of these techniques may help rule out source of information as a confounding factor.

One approach entailed stratifying analyses in a case-control study by information source and then estimating the effect attributable to the proxy stratum by dividing estimates of the effects derived from proxies by estimates obtained from information derived directly from cases and controls at multiple exposure levels (Walker et al, 1988). With large differences across strata, stratum-specific estimates would be presented. If the effects do not differ across strata, then pooling data without regard to information source would be appropriate. A similar strategy, which is applicable in survey and case-control studies, would be to use multiple regression with interaction terms for source of information and each independent variable or exposure. Two related strategies have also been employed in case-control studies. One (McLaughlin et al, 1984) relied on two control groups, one of which was living and was interviewed directly; the other was of deceased persons. For this group a proxy respondent was interviewed. Results were then compared using two separate control groups. Another (Heyman et al, 1984) entailed obtaining information from subjects and their proxies within a control group for a study of Alzheimer's disease patients. By necessity, information about Alzheimer's disease patients came from proxies. Information on the degree of agreement between control subjects and their proxies was presented for each of the items in this study and became a part of the interpretation of study results.

As pointed out by Kelsey et al (1989), to use these analytical strategies for evaluating the effects of using proxies in case control studies, it is necessary to include a sufficient number of proxies in the study to create separate strata. The same, of course, would apply with survey data in which a term for information source or its interaction with a study variable is included within the multivariate regression analysis. Further, if a large enough number of proxies is included, it might be possible to extend the analysis to include selected proxy and subject characteristics within the analyses. Although these strategies may be cumbersome and may yield results that are difficult to interpret, it is important to employ them so that results that rely on subject and proxy reports can be interpreted with an understanding of the relative lack of precision and bias.

SUMMARY AND CONCLUSIONS

The use of proxies in epidemiologic studies of the elderly is essential to reduce nonresponse. The need for proxies increases with subject age and disability. Surprisingly little is known about the use of proxies, and the standard operating procedure is to obtain information from any source available and to use this information in a combined analytical framework without regard to the source of information. In light of the existing evidence, it seems that to continue with this strategy without assessing the potential impact it may have on study results is inappropriate. The use of proxies may, in fact, introduce considerable measurement error. Given evidence on the possibility for diminished precision and increased bias resulting from proxy-derived data, and the fact that these associations are neither simple nor predictable a priori, scientists have an obligation to evaluate these potential sources of error. Additional research is needed to address these issues directly. In the absence of definitive answers, researchers must follow a practical strategy designed to minimize imprecision and bias and to evaluate and report imprecision and bias. Such efforts will permit the scientific community to benefit from any uncertainty that exits.

ACKNOWLEDGMENTS

This work was supported by NIH grant R01 AG04366. The author would like to acknowledge the thoughtful review and critique by J. Richard Hebel, Ph.D., Jean C. Scott, M.P.H., R.N., and Sheryl Zimmerman, Ph.D., and expert typing by Doris Scheihing.

REFERENCES

Bassett SS, Magaziner J, Hebel JR (1990). Reliability of proxy response. Psychol Age 5: 127–132.

Burnam A, Leaf PJ, Skinner EA, Cottler L, Melville ML, Thompson JW (1985). Proxy interviews. In Eaton WW, Kessler LG (eds), Epidemiologic Field Methods in Psychiatry: The NIMH Epidemiologic Catchment Area Program. New York, Academic Press.

Clipp EC, Elder GH (1987). Elderly confidants in geriatric assessment. Compr Gerontol B 1:35–40.

Cohen J (1977). Statistical Power Analysis for the Behavioral Sciences. New York, Academic Press.

Cornoni-Huntley J, Brock DB, Ostfield AM, Taylor JO, Wallace RB (1986). Established populations for epidemiologic studies of the elderly: Resource data book. NIH Pub. No. 86-2443. Washington, DC, National Institute on Aging.

Enterline PE, Capt KG (1959). A validation of information provided by household respondents in health surveys. Am J Public Health 49:205–212.

Epstein AM, Hall JA, Tognetti J, Son LA, Conant L (1989). Using proxies to evaluate quality of life. Med Care 27:S91–S98.

Fitti JE, Kovar MG (1987). The supplement on aging to the 1984 National Health Interview Study. Vital and Health Statistics, Ser. 1, No. 21. DHHS Pub. No. (PHS) 87-1323. Washington, DC, U.S. Government Printing Office.

Fleiss JL (1973). Statistical methods for rates and proportions. New York, Wiley.

Gordis L (1982). Should dead cases be matched to dead controls? Am J Epidemiol 115:1–5.

Herrmann N (1985). Retrospective information from questionnaires. I. Comparability of primary respondents and their next-of-kin. Am J Epidemiol 121:937–947.

Herzog AR, Rogers WL (1988). Age and response rates to interview sample surveys. J Gerontol 43:200–205.

Heyman A, Wilkinson WE, Stafford JA, Helms MJ, Sigmon AV, Weingerg T (1984). Alzheimer's disease: A study of epidemiological aspects. Ann Neurol 15:335–341.

Hing E, Sekscenski E, Strahan G (1989). The National Nursing Home Survey: 1985 Summary of the United States. Vital and Health Statistics, Ser. 13, No. 97. DHHS Pub. No. (PHS) 89-1758. Public Health Service, Washington, DC.

Humble CG, Samet JM, Skiller BE (1984). Comparison of self- and surrogate-reported dietary information. Am J Epidemiol 119:86–98.

Kelsey JL, O'Brien LA, Grisso JA, Hoffman S (1989). Issues in carrying out epidemiologic research in the elderly. Am J Epidemiol 130:857–866.

Kolonel LN, Hirohata T, Nomura AMY (1977). Adequacy of survey data collected from substitute respondents. Am J Epidemiol 106:476–484.

Lerchen ML, Samet JM (1986). An assessment of the validity of questionnaire responses provided by a surviving spouse. Am J Epidemiol 123:481–489.

Maclean M, Genn H (1979). Proxy response in social surveys. In Atkinson J, Harris D, Hartwell R (eds.) Methodological Issues in Social Surveys. Atlantic Highlands, NJ, Humanities Press, pp. 58–77.

Magaziner J, Hebel JR, Warren JW (1987). The use of proxy responses for aged patients in long-term care settings. Compr Gerontol B1:118–121.

Magaziner J, Simonsick EM, Kashner TM, Hebel JR (1988). Patient–proxy response comparability on measures of patient health and functional status. J Clin Epidemiol 41:1065–1074.

Marshall J, Priore R, Haughey B, et al. (1984). Spouse-subject interviews and the reliability of diet studies. Am J Epidemiol 112:675–683.

McLaughlin JK, Mandel JS, Blot WJ, Schuman LM, Mehl ES, Fraumeni, Jr, JF (1984). A population-based case-control study of renal cell carcinoma. JNCL 72:275–284.

Moore JC (1988). Self/proxy response status and survey response quality. J Off Stat 4:155–172.

Mosely RR, Wolinsky FD (1986). The use of proxies in health surveys. Med Care 24:496–510.

Norris FH (1985). Characteristics of older nonrespondents over five waves of a panel study. J Gerontol 40(5):627–636.

Pickle LW, Brown LM, Blot WJ (1983). Information available from surrogate respondents in case-control interview studies. Am J Epidemiol 118:99–108.

Rocca WA, Fratiglioni L, Bracco L, Pedone D, Groppi C, Schoenberg BS (1986). The use of surrogate respondents to obtain questionnaire data in case-control studies of neurologic diseases. J Chronic Dis 39:907–912.

Rogers WL (1988). The relative validities of self and proxy reports. Paper presented at the 41st Annual Scientific Meeting of the Gerontological Society of America, San Francisco.

Rogers WL, Herzog AR (1989). The consequences of accepting proxy respondents on total survey error for elderly populations. Paper presented at the Fifth Conference on Health Survey Research Methods, Keystone, Colorado.

Rogers WL, Herzog AR (in press). Collecting data about the oldest-old: Problems and procedures. In Suzman RM, Willis DP, Manton KG (eds), The Oldest-Old. New York, Oxford.

Rubenstein LZ, Schairer C, Wieland GD, Kane R (1984). Systematic biases in functional status assessment of elderly adults: Effects of different data sources. J Gerontol 39:686–691.

Walker AM, Velema JP, Robins JA (1988). Analysis of case-control data derived in part from proxy respondents. Am J Epidemiol 127:905–914.

9

Epidemiologic Studies of Cognitive Function in the Elderly: Rationale, Methods, and Findings

PATRICIA L. COLSHER

Despite recognition that age-associated cognitive dysfunction represents a significant and increasing public health problem (Kane, 1986), relatively little is known about population distributions of cognitive functions (Cutler and Grams, 1988). With the exception of the recent Established Populations for Epidemiologic Studies of the Elderly (Cornoni-Huntley et al, 1986), the Epidemiologic Catchment Area study (Holzer et al, 1984), the Framingham study (Farmer et al, 1987), and a handful of smaller cohort studies (Busse and Maddox, 1985; Cunningham and Ownes, 1983; Jarvik and Bank, 1983; Shaie, 1983; Siegler, 1983), most knowledge of and theorizing about age-associated changes in cognitive function have derived from small experimental and clinical investigations.

However, as may be seen in Table 9-1, which summarizes the characteristics of all cognitive function papers published in four major gerontologic and geriatric journals during 1986 and 1987, participants in these studies are not representative of the elderly as a group. For example, of the 33 studies in both 1986 and 1987 that specified maximum ages, one third did not include persons over the age of 75. Participants were better educated than most elderly persons: In 1984, 54 percent of persons 65 years of age and older had less than a high school education, and 25 percent had only a high school diploma (U.S. Bureau of the Census, 1989). Moreover, a number of studies do not provide any information on educational attainment. Recruitment sources, including alumni organizations, senior centers, and retirement communities, may bias the sample further. Finally, although some studies explicitly specify health-related exclusionary criteria, others simply describe participants as "healthy" without reporting how this determination was made and whether "unhealthy" persons were excluded or simply did not volunteer; still other studies provide no health information at all. Because many measures of cognitive function are sensitive to education, health status, and level of physical, recreational, and social function (Perlmutter, 1987), it is difficult to generalize from experimental and clinical studies to the general population.

Table 9-1 Characteristics of Cognitive Function Papers Published in 1986 and 1987 in Four Gerontologic and Geriatric Journals[a]

	1986	1987
Number of articles	53	39
Sample size:		
Range	5–1203	1–825
Mean	79.1	86.8
Median	25.5	27.0
Age (in years):		
Range of means	47.5–83.8	53.0–76.4
Mean of means	68.9	68.8
Median of means	69.6	69.9
Only median or distribution given (%)	9 (17.0)	5 (12.8)
Not specified (%)	2 (3.8)	0
Specifying maximum age (%)	33 (62.3)	33 (84.6)
With maximum <76 (%)	11 (20.8)	11 (28.2)
Educational attainment (in years):		
Range of means	8.0–17.0	9.4–16.5
Mean of means	13.6	13.3
Median of means	14.1	13.4
Only median or distribution given (%)	3 (5.7)	5 (12.8)
No information given (%)	23 (43.4)	11 (28.2)
Participant source: number (%):		
Clinic, hospital, nursing home	15 (28.3)	10 (25.6)
Organizations[b]	17 (32.1)	13 (33.3)
Community volunteers	16 (30.2)	13 (33.3)
Advertisements	5 (9.4)	5 (12.8)
Population-based	4 (7.5)	2 (5.1)
Other[c]	3 (5.7)	(7.7)
No information	5 (9.4)	3 (7.7)
Health information: number (%):		
Health as independent variable	6 (11.3)	6 (15.4)
Sensory function exclusions	6 (11.3)	10 (25.6)
Other health exclusions[d]	10 (18.9)	10 (25.6)
Health history, physical examination[e]	8 (15.1)	6 (15.4)
Self-perceived health status	15 (28.3)	12 (30.8)
"Healthy"	4 (7.5)	2 (5.1)
No health information	16 (30.2)	9 (23.1)

[a]Journals included *Journal of Gerontology, Psychology and Aging, Journal of the American Geriatrics Society,* and *Age and Ageing.* Values in the table are, whenever possible, restricted to the groups of participants described by the authors as "old." Younger groups of respondents are not included in sample size, age, or educational attainment calculations.

[b]Includes alumni organizations, senior centers, retirement groups, retirement communities, religious organizations, volunteer groups, and other clubs.

[c]Includes personal contact and subject pools.

[d]Includes history of substance abuse, neurologic and psychiatric illness, major illness, medication use.

[e]Includes explicit mention of taking systematic health history or performing physical examination.

[f]Participant source and health information percentages sum to more than 100 because multiple sources of participants or types of health information may be included.

Knowledge of the population distributions of cognitive functions would be useful in developing screens for *nascent* cognitive dysfunction, describing age-associated changes in cognitive functions, and determining risk factors for cognitive morbidity. This chapter addresses some of the major methodologic issues in population-based studies of cognitive function, including test selection, cohort selection, and possible confounding variables.

TEST SELECTION

There is a large pool of cognitive function tests from which to select, including tests of psychometric intelligence, aptitude, and achievement; mental status screening examinations; neuropsychological batteries and specialized tests (e.g., dementia screens and clinical memory tests); and laboratory-based measures. These tests have been developed by different disciplines for different purposes and vary in their adaptability for epidemiologic investigations. This section will review the general categories of tests, provide specific examples, and discuss their use in epidemiologic investigations.

Psychometric Intelligence

Tests of psychometric intelligence were originally intended to screen schoolchildren for special academic services (Anastasi, 1976). Although tests suitable for adults have been developed, they remain closely related to a conceptualization of intelligence rooted in Western academic success (Gardner, 1983) and correlate best with academic achievement (Anastasi, 1976). There are both group tests that can be administered easily to large numbers of examinees simultaneously and individual tests of intelligence, such as the Stanford-Binet (Terman and Merrill, 1973) and Wechsler (Wechsler, 1983) tests, which are administered by a skilled examiner to a single examinee at a time.

Most group intelligence tests were developed for use in academic settings with children or adolescents and are not suitable for use with normal-functioning adults. Two major exceptions are the Armed Forces Qualification Test and the Primary Mental Abilities test battery.

The Armed Forces Qualification Test (Army Behavior and Systems Research, 1970) is the contemporary version of the Army Alpha and Beta (an adaptation of the Alpha for persons with limited English language skills), which were developed to classify World War I U.S. military inductees (Yerkes, 1921). The Army Alpha includes multiple-choice vocabulary, arithmetic, and spatial skills (determining the number of same-size blocks in a stack) questions. Yerkes's (Yerkes, 1921) analyses of the performance of 15,385 inductees on the Army Alpha is one of the first large-scale demonstrations of cross-sectional age-associated differences in cognitive function. In general, however, the military classification tests do not seem to be used frequently in current civilian research.

The Primary Mental Abilities (Thurstone and Thurstone, 1949; Thurstone, 1958) was developed by Thurstone and is based on a multiple-factor conceptualization of intelligence. The subtests of the PMA are summarized in Table 9-2.

Table 9-2 Sections of Primary Mental Abilities Test Battery

Vocabulary: Multiple-choice synonyms
Spatial skills: Imagining how objects would appear when rotated in space
Reasoning: Determining what should come next in a series
Arithmetic skills: Checking sums for accuracy
Verbal fluency: Ability to generate words beginning with a specified letter

Schaie (1983) used the PMA in the Seattle Longitudinal Study, which examined cognitive function and related psychobehavioral measures in 4504 members of a health maintenance organization. Only modest longitudinal decrements in function occurred prior to age 60. After age 75, however, larger decrements occurred and virtually all respondents had experienced a decrement in at least one of the five PMA tests (Schaie, 1983). The occurrence of physical illnesses, especially cardiovascular conditions, was an important determinant of cognitive morbidity (Hertzog, Schaie, and Gribbin, 1978; Schaie, 1989), whereas preservation of cognitive function was associated with above-average success and life satisfaction (Schaie, 1989).

The classic individual tests of psychometric intelligence are the Simon-Binet (Binet and Simon, 1905) and the Stanford-Binet (Terman and Merrill, 1973), an adapted version of the Simon-Binet. The Stanford-Binet consists of a series of subtests that are summarized in Table 9-3. Although the Stanford-Binet has been modified to include items of adult difficulty, it is not regarded as an appropriate clinical test for adults functioning in the superior range (Anastasi, 1976; Kennedy, 1960). It may still be useful, however, in epidemiologic investigations when there is no interest in discriminating among those who function at very high levels.

The Wechsler Adult Intelligence Scale (WAIS) and the more recent WAIS-Revised (Wechsler, 1983) consist of a series of subtests that are classified as verbal or performance tests and yield verbal, performance, and full-scale intelligence quotients. The

Table 9-3 Sections of Stanford-Binet Intelligence Scale

Vocabulary: Define words
Proverbs: Interpret common proverbs
Problem solving and reasoning: Logic problems
Reasons: Tell why certain practices are followed (e.g., criminals are punished)
Essential differences and similarities: How two things are different (e.g., work and play) or similar (e.g., egg and seed)
Opposite analogies: Fill-in-the-blank analogies (e.g., "ability is native; education is . . .")
Reconciliation of opposites: Finding the common dimension of opposites (e.g., winter and summer)
Memory for prose: Ability to recall ideas in a paragraph
Digit span: Number of digits that can be repeated
Sentence building: Construct sentence using specified words (e.g., "ceremonial, dignity, impression")
Sentence completion: Fill-in-the-blank in sentences (e.g., "_____ either of us could speak, we were at the bottom of the stairs.")
Paper cutting: Examiner folds paper and cuts it; examinee repeats.
Spatial orientation: What direction would a person have to face so that their (right/left) hand was toward a specified direction
Abstract words: Define abstract words, tell difference between pairs of abstract words
Coding: Examinee is shown a phrase in English and in code; must determine the rule underlying the code and write a word that has no letters in common with the original phrase in the code.

subtests of the WAIS are summarized in Table 9-4. The WAIS and WAIS-R are frequently used in both clinical and research settings, and both the Duke Longitudinal Study (Busse and Maddox, 1985; Siegler, 1983) and the Framingham Study (Farmer et al, 1987) included portions of the WAIS.

The Duke Longitudinal Study consisted of an initial sample of community volunteers ($N = 267$) and a second sample randomly selected from a listing of persons covered by major health insurance ($N = 502$). The initial sample was similar to the community in age, gender, educational attainment, and socioeconomic status, but was healthier and more active than older persons in general (Busse and Maddox, 1985). The second sample was better educated and of higher socioeconomic status than the general population (Busse and Maddox, 1985; Siegler, 1983). Declines in psychometric intelligence began occurring when respondents were in their 70s. Cardiovascular disease, including coronary artery disease and untreated hypertension, was an important predictor of decline (Wilkie and Eisdorfer, 1971). In addition, "distance from death" was found to be an important determinant of cognitive decline (Siegler et al, 1983). That is, the decline among persons who survived the follow-up period was less than that among nonsurvivors, a phenomenon termed the *terminal drop.*

In the Framingham Study, the WAIS has been used to assess the impact of cardiovascular disease on cognitive function. For example, Farmer and colleagues (1987) examined the relationship between blood pressure and psychometric intelligence in 2032 persons 55–89 years of age. Only the digit span test was significantly related to blood pressure: Persons younger than 75 years of age who were definite or borderline hypertensives performed less well than same-age normotensives, and persons 75 years of age and older who were definite or borderline hypertensives performed better than same-age normotensives.

To summarize, several groups of investigators have used tests of psychometric intelligence in epidemiologic investigations. Although some of these tests are easily administered paper-and-pencil tests (e.g., the Primary Mental Abilities battery), others (e.g., the Wechsler Adult Intelligence Scale) require that a trained administrator test individual subjects using special equipment. Both types of tests, however, have indicated declines in psychometric intelligence beginning in the 70s and a relationship between psychometric intelligence and physical health.

Table 9-4 Subtests of Wechsler Adult Intelligence Scale

Verbal
Vocabulary: Define words
Information: Give information known in this culture, ranging in difficulty from commonly known (e.g., colors of flag) to less well known (e.g., authors of literary works)
Comprehension: Interpret proverbs and tell why practices are followed (e.g., why marriage licenses are required)
Arithmetic: Solve simple mental word problems
Similarities: Explain how two things are alike
Digit span: Repeat forwards and backwards an increasing number of digits until limit is reached
Performance
Digit–symbol: Substitute simple symbols for numerals
Picture completion: Tell what is missing from a drawing
Block design: Use colored blocks to copy a design
Picture arrangement: Arrange a series of pictures so that they tell a coherent story
Object assemble: Assemble jigsaw puzzles shaped like familiar objects

Mental Status Screening Examinations

Mental status screening examinations were developed as bedside tools for use by clinicians and provide a systematic, quantitative assessment of basic cognitive function. These tests were not intended to be sensitive to higher levels of function; rather, they were meant to provide a screen for gross cognitive dysfunction and disorientation.

Table 9-5 summarizes the components of several widely used mental status screening examinations: the Mini-Mental State Examination (Folstein, Folstein, and McHugh, 1975), the Short Portable Mental Status Questionnaire (Pfeiffer, 1975), the Mental Status Questionnaire (Kahn et al., 1960), and the Orientation–Memory–Concentration Test (Katzman et al., 1983). All four batteries include questions about the current date, and three of the four (all but OMC) ask where the interview is being conducted (orientation in time and place). Both the SPMSQ and MSQ include requests for personal (e.g., birthdate, age, mother's maiden name, address, and phone number) and public (recent presidents) information. The MMSE, SPMSQ, and OMC include tests of concentration, and the MMSE and OMC include brief memory tests.

Several groups have included mental status screening examinations in epidemiologic investigations. Holzer and colleagues (1984) described the use of the MMSE in the Yale cohort of the Epidemiological Catchment Area Program. They reported that one item (asking on which floor of the building the interview was conducted), was regarded by community-dwelling respondents as "silly." As a result, only institutionalized respondents were asked that question, and community-dwelling respondents were given credit for a correct response. Of the 5035 respondents, 118 (2.3 percent) answered five or fewer questions, and 69 (1.4 percent) answered between 6 and 25 questions. Respondents in the former group were described as very ill, having language problems, or unwilling to continue the interview. Respondents in the latter group included persons who got most of the items they attempted correct but did not seem to take the cognitive testing seriously and/or persons who were not willing to be tested. The authors reported significant declines in MMSE scores across age groups and an

Table 9-5 Comparison of Mental Status Screening Examinations

	MMSE	SPMSO	MSQ	OMC[a]
Orientation:				
Place	X	X	X	
Time	X	X	X	X
Memory performance test	X			X
Concentration/attention[b]	X	X		X
Information:				
Public		X	X	
Personal		X	X	
Other[c]	X		X	

Notes:

[a]MMSE = Mini-Mental State Examination; SPMSQ = Short Portable Mental Status Examination; MSQ = Mental Status Questionnaire; OMC = Orientation-Memory-Concentration.

[b]Serial subtraction, spelling words backward, counting backward, saying months in reverse order.

[c]Information about examiner, naming objects, repetition, following commands, writing sentence, copying design.

increase in the percentage of persons who scored in the impaired range. There were also age-associated declines in the percentage of respondents who got individual items correct, although for some items (e.g., naming a watch and pencil, reporting the town and state) the declines were slight.

Magaziner, Bassett, and Hebel (1987) used the MMSE in a study of 783 women randomly selected from a metropolitan area who were 65 years of age and older. They found that age and educational attainment interacted, so that younger women with more education had the highest scores and older women with less education had the lowest scores, but older women with more education scored higher than did younger women with less education.

Clarke, Lowry, and Clarke (1986) examined gross cognitive function in persons served by a 12-physician practice in an English town. They used the Information and Orientation sections of the Clifton Assessment Schedule, a psychogeriatric assessment instrument that includes orientation in time and place; basic personal and public information; ability to recite the alphabet, count from 1 to 20, write one's own name, and read; and performance of a maze (Pattie and Gilleard, 1975). Thus, their assessment was similar to a mental status screening examination. All community-dwelling and institutionalized persons 75 years of age and older were included in the target group, and the authors reported a 94 percent participation rate, with 5 percent refusals and 1 percent not traceable. Most of the refusals were the result of a family member refusing on behalf of the elder. Interestingly, the physicians treating persons who refused to participate did not view them as having special health problems. Of the 1124 community-dwelling elders, 28 (2.5 percent) were classified as having marked impairment; 26 of the 79 institutionalized elders (32.9 percent) had marked impairments. The rates among men and women were similar, with 3.1 percent of men and 3.6 percent of women classified as impaired, and the rates increased with age, from 2.0 percent among 75- to 79-year-olds, to 3.7 percent among 80- to 84-year-olds, to 13.0 percent among persons 85 years of age and older.

To summarize, mental status screening examinations are brief and easily administered, provide a quantitative index of cognitive function, and can be used to categorize persons as cognitively impaired. These characteristics make them attractive for use in studies of large numbers of persons where the goal is to estimate rates of cognitive impairment. However, mental status screening examinations are not suitable for discriminating among persons functioning at normal or superior levels and are thus not adequate for a full characterization of the population distribution of cognitive function.

Neuropsychological Batteries

Neuropsychological batteries are lengthy, complex tests of a variety of functions, including sensory-perceptual function, psychomotor skills, memory, intelligence, and complex cognitive functions, such as problem solving and planning. They may take between 6 and 8 hours to administer to persons who are functioning relatively well, and much longer for those with cognitive impairments or even with persons who have physical problems but are cognitively intact. Examiners must be highly skilled in the administration of the tests.

One of the most widely used batteries, the Halstead-Reitan (Golden et al, 1981), is summarized in Table 9-6. In addition to the tests listed, the WAIS-R is often included

Table 9-6 Components of Halstead–Reitan Battery

Category test: Examinee is shown 208 illustrations that suggest a number between 1 and 4 (e.g., the Roman numeral III, a group of three circles and one square, and a square with three solid sides and one dashed side; seven subtests each with different organizing principles.
Tactual performance test: Examinee is blindfolded and places blocks in formboard. Blindfold is removed and examinee draws forms and arrangement of holes. Tested with preferred, nonpreferred, and both hands.
Rhythm test: Examinee is presented with 30 pairs of rhythmic passages, which are judged as same or different.
Speech sounds: Sixty nonsense words are read to examinee, who must pick each from among four alternatives.
Finger tapping: Examinee presses a lever as quickly as possible.
Trail-making test: Examinee is to "connect-the-dots" with numbers and alternating between numbers and letters.
Grip strength: Examinee uses dynamometer with both preferred and nonpreferred hands.
Sensory-perceptual: Examinee identifies side on which tactile, visual, and auditory stimuli are presented.
Tactile perception: Examinee identifies which finger is touched, numbers written on finger, and forms.
Aphasia screening test: Examinee shows ability to name objects, read, spell, identify letters and numbers, write, calculate, identify body parts, pantomime actions, understand spoken language, differentiate left and right, follow verbal directions.

in the Halstead-Reitan. When used clinically, the battery yields scores for each of the component tests as well as a composite score called the Average Impairment Index. Because of the length of the full battery, it is not uncommon for experimental and clinical studies to report only a handful of the tests. The most commonly used are the Category Test, the Tactual Performance Test, the Trail Making Test, and Finger Oscillation. Although these tests do not appear to have been used in epidemiologic studies, they may be adaptable. For example, although the Category Test was designed to be administered using slides and is rather lengthy, a booklet form of portions of the test could be used. The Trail Making Test is a paper–pencil test and thus is portable, but examiners must correct errors as they are made. Because the amount of time taken to complete the trail is measured, unskilled or inattentive examiners can easily distort the scores.

The other major neuropsychological battery is the Standardized Version of Luria's Neuropsychological Techniques, more commonly called the Luria-Nebraska (Christensen, 1974). It consists of 269 items that assess motor function, tactile perception, visual function, receptive and expressive speech, writing, reading, arithmetic skills, memory, and other intellectual skills. The Luria-Nebraska stresses a qualitative not quantitative approach, but yields a summary score called the Summary Pathognomic, scores reflecting left and right hemisphere function, and a summary profile. Administration of the Luria-Nebraska requires a high degree of skill and the exercise of clinical judgment, which may not be feasible in large investigations.

There are also a number of individual neuropsychological tests that have been used in experimental and clinical investigations and that may be adaptable for use in epidemiologic investigations. The Benton Visual Retention Test (Benton, 1974) and Bender-Gestalt test (Bender, 1938) require the reproduction of geometric figures. In Raven's Progressive Matrices (Raven, 1943), the examinee must determine which design fits into a pattern. Gollin figures (Gollin, 1960) are incomplete outlines of figures (e.g., an umbrella) that the examinee must identify. Porteus mazes (Porteus, 1959) are paper–pencil mazes of increasing difficulty, and the Wisconsin Card Sorting Test (Berg, 1948; Nelson, 1976) is a concept formation test.

Specialized Batteries

A number of specialized test batteries have been developed to assess specific domains of function (e.g., memory) or detect specific conditions (e.g., dementia screens). Because they are often relatively brief, portable, and straightforward in administration, they may be useful in epidemiologic investigations.

Table 9-7 summarizes three clinical memory batteries—the Wechsler Memory Scale (Wechsler, 1945), Cronholm and Molander Memory Test Battery (Cronholm and Molander, 1957; Cronholm and Ottoson, 1963), and Randt Memory Test Battery (Randt, Brown, and Osborne, 1980)—which have also been used in experimental studies. All three tests ask for general information of a public and/or personal nature and contain memory performance tests. The Wechsler and Randt batteries include tests of memory span (the number of items that can be held briefly in memory) and memory for prose (a paragraph). The Wechsler and Cronholm-Molander batteries include tests of visual memory and paired-associates learning, in which the examinee learns pairs of words, one of which is later presented to serve as a recall cue for the other. The Randt battery also includes memorization of a list of words and an incidental memory test. Incidental memory is memory for information the examinee was not forewarned that he or she would be asked to remember.

The previously described Duke Longitudinal Study (Siegler, 1983; Siegler et al, 1982) included the Wechsler Memory Scale (Wechsler, 1945). There was relatively little age-associated decline in the easy paired-associates learning test, somewhat more in the hard paired-associates, and a relatively large decline in the visual memory test (McCarty, Siegler, and Logue, 1982). Survivorship was also related in an important way to memory performance, with performance among respondents who were to survive a longer time superior to that of respondents who were to survive a shorter time (Siegler, McCarty and Logue, 1982).

Table 9-7 Comparison of Memory Batteries[a]

	WMS	C–M	Randt
General information	X	X	X
Orientation	X		
Attention/concentration	X		
Memory span	X		X
Memory performance:			
Prose	X		X
Visual	X	X	
Paired-associates	X	X	
List of words			X
Incidental memory			X

[a]WMS = full version of Wechsler Memory Scale; C–M = Cronholm and Molander Memory Test Battery; Randt = Randt Memory Test Battery.

Scherr and colleagues (1988) reported on the use of a memory test that is similar to the prose memory section of the Wechsler Memory Scale in the East Boston Senior Health Project ($N = 3812$), one of the four Established Populations for Epidemiologic Studies of the Elderly. The test consisted of a brief paragraph containing six ideas that were to be recalled whether verbatim or in gist. Cross-sectional correlates of memory performance included age, educational attainment, ability to perform routine activities, and social participation.

Dementia screening batteries, summarized in Table 9-8, include a variety of information obtained from different sources. The Blessed Dementia Scale (Blessed, Tomlinson, and Roth, 1968) and Alzheimer's Disease Assessment Scale (Rosen, Mohs, and Davis, 1984) include both performance tests and behavior ratings, as do the interrelated Brief Cognitive Rating Scale (Reisberg et al, 1983) and the Global Deterioration Scale (Reisberg et al, 1982). The Hachinski Ischemia Scale (Hachinski et al, 1975) includes behavior ratings and health history; the Sandoz Clinical Assessment—Geriatric (Shader, Hermatz, and Salzman, 1974) and the Clinical Dementia Rating (Hughes et al, 1982) include behavior ratings; and the Iowa Test of Abnormal Decline in Older Persons (Eslinger et al, 1985) includes performance testing.

Dementia batteries that include both performance testing and behavior ratings may be especially useful in studies of very old or frail persons. Clarke, Lowry, and Clarke (1986), for example, attributed the bulk of their refusals to family members seeking to protect an elder. Family members might be more willing to allow the participation of an elder if response demands on the elder were slight and the bulk of information were obtained from proxies. The combination of self-

Table 9-8 Comparison of Dementia Scales[a]

Measure	Blessed	Hach	ADAS	BCRS	GDS	SCAG	Iowa	CDR
Performance tests:								
Orientation	X			X	X		X	
Information	X			X	X			
Memory	X		X	X	X		X	
Concentration	X			X	X		X	
Language skill			X				X	
Visuo-spatial skill							X	
Behavior ratings:								
Affective status	X	X	X			X		
Delusions/hallucinations			X					
Interpersonal behavior	X		X			X		X
Activities of daily living	X			X	X	X		X
Instrumental activities	X			X	X	X		X
Cognition	X					X		X
Motor activity			X					
Appetite changes			X			X		
Health information:								
History of illness		X						

[a] Blessed = Blessed Dementia Scale; Hach = full Hachinski Ischemia Score; ADAS = Alzheimer's Disease Assessment Scale; BCRS = Brief Cognitive Rating Scale; GDS = Global Deterioration Scale; SCAG = Sandoz Clinical Assessment—Geriatric; Iowa = Iowa Test of Abnormal Mental Decline in Older Persons; CDR = Clinical Dementia Rating.

response and proxy response may also be more appropriate for institutionalized populations.

General Comments on Standardized Tests of Cognitive Function

Standardized tests of cognitive function have been widely used in academic and clinical settings. There is substantial precedent for their use in both basic and applied research. They typically offer a well-structured testing procedure that can be replicated by trained examiners. However, the amount of training that is required varies, from modest for simple tests (e.g., mental status screening examinations) to extensive for individual tests of psychometric intelligence and neuropsychological batteries. Similarly, some tests require only that the examiner have a copy of the questions and an answer blank; others require equipment that may be both expensive and cumbersome.

One of the more serious questions about the use of standardized tests relates to the conceptualization of neuropsychological function prevalent at the time the tests were developed. As cognitive neuropsychology has developed, conceptualizations of nervous system function have also evolved. Tests that were developed several decades ago may be updated, but this typically involves obtaining new norms and rewording questions to reflect contemporary language habits (e.g., substituting *cafeteria worker* for *scrub woman* in a memory test). The underlying conceptualization of the tests remains unaltered.

There may be questions about the reliability and validity of some of the standardized tests (Morrison, 1987). If reliability and validity estimates were obtained with relatively small samples of well-functioning elders, they may not generalize to the general population of elderly persons. The criteria against which tests were validated may also be an issue. As was noted, tests of psychometric intelligence may correlate well with educational attainment but not as well with job success (Anastasi,1976). The characteristics of samples used in estimating the sensitivity and specificity of clinical tests may inflate these values. For example, in a recent evaluation of "clock drawing" as a screen for Alzheimer's disease (Wollf-Klein et al, 1989), the normal controls had a mean Mini-Mental State Exam (Folstein et al, 1975) of 27.7 and the Alzheimer's patients had a mean score of 12.8. The obtained sensitivity of 86.7 percent and specificity of 92.7 percent might have been lower had the patient group been less impaired. This issue is especially important in selecting tests for community studies of nascent pathologic changes in cognitive function.

The appropriateness of the norms for some tests may also be questioned (Morrison, 1987). Specific norms for the elderly may not even be available. In some cases, persons over 65 or even 50 years of age are treated as a monolithic group, despite evidence that many changes in cognitive function may not become marked until the 70s (Schaie, 1983; Siegler, 1983). Norms for the elderly may be extrapolated from the norms for younger persons. As noted by Magaziner (Katzman et al, 1983), age and educational attainment may interact, and failure to consider educational differences may result in misclassification. Finally, the increasing overall level of education among the elderly may render some norms outdated. That is, many tests of cognitive function are sensitive to the effects of education. If the elderly normative sample was less educated than the elderly persons being tested, use of the norms may result in an *underestimation* of the prevalence of cognitive dysfunction.

Finally, standardized tests were developed under the assumption that they would be administered in a well-controlled setting. Distractions and interruptions can easily invalidate a test, and the impact of less than ideal circumstances on the reliability and validity of tests is typically unknown. The extent to which testing conditions can be controlled in the field is thus an important consideration in test selection.

Laboratory Tests of Cognitive Function

Cognitive neuropsychologists have proposed a number of putative cognitive functions and processes and developed a variety of laboratory measures for these functions and processes. Weingartner, Grafman, and Newhouse (1987) recently proposed the development of a "psychobiological taxonomy of cognitive impairments" based largely on conceptualizations of cognitive functions that have been explored in the laboratory but are not yet typically included in standardized tests. The following discussion of functions and processes includes those discussed by Weingartner and several additional candidates. Definitions and examples of the functions are provided and laboratory findings of age-associated differences are reviewed.

Pavlovian and Instrumental Conditioning

In Pavlovian (or classical) conditioning (Hulse et al, 1975) presentation of the unconditioned stimulus (e.g., food) is contingent upon presentation of the conditioned stimulus (e.g., a bell), regardless of what the subject does. In instrumental conditioning, presentation of the reinforcer (e.g., food) is contingent on the behavior of the subject (e.g., pressing a lever). Pavlovian conditioning appears to be less efficient in the elderly (Woodruff-Pak and Thompson, 1988).

Controlled and Automatic Processes

Controlled processes (Hasher and Zacks, 1979) are those that are attention demanding and effortful. Automatic processes demand little attention or effort and, once started, tend to be completed. With training and experience, a controlled process may become automatic. It has been argued that automatic processes are not as sensitive to age-related declines as are controlled processes (Hasher and Zacks, 1979; Hess and Slaughter, 1986). Although some studies have failed to find age differences in automatic processes (Attig and Hasher, 1980; Perlmutter et al., 1981), other studies using the same (Kausler et al, 1982; Kausler et al, 1981) or different tests (Kausler and Puckett, 1980; Kausler and Puckett, 1981) have found that younger adults are superior to older adults.

Acquisition, Retention, and Retrieval

Acquisition is the process whereby new material is learned; it is often measured by the number of trials taken to achieve a specified criterion. Retention is measured by performance of a previously learned task at a given interval. Retrieval is the process by which the subject gains access to previously learned material. Rate of acquisition is slower among the elderly (Canestrari, 1968). Some studies have suggested that, after controlling for initial learning, retention is similar in older and younger persons (Hulicka and Weiss, 1965; Rybarczyk et al., 1987), although others have suggested that the elderly do not retain newly learned information as long as do younger persons (Harwood and Naylor, 1969; Hulicka and Rust, 1964; Park et al, 1989).

Because information is rarely learned in isolation, the *context* in which learning takes place may be important (Hunt and Ellis, 1974). Reinstatement of the original context may aid persons in recalling information. The use of contextual information by the elderly seems to be similar to its use by younger persons (Park et al, 1987; Zelinski and Light, 1988).

When the "context" is internal, it is referred to as a state, and the learning that occurs is referred to as state-dependent learning (Seiden and Dysktra, 1977). In the state-dependent learning paradigm, half of the subjects learn a task under, for example, the influence of alcohol, and the other half are given a placebo. During testing, half of the subjects in the alcohol group are tested under the influence of alcohol and the other half are tested with a placebo. Similarly, half of the group that was trained with a placebo are tested under the influence of alcohol and half are tested with a placebo. Groups that are trained and tested under the same conditions (i.e., the alcohol–alcohol and placebo–placebo groups) perform better than the mixed-condition groups.

Recall and Recognition Memory

Recall and recognition memory tests both begin with the subject learning information such as a list of words. The subject must then generate the list of words either without external cues ("free recall") or with hints of some sort ("cued recall"). In recognition memory tests, the subject is given an original list of words embedded in a list of new words and must select those that were previously presented. Recognition memory seems to be more robust than recall memory (Perlmutter, 1979). That is, it is less sensitive to the effects of age and illness.

Sensory, Primary, and Secondary Memory

Sensory memory (Poon, 1985) is the auditory (echoic) or visual (iconic) image that is retained briefly after something is heard or seen. Primary memory is of limited capacity and duration, and secondary memory is of unlimited capacity and duration. There are modest changes in sensory memory with age (Gilmore et al, 1986; Poon, 1984). Primary memory remains largely intact (Fozard, 1980), but there are relatively large age-associated differences in secondary memory (Poon, 1985). In a recent comparison of age-associated changes in primary and secondary memory, the decrements in secondary memory were larger than those in primary memory (Coyne et al, 1986).

Episodic and Semantic Memory and Declarative and Procedural Memory

Episodic memory is memory for personal experiences and semantic memory is memory for public facts (Tulving, 1987; Tulving, 1983). Declarative memory is memory for specific pieces of information, and procedural memory is memory for how things are done. Different types of memory may be differentially affected by neurologic damage (Tulving, 1987; Tulving, 1983). For example, procedural memory may be preserved when declarative memory is impaired.

Elaborate and Superficial Processing

The distinction between elaborate and superficial processing (Craik and Tulving, 1975) refers to how thoroughly information is processed when it is being learned. For example, in learning a list of words, a subject could simply read the words (relatively superficial) or try to make up sentences using the words (relatively elaborate). The elderly seem to be less likely to engage in elaborate processing (Puglisi and Park, 1987; Smith, 1980).

Incidental Learning

When subjects are not told that they will be expected to remember certain information but are later asked to remember it, incidental learning (Montague, 1972) is being assessed. For example, a "routine" health history may be taken prior to the nominal test and subjects may be asked to remember what was included in the health history. Less incidental learning appears to occur among the elderly (Eysenck, 1974; Sinnott, 1986).

Language and Pattern Processing

The distinction between language and pattern processing refers to the processing of verbal and nonverbal information. There seem to be age-associated differences in memory for both verbal and nonverbal information (Poon, 1985; Salthouse, 1982).

Inductive and Deductive Reasoning

Psychological tests of problem solving and concept formation typically require inductive (formulating a general rule from specific examples) and deductive (deriving specific examples from a general rule) reasoning (Salthouse, 1982). Age-associated declines have been reported in both concept formation and problem solving (Cornelius and Capi, 1987; Hess and Slaughter, 1986; Salthouse, 1987).

Abstract and Concrete Thought

Abstract thought is regarded as relatively high level functioning and may be measured by proverb interpretation tests; concrete thought involves the literal interpretation of information (Salthouse, 1982). It has been suggested that age-associated differences in problem solving and concept formation are a result of the relatively abstract nature of the problems. Although some studies have indicated performance decrements even when concrete problems are posed (Harley, 1981), others have indicated that the elderly are superior to younger persons (Cornelius and Capi, 1987).

Metacognition

The ability to think about and evaluate one's own cognitive processes is metacognition (Flavell and Wellman, 1976). It has received considerable attention from developmental psychologists, who argue that it is a relatively advanced cognitive process. A number of metacognition measures exist, including the Metamemory Questionnaire (Zelinski et al, 1980), Cognitive Failures Questionnaire (Broadbent et al, 1982), Everyday Memory Questionnaire (Sunderland et al, 1983), and Memory Questionnaire (Perlmutter, 1978). Metamemory studies have often yielded conflicting results (Perlmutter, 1987; Salthouse, 1982).

Several "laboratory" measures of cognitive function were included in the Iowa 65+ Rural Health Study (Cornoni-Huntley et al, 1986), a population-based (baseline N = 3673) study of community-dwelling persons 65 years of age and older residing in two rural Iowa counties. The RHS is one of the four National Institute on Aging-sponsored Established Populations for Epidemiologic Studies of the Elderly (EPESE). At baseline and the three-year follow-up interview, a 20-word free-recall memory test was administered. In longitudinal analyses (Colsher and Wallace, 1989a), performance on the recall test was related to the occurrence of selected illnesses (including stroke, myocardial infarction, cancer, and diabetes), subsequent two-year survivorship, ability to perform routine activities, and health habits, including alcohol consumption, cigarette smoking, and participation in physically active and mentally stimulating recreation pursuits. Advanced age was also associated with accelerated decline. In cross-sectional analyses (Wallace et al, 1985), diastolic hypertension was associated with significantly poorer recall memory performance after adjustment for age, educational attainment, use of antihypertensive medications, general health status, depressive symptoms, and alcohol consumption.

Measures of metamemory, including self-rated memory (Hulse et al, 1975) and self-reported memory problems (Cornoni-Huntley et al, 1986), were also included in the RHS. In a cross-sectional study of the impact of affect on cognitive function, the metamemory measures were significantly related to the presence of clinical depression but recall memory performance was not (O'Hara et al, 1986).

The recall memory tests, metamemory measures, and a modified version of the Short Portable Mental Status Examination were included in an RHS analysis on the effects of vision and hearing problems on cognitive function (Colsher and Wallace, 1990). After adjustment for age, educational attainment, physical health, and depressive symptoms, the measures of metamemory were significantly related to self-reported hearing impairment, but performance on the recall test and the mental status examination were not. The relationship between vision and metamemory, recall memory performance, and performance on the mental status examination was largely accounted for by age, educational attainment, physical health, and depressive symptoms.

In general, however, laboratory measures of cognitive function have not been used in epidemiologic research. This may be in part due to the lack of standardization or norms as well as the lack of communication between cognitive neuropsychologists and epidemiologists. Often there are several tests of the same function and the experimental literature may report only modest correlations among the alternative measures. Some laboratory tests are heavily instrumented (e.g., some Pavlovian learning paradigms) and may not be practical or appropriate for field use. Like standardized tests, laboratory tests of cognitive function typically require a well-controlled testing environment. However, the adaptation of laboratory techniques that reflect current understanding of cognitive function for use in epidemiologic studies may be especially important to understanding the population distributions of cognitive function.

COHORT SELECTION

One of the major criticisms of many experimental studies of cognitive function is that the participants are not representative of the general population. As was shown in Table 9-1, persons included in these studies are relatively young, well-educated, and healthy. Participants included elderly students recruited from university classes, members of alumni and professional organizations, and residents of affluent private retirement communities.

The representatives of participants in an epidemiologic study will also obviously depend on the characteristics of the parent population. Although much useful epidemiologic information may be obtained from the members of alumni and professional organizations, the cognitive characteristics of the graduates of prestigous universities and health care professionals would reasonably be expected to differ from those of the general population. A geographically defined population, such as residents of a private retirement community, may be similarly unsuitable for making inferences about the elderly population as a whole.

Even when a suitably representative study cohort has been developed, selective nonparticipation may lead to bias. For example, in the previously described Iowa 65+ Rural Health Study, the percentage of persons who refused to attempt the recall test increased with age and decreased with educational attainment (Colsher and Wallace, 1989b). Thus, persons who would be expected to perform more poorly on the test were more likely to refuse to attempt the test. Similarly, longitudinal studies may be biased by the selective attrition of persons who perform relatively poorly on the tests of cognitive function (Cooney et al, 1988).

The selection of an appropriate sample size may be especially challenging in studies of cognitive function. Formulas for the computation of sample size require an estimate of the variability of the test. In many cases, estimates of the variability of a test will not be available at all and pilot investigations will be necessary. In other cases, although these estimates may be available (e.g., from normative data for standardized tests), they may be inappropriate for the study sample and conditions. That is, the variability of a test administered to healthy young people under optimal testing conditions may differ considerably from that which is obtained with chronically ill elderly persons tested in their homes.

POTENTIAL CONFOUNDERS

One of the most commonly encountered covariates of cognitive function, educational attainment, has already been discussed. Different age groups differ in formal education attainment, and many tests of cognitive function are significantly related to educational attainment. A self-report of educational attainment is easy to obtain and may provide important information about cognitive function.

The terminal drop, or accelerated decline in cognitive function observed prior to death (Kleemeier, 1962; Riegel and Riegel, 1972; Rotwinick, 1978; White and Cunningham, 1988) may have a significant impact on estimates of cognitive function among the elderly. By including mortality surveillance, it may be possible to separate the effects of terminal drop from other potential causes of cognitive decline.

Physical health status may be a particularly important determinant of cognitive function in the elderly. Certainly the presence of neurologic conditions may result in cognitive impairment. A number of other illnesses, including hypertension (Elias et al, 1989; Franceschi et al, 1982; Mazzucchi et al, 1986; Wallace et al, 1985; Wilkie et al, 1976), other cardiovascular conditions (Garcia et al, 1984; Lagergren, 1974; Reich et al, 1983), cancer (Folstein et al, 1983; Levin et al, 1978; Siberfarb et al, 1981), diabetes (Bale, 1973; Francheschi et al, 1984; Perlmutter et al, 1984), chronic renal insufficiency (English et al, 1978; Ryan et al, 1981; Ziesat et al, 1980), chronic liver disease (Gilberstadt et al, 1980; Tarter et al, 1984), chronic obstructive pulmonary disease (Grant et al, 1981; McSweeny et al, 1985; Prigatano et al, 1983), and thyroid disorders (Alvarez et al, 1983; Levander and Rosenquist, 1979; MacCrimmons et al, 1979; Whybrow et al, 1969) may be associated with altered cognitive function. Obtaining a self-reported health history may be useful in assessing the impact of illness on cognitive function. Unfortunately, of course, those persons whose cognitive function is the most affected by illness may deny history of a specific illness because they do not understand the question or because they have forgotten that they have that illness.

An assessment of sensory function may also be desirable (Sands and Meredith, 1989). Commonly used tests of cognitive function are not appropriate for use with persons with severe sensory impairments, and special tests have been developed for these populations (Hayes, 1942; Hayes, 1943; Sattler, 1974). It is less clear, however, how mild impairments that do not substantially interfere with everyday function might affect scores on relatively complex, timed tests. Finally, there is some evidence that sensory impairment is associated with accelerated cognitive decline in certain groups such as persons with Alzheimer's disease (Avorn, 1983; Herbst and Humphrey, 1980; Jones et al, 1984; Thomas et al, 1983; Uhlman et al, 1986), although this conclusion has been disputed (Eastwood and Rifat, 1986; Eastwood et al, 1985; Weinstein and Amsel, 1986a, b). A systematic assessment of sensory function will allow an examination of these issues.

Physical flexibility and motor skills also may have an impact on performance (Whitebourne, 1985). Again, special tests have been developed for persons with severe impairments (Allena and Collins, 1955). Even very mild impairments (e.g., mild arthritis affecting the hands that might result in slowed writing and difficulty turning pages), however, may result in inaccurate scores.

Affective status, including depression (National Institute on Aging, 1980; Sydne-Smith and Kiloh, 1981; Niederhe and Yoder, 1989) and anxiety (Yesavage, 1983), may be related to performance on tests of cognitive function. A number of standardized measures of depression exist, including both self-administered questionnaires such as the Geriatric Depression Scale (Brink et al, 1982), Beck Depression Inventory (Beck et al, 1961), Zung Self-Rating Depression Scale (Zung, 1965), and Center for Epidemiologic Studies Depression Scale (Radloff, 1977), and interviewer-administered questionnaires such as the Hamilton Rating Scale (Hamilton, 1967) and the Montgomery and Asberg Depression Scale (Montgomery and Asberg, 1979). Structured interviews, such as the Schedule for Affective Disorders and Schizophrenia (Endicott and Spitzer, 1968), Structured Clinical Interview for DSM III (Spitzer and Williams, 1983), Diagnostic Interview Survey (Robbins et al, 1981), and Longitudinal Interval Follow-up Evaluation (Keller et al, 1987), are more time-consuming and may not be appropriate. Several anxiety scales, including the Spielberger State-Trait Anxiety Scale (Spielberger, 1973), the Taylor Manifest Anxiety Scale (Taylor, 1955), and the Profile of Mood States (McNair et al, 1971) have been reported in the experimental and clinical literature.

Alcohol intake may also be associated with cognitive impairment. Certainly, alcoholism may be associated with severe cognitive impairment (Mishara and Kastenbaum, 1980; Willenbring, 1988), but modest alcohol consumption may also impair function (Loftus, 1980). Because of age-associated changes in alcohol metabolism (Wood, 1985), the elderly may be particularly vulnerable to temporary decrements in cognitive function associated with alcohol intake.

Exposure to chemicals, including organophosphate pesticides and hydrocarbons, has also been associated with a variety of cognitive deficits (Eskenazi and Maizlish, 1988). Because elderly persons may have worked with these substances at a time when their effects were less well understood, their exposure histories may differ from those of younger persons.

In summary, contemporary tests of cognitive function are sensitive to a number of factors in addition to age, including educational attainment, subsequent mortality, physical illnesses, sensory impairments, mobility impairments, depression, anxiety, alcohol intake, and exposure to various chemicals. The elderly may differ from younger persons on a number of these characteristics, and thus their assessment is an important component of epidemiologic investigations of cognitive function.

SUGGESTIONS FOR FURTHER RESEARCH

One of the fundamental issues to be addressed in the epidemiology of cognitive function is the development of suitable tests of cognitive function. Although it is clear that mental status screening examinations can be included in large field studies and that simple memory tests are also feasible, the use of more sophisticated tests may be problematic. For example, with the exception of the Framingham Study, the use of individual psychometric tests of intelligence has been limited to relatively small studies.

Ideally, a test battery for epidemiologic studies of cognitive function should be portable, relatively easy to administer, and of a length that is acceptable to respondents; should have acceptable reliability and validity in a variety of settings, including the home and clinic; should be sensitive to normal and superior levels of cognitive function; should be suitable for repeated administration; and should reflect contemproary conceptualizations of cognitive function. The battery should also be related clearly to the ability to perform both simple and complex everyday activities and clinical evaluations of cognitive function.

Faust and Fogel (1989) recently proposed the High Sensitivity Cognitive Screen for use in epidemiologic and experimental investigations and in routine clinical assessment of cognitive function. It takes 20–30 minutes to administer and consists of 15 subtests, which are summarized in Table 9-9. The initial report on this test battery involved patient groups, but it does appear to have promise for use in epidemiologic studies.

Additional research using already-existing measures of cognitive function is also important. Replication of previous findings with different populations would be of interest, especially when the original studies used relatively privileged respondents. Studies of minority elderly should be undertaken with appropriate tests. The cultural bias of common tests of psychometric intelligence (Anastasi, 1976), for example, might result in inaccurate descriptions of age-associated changes.

Finally, the relationship between existing measures of cognitive function and ability to perform everyday activities should be explored further. For example, Soderback

Table 9-9 Components of the High-Sensitivity Cognitive Screen

Sentence recall, immediate and delayed: Repeat two sentences. Three attempts allowed on immediate recall test; delayed test is given later in the battery.
Paired-associates learning, immediate and delayed: Six pairs of words are read. On testing, the first word in each pair is a recall cue for the second. Three trials are allowed on the immediate test; delayed test is given later in the battery.
Repetition: Repeat a six-word sentence (three attempts allowed).
Word fluency: Produce words beginning with *s* and *t*.
Naming: Identify objects from verbal descriptions.
Reading: Read a 12-word sentence at the eight-grade level.
Writing: Write a 10-word sentence from dictation.
Visual-motor skills: Copy figures from the Bender-Gestalt.
Spatial skills: Shown geometric figures in parts, identify figure.
Alternating numbers: Begin with 10 and alternately add 3 and 6.
Signaling to numbers: Tap table to odd but not even numbers in list of 30 numbers.
Conflicting stimuli: Raise arm rapidly if told to do so softly and slowly if told to do so loudly; 20 repetitions.
Sentence construction: Construct sentences from three sets of three words. each.

related Luria's conceptualization of cognitive function to ability to shop, cook, and clean (Soderbak, 1988). Several authors have reported that impaired performance on mental status screening examinations is associated with impaired ability to perform basic self-care activities (Skurla et al, 1988; Winograd, 1984). It is less clear how very mild cognitive changes might relate to the performance of relatively complex activities, yet for many persons, such mild changes may have an important impact on quality of life. Recently, for example, there has been increasing interest in the relationship between cognitive function and driving skills (Irwin, 1989).

In conclusion, population-based studies of age-associated changes in cognitive function promise to be fairly complex undertakings: There is no simple unitary measure that will be sensitive to the full range of function (Anonymous, 1987), and there are many potential confounders. Such studies are critical, however, to understanding cognitive function throughout the lifespan.

ACKNOWLEDGMENT

This work was supported by National Institute on Aging Grants AG-07094 and AG-06785.

REFERENCES

Allen RM, Collins MG (1955). Suggestions for the adaptive administration of intelligence tests for those with cerebral palsy. Cerebral Palsy Rev 16:11–14.

Alvarez MA, Gomez A, Alavez E, Navarro D (1983). Attention disturbance in Grave's disease. Psychoneuroendocrinology 8:451–454.

Anastasi A (1976). Psychological testing. New York, Macmillan.

Anonymous (1987). Memory testing: No thermometers available. Lancet ii:605–606.

Army Behavior and Systems Research (1970). Armed Forces Qualification Test. Arlington, VA, US Army.

Attig M, Hasher L (1980). The processing of frequency of occurrence of information by adults. J Gerontol 35:66–69.

Avorn J (1983). Biomedical and social determinants of cognitive impairments in the elderly. J Am Geriatr Soc 31:137–143.

Bale RN (1973). Brain damage in diabetes mellitus. Br J Psychiatr 122:337–341.

Beck AT, Ward CH, Mendelsohn M, Mock J, Erbaugh J (1961). An inventory for measuring depression. Arch Gen Psychitr 4:53–63.

Bender LA (1938). A visual-motor Gestalt test and its clinical use. Am Orthopsychiatric Association Research Monogr. No. 3.

Benton AL (1974). Revised visual retention test: Manual. New York, Psychological Corporation.

Berg EA (1948). Simple objective technique for measuring flexibility in thinking. J Gen Psychol 39:15–22.

Binet A, Simon T (1905). Méthodes nouvelle pour le diagnostic du niveau intellectuel des anormaux. Ann Psychol 11:191–244.

Blessed G, Tomlinson BE, Roth M (1968). The association between quantitative measures of dementia and senile changes in the cerebral gray matter of elderly subjects. Br J Psychiatr 114:797–811.

Botwinick J, West R, Storandt M (1978). Predicting death from behavioral performance. J Gerontol 33:755–762.

Brink TL, Yesavage JA, Lum O, Heersema P, Adey M, Rose TL (1982). Screening test for geriatric depression. Clin Gerontol 1:37–43.

Broadbent DE, Cooper PF, Fitzgerald P, Parkes KR (1982). The Cognitive Failures Questionnaire (CFQ) and its correlqtes. Br J Soc Clin Psychol 21:1–16.

Busse EW, Maddox GL (1985). Duke longitudinal studies of normal aging. New York, Springer.

Canestrari RE (1968). Age changes in acquisition. In GA Talland (ed), Human aging and behavior. New York, Academic Press.

Christensen AL (1974). Luria's neuropsychological investigation: Text. Copenhagen, Munksgaard.

Clarke M, Lowry R, Clarke S (1986). Cognitive impairment in the elderly—a community survey. Age and Ageing 15:278–284.

Colsher PL, Wallace RB (1989a). Longitudinal changes in memory function. Findings from a population-based study of community-dwelling elders. Paper presented at the World Congress of Gerontology, Acapulco, Mexico, June.

Colsher PL, Wallace RB (1989b). Data quality and age: Health and psychobehavioral correlates of item nonresponse and inconsistent responses. J Gerontol: Psychol Sci 44:P45–P52.

Colsher PL, Wallace RB (1990). Are hearing and visual dysfunction associated with cognitive impairment: A population-based approach. J Appl Gerontol 9:91–105.

Cooney TM, Schaie KW, Willis SL (1988). The relationship between prior functioning on cognitive and personality dimensions and subject attrition in longitudinal research. J Gerontol: Psychol Sci 43:P12–P17.

Cornelius SW, Capi A (1987). Everyday problem solving in adulthood and old age. Psychol Aging 2:144–153.

Cornoni-Huntley J, Brock D, Ostfeld AM, Taylor JO, Wallace RB (1986). Established Populations for Epidemiologic Studies of the Elderly. Resource data book. (NIH Pub. No. 86-2443). Bethesda, MD, National Institutes of Health.

Coyne AC, Allen PA, Wickens DD (1986). Influence of adult age on primary and secondary memory search. Psychol Aging 1:187–194.

Craik FIM, Tulving E (1975). Depth of processing and the retention of words in episodic memory. J Exp Psychol: Gen 104:268–294.

Cronholm B, Molander L (1957). Memory disturbances after electro-convulsive therapy. Acta Psychiatr Neurol Scand 32:218–234.

Cronholm B, Ottoson J (1963). Reliability and validity of a memory test battery. Acta Psychiatr Scand 39:218–234.

Cunningham WR, Ownes WA (1983). The Iowa State Study of adult development in intellectual abilities. In Scahie KW (ed), Longitudinal studies of adult psychological development. New York, Guilford Press.

Cutler SJ, Grams AE (1988). Correlates of self-reported everyday memory problems. J Gerontol (Soc Sci) 43:582–590.

Eastwood MR, Rifat S (1986). More on the association between hearing and cognitive impairment: Letter to the editor. J Am Geriatr Soc 35:888.

Eastwood MR, Corbin SL, Reed M, Nobbs H, Kedward HB (1985). Acquired hearing loss and psychiatric illness: An estimate of prevalence and co-morbidity in a geriatric setting. Br J Psychiatry 147:552–556.

Elias MF, Schultz NR, Robbins MA, Elias PK (1989). A longitudinal study of neuropsychological performance by hypertensives and normotensives: A third measurement point. J Gerontol: Psychol Sci 44:P25–P28.

Endicott J, Spitzer RL (1968). A diagnostic interview: The Schedule for Affective Disorders and Schizophrenia. Comp Psychiatry 9:138–147.

English A, Savage RD, Britton PG, Ward MK, Kerr DNS (1978). Intellectual impairment in chronic renal failure. Br Med J 1:888–890.

Eskenazi B, Maizlish NA (1988). Effects of occupational exposures to chemicals on neurobehavioral functioning. In Tarter RE, Van Thiel DH, and Edwards KL (eds), Medical Neuropsychology: The impact of Disease on Behavior. New York, Plenum.

Eslinger PJ, Damasio AR, Benton AL, Van Allen M (1985). Neuropsychologic detection of abnormal mental decline in older persons. J Am Med Assoc 253:670–674.

Eysenck MW (1974). Age differences in incidental learning. Dev Psychol 10:936–941.

Farmer ME, White LR, Abbott RD, Kittner SJ, Kaplan E, Wolz MM, Brody JA, Wolf PA (1987). Blood pressure and cognitive performance. The Framingham Study. Am J Epidemiol 126:1103–1114.

Faust D, Fogel BS (1989). The development and initial validation of a sensitive bedside cognitive screening test. J Nerv Ment Dis 177:25–31.

Flavell JH, Wellman HM (1976). Metamemory. In Kail RV, Hagen JW (eds), Memory in Cognitive Development. Hillsdale, NJ, Erlbaum.

Folstein MF, Folstein SE, McHugh PR (1975). "Mini-mental state": A practical method for grading the cognitive state of patients for clinicians. J Psychiatr Res 12:189–198.

Folstein MF, Fetting JH, Lobo A, Niaz U, Capozzili KD (1983). Cognitive assessment of cancer patients. Cancer (Suppl.) 53:2250–2257.

Fozard JL (1982). The time for remembering. In LW Poon, JL Fozard, LS Cermak, D Arenberg, LW Thompson (eds), New Directions in Memory and Aging: Proceedings of the George A. Talland Memorial Conference. Hillsdale, NJ, Erlbaum, 1980.

Franceschi M, Tancredi O, Smirne S, Mercinelli A, Canal N (1982). Cognitive processes in hypertension. Hypertension 4:226–229.

Francheschi M, Cecchetto R, Minicucci F, Smizne S, Baio G, Canal N (1984). Cognitive processes in insulin-dependent diabetics. Diabetes Care 7:228–231.

Garcia CA, Tweedy JR, Blass JP (1984). Underdiagnosis of cognitive impairment in a rehabilitation setting. J Am Geriatr Soc 32:339–342.

Gardner H (1983). Frames of mind. New York, Basic Books.

Gilberstadt SJ, Gilberstadt H, Zieve L, Buegel B, Collier RO, McClain CJ (1980). Psychomotor performance deficits in cirrhotic patients without overt encephalopathy. Arch Intern Med 140:519–521.

Gilmore GC, Allan TM, Royer FL (1986). Iconic memory and aging. J Gerontol 41:183–190.
Golden CJ, Osmon DC, Moses JA, Berg RA (1981). Interpretation of the Halstead–Reitan Neuropsychological Test Battery. New York, Grune & Stratton.
Gollin ES (1960). Developmental studies of visual recognition of incomplete objects. Percept Motor Skills 11:289–298.
Grant I, Heaton RK, McSweeny AJ, Adams KM, Timms RM (1981). Neuropsychological findings in hypoxemic chronic obstructive pulmonary disease. Arch Intern Med 142:1470–1476.
Hachinski VC, Iliff LD, Zilhka E, Du Bolay GH, McAllister VL, Marshall J, Russell RWR, Symon L (1975). Cerebral blood flow in dementia. Arch Neurol 32:632–637.
Hamilton M (1967). Development of a rating scale for primary depressive illness. Br J Soc Clin Psychol 6:278–296.
Hartley AA (1981). Adult age differences in deductive reasoning processes. J Gerontol 36:700–706.
Harwood E, Naylor GFK (1969). Recall and recognition in elderly and young subjects. Aust J Psychol 21:251–257.
Hasher L, Zacks RT (1979). Automatic and effortful processes in memory. J Exp Psychol Gen 108:356–388.
Hayes SP (1942). Alternative scales for mental measurement of the visually handicapped. Outlook for Blind 36:225–230.
Hayes SP (1943). A second test scale for the mental measurement of the visually handicapped. Outlook for Blind 37:37–41.
Herbst KG, Humphrey C (1980). Hearing impairment and mental state in the elderly living at home. Br Med J 281:903–905.
Hertzog C, Schaie KW, Gribbin K (1978). Cardiovascular disease and changes in intellectual functioning from middle to old age. J Gerontol 33:872–883.
Hess TM, Slaughter SJ (1986). Aging effects on prototype abstraction and concept identification. J Gerontol 41:214–221.
Holzer CE, Tischler GL, Leaf PJ, Myers JK (1984). An epidemiologic assessment of cognitive impairment in a community population. Res Commun Mental Health 4:3–32.
Hughes CP, Berg L, Danziger WL, Coben LA, Martin RL (1982). A new clinical scale for the staging of dementia. Br J Psychiatr 140:566–572.
Hulicka IM, Ruse LD (1964). Age-related retention deficit as a function of learning. J Am Geriatr Soc 11:1061–1065.
Hulicka IM, Weiss R (1965). Age differences in retention as a function of learning. J Consult Psychol 29:125–129.
Hulse SH, Deese J, Egeth H (1975). The psychology of learning. New York, McGraw-Hill.
Hunt RR, Ellis HD (1974). Recognition memory and degree of semantic contextual change. J Exp Psychol 103:1153–1159.
Irwin L (1989). Elderly drivers' perceptions of their driving abilities compared to their cognitive skills and driving performance. In ED Taira (ed), Assessing the Driving Ability of the Elderly. New York, Haworth.
Jarvik LF, Bank L (1983). Aging twins: Longitudinal psychometric data. In KW Scahie (ed), Longitudinal Studies of Adult Psychological Development. New York, Guilford Press.
Jones DA, Victor CA, Vetter NJ (1984). Hearing difficulty and its psychological implications for the elderly. J Epidemiol Commun Health 38:75–78.
Kahn RL, Goldfarb AI, Pollack M, Peck A (1960). Brief objective measures for the determination of mental status in the aged. Am J Psychiatr 117:326–328.
Kane RA (1986). Senile dementia and public policy. In MLM Gilhooly, SH Zarit, JE Birren (eds.), The Dementias: Policy and Management. Englewood Cliffs, NJ, Prentice-Hall.
Katzman R, Brown T, Fuld P, Peck A, Schechter R, Schimmel H (1983). Validation of a short

orientation-memory-concentration test of cognitive impairment. Am J Psychiatr 140:734–739.

Kausler DH, Puckett JM (1980). Adult age differences in recognition memory for a non-semantic attribute. Exp Aging Res 6:349–356.

Kausler DH, Puckett JM (1981). Adult age differences in memory for modality attributes. Exp Aging Res 7:117–125.

Kausler DH, Hakami MK, Wright RE. Adult age differences in frequency judgments of categorical representations. J Gerontol 37:365–371.

Kausler DH, Wright RE, Hakami MK (1981). Variation in task complexity and adult age differences in frequency-of-occurrence judgments. Bull Psychonom Soc 18:195–197.

Keller MB, Lavori PW, Friedman B (1987). The Longitudinal Interview Follow-up Evaluation: A comprehensive method for assessing outcome in prospective longitudinal studies. Arch Gcn Psychiatr 44:540–548.

Kennedy WA (1960). The ceiling of the new Stanford-Binet. J Clin Psychol 17:284–286.

Kleemeier RW (1962). Intellectual changes in the senium. Proc Am Stat Assoc 1:181–190.

Lagergren K (1974). Effect of exogeneous changes in heart rate upon mental performance in patients treated with artificial pacemakers for complete heart block. Br Heart J 36:1126–1132.

Levander S, Rosenquist U (1979). Cerebral function in hypothyroid patients. Neuropsychobiology 5:274–281.

Levine PM, Silberfarb PM, Lipowski ZJ (1978). Mental disorders in cancer patients. A study of 100 psychiatric referrals. Cancer 42:1385–1391.

Loftus E (1980). Memory. Reading, MA, Addison-Wesley.

MacCrimmon DJ, Wallace JE, Goldberg WM, Streiner DL (1979). Emotional disturbance and cognitive deficits in hypo-thyroidism. Psychosom Med 41:331–340.

Magaziner J, Bassett SS, Hebel JR (1987). Predicting performance on the Mini-Mental State Examination. Use of age- and education-specific equations. J Am Geriatr Soc 35:996–1000.

Mazzucchi A, Mutti A, Poletti A, Ravanetti C, Novarini A, Parma M (1986). Neuropsychological deficits in arterial hypertension. Acta Neurol Scand 73:619–627.

McCarty SM, Siegler IC, Logue PE (1982). Cross-sectional patterns of Three Wechsler Memory Scale Subtests. J Gerontol 37:169–175.

McNair DM, Lorr M, Droppleman LF (1971). Profile of Mood States: Manual. San Diego: Educational and Industrial Testing Services.

McSweeny AJ, Grant I, Heaton RK, Prigatano GP, Adams KM (1985). Relationship of neuropsychological status to everyday functioning in healthy and chronically ill persons. J Clin Exp Neuropsychol 7:281–291.

Mishara B, Kastenbau R (1980). Alcohol and Old Age. New York, Grune & Stratton.

Montague WE (1972). Elaborative strategies in verbal learning and memory. In GH Bower (ed.), Psychology of Learning and Motivation, Vol. 6. New York, Academic Press.

Montgomery SA, Asberg M (1979). A new depression scale designed to be sensitive to change. Br J Psychiatr 134:382–389.

Morrison HL (1987). Neuropsychiatric assessment of dementia: Inadequacy of test protocols. In R Rosner, HI Schwartz (eds.), Geriatric Psychiatry and the Law. New York, Plenum Press.

National Institute on Aging (1980). Senility reconsidered. JAMA 244:259–263.

Nelson HE (1976). A modified card sorting test sensitive to frontal lobe defects. Cortex 12:313–324.

Niederhe G, Yoder C (1989). Metamemory perceptions in depressions of young and older adults. J Nerv Ment Disorders 177:4–14.

O'Hara MW, Hinrichs JV, Kohout FJ, Wallace RB, Lemke JH (1986). Memory complaint and memory performance in the depressed elderly. Psychol Aging 3:208–214.

Park DC, Puglisi JT, Smith AD (1989). Memory for pictures: Does an age-related decline exist? Psychol Aging 1:11–17.

Park DC, Puglisi JT, Smith AD, Dudley WN (1987). Cue utilization and encoding specificity in picture recognition by older adults. J Gerontol 42:423–425.

Pattie AH, Gilleard GJ (1975). A brief psychogeriatric assessment schedule. Validation against psychiatric diagnosis and discharge from hospital. Br J Psychiatr 127:489–493.

Perlmutter M, Metzger R, Nezworski T, Miller K (1981). Spatial and temporal memory in 20 and 60 year olds. J Gerontol 36:59–65.

Perlmutter LC, Hakami MK, Hodgson-Harrington C, Ginsberg J, Katz J, Singer DE, Nathan DM (1984). Decreased cognitive function in aging non-insulin-dependent diabetic patients. Am J Med 77:1043–1048.

Perlmutter M, Adams C, Berry J, Kaplan M, Person D, Verondik F (1987). Aging and memory. In KW Scahie (ed.), Annual Review of Gerontology and Geriatrics, Vol. 7. New York, Springer.

Perlmutter M (1978). What is memory aging the aging of? Dev Psychol 14:330–345.

Perlmutter M (1979). Age differences in adults' free recall, cued recall, and recognition. J Gerontol 34:533–539.

Perlmutter M (1987). Metamemory. In GL Maddox (ed.), The Encyclopedia of Aging. New York, Springer.

Pfeiffer E (1975). A short portable mental status questionnaire for the assessment of organic brain deficits in elderly patients. J Am Geriatr Soc 23:433–441.

Poon LW (1985). Differences in human memory with aging: Nature, causes, and clinical implications. In JE Birren, KW Schaie (eds.), Handbook of the Psychology of Aging. New York, Van Nostrand Reinhold.

Porteus ST (1959). The Maze Test and Clinical Psychology. Palo Alto, CA, Pacific Books.

Prigatano GP, Parsons OA, Wright E, Levin DC, Hawryluk G (1983). Neuropsychological test performance in mildly hypoxemic patients with chronic obstructive pulmonary disease. J Consult Clin Psychol 51:108–116.

Puglisi JT, Park DC (1987). Perceptual elaboration and memory in older adults. J Gerontol 42:160–162.

Radloff LS (1977). The CES-D Scale: A self-report depression scale for research in the general population. Appl Psychol Meas 1:385–401.

Randt D, Brown E, Osborne D (1980). A memory test for longitudinal measurement of mild to moderate deficits. Clin Neuropsychol 2:184–190.

Raven JC (1943). Progressive Matrices. London, Lewis.

Reich P, Regestein QR, Murawski BJ, DeSilva DA, Lown B (1983). Unrecognized organic mental disorders in survivors of cardiac arrest. Am J Psychiatr 140:1194–1197.

Reisberg B, Schneck MK, Ferris SH, Schwartz GE, deLeon MJ (1983). The Brief Cognitive Rating Scale (BCRS): Findings in primary degenerative dementia (PDD). Psychopharmacol Bull 19:47–51.

Reisberg B, Ferris SH, deLeon MJ, Crook T (1982). The Global Deterioration Scale for assessment of primary degenerative dementia. Am J Psychiatr 139:1136–1139.

Riegel KF, Riegel RM (1972). Development, drop, and death. Dev Psychol 6:309–316.

Robbins LN, Helzer JE, Croughan J (1981). National Institute of Mental Health Diagnostic Interview Survey: Its history, characteristics, and validity. Arch Gen Psychiatr 38:381–389.

Rosen WG, Mohs RC, Davis KL (1984). A new rating scale for Alzheimer's disease. Am J Psychiatr 141:1356–1364.

Ryan JJ, Souheaver GT, DeWolfe AS (1981). Halstead–Reitan test results in chronic hemodialysis. J Nerv Ment Disorders 169:311–314.
Rybarczyk BD, Hart RP, Harkins SW (1987). Age and forgetting rate with pictorial stimuli. Psychol Aging 2:404–406.
Salthouse TA (1982). Adult cognition. An experimental psychology of human aging. New York, Springer-Verlag.
Salthouse TA (1987). The role of representations in age differences in analogical reasoning. Psychol Aging 2:357–362.
Sands LP, Meredith W (1989). Effects of sensory and motor functioning on adult intellectual performance. J Gerontol (Psychol Sci) 44:56–58.
Sattler JM (1974). Assessment of children's intelligence. Philadelphia, Saunders.
Schaie KW (1983). The Seattle Longitudinal Study: A 21-year experience of psychometric intelligence in adulthood. In KW Scahie (ed.), Longitudinal Studies of Adult Psychological Development. New York, Guilford Press.
Schaie KW (1989). The hazards of cognitive aging. Gerontologist 29:484–493.
Schaie KW (1989). Individual differences in rate of cognitive change in adulthood. In VL Bengtson, KW Scahie (eds.), The Course of Later Life. Springer, New York.
Scherr PA, Albertt M, Funkenstein HH, Cook NR, Hennekens CH, Branch LG, White LR, Taylor JO, Evans DA (1988). Correlates of cognitive function in an elderly community population. Am J Epidemiol 128:1084–1101.
Seiden LS, Dykstra LA (1977). Psychopharmacology: A Biochemical and Behavioral Approach. New York, Van Nostrand Reinhold.
Shader RI, Harmatz JS, Salzman C (1974). A new scale for clinical assessment in geriatric populations: Sandoz Clinical Assessment—Geriatric (SCAG). J Am Geriatr Soc 22:107–113.
Siegler IC (1983). Psychological aspects of the Duke Longitudinal Study. In KW Schaie (ed.), Longitudinal Studies of Adult Psychological Development. New York, Guilford Press, 1983.
Siegler IC, Harkins SW, Thompson LW (1983). Stability and change in intellectual performance: An examination of the terminal drop in the later years of life. Paper presented at the meeting of the Gerontological Society, Portland, November, 1974. Reported in IC Siegler, Psychological aspects of the Duke Longitudinal Study. In KW Schaie (ed.), Longitudinal Studies of Adult Psychological Development. New York, Guilford Press, pp. 136–190.
Siegler IC, McCarty SM, Logue PE (1982). Wechsler Memory Scale scores, selective attrition, and distance from death. J Gerontol 37:176–181.
Silberfarb PM, Philibert D, Levine PM (1981). Psychosocial aspects of neoplastic disease: II. Affective and cognitive effects of chemotherapy in cancer patients. Am J Psychiatr 137:597–601.
Sinnott JD (1986). Prospective/intentional and incidental everyday memory: Effects of age and passage of time. Psychol Aging 1:110–116.
Skurla E, Rogers JC, Sunderland T (1988). Direct assessment of activities of daily living in Alzheimer's disease. A controlled study. J Am Geriatr Soc 36:97–103.
Smith AD (1980). Age differences in encoding, storage, and retrieval. In LW Poon, JL Fozard, LS Cermack, D Arenberg, LW Thompson (eds.), New Directions in Memory and Aging: Proceedings from the George A. Talland Memorial Conference. Hillsdale, NJ, Erlbaum.
Soderback I (1988). A housework-based assessment of intellectual functions in patients with acquired brain damage. Scand J Rehabil Med 20:57–69.
Spielberger CD (1973). Preliminary Manual for the State-Trait Anxiety Scale. Palo Alto, CA, Consulting Psychologists Press.

Spitzer RL, Williams JBW (1983). Structured Clinical Interview for DSM-III—Upjohn Version. New York, New York State Psychiatric Institute.

Sunderland A, Harris JE, Baddley AD (1983). Do laboratory tests predict everyday memory? A neuropsychological study. J Learning Verbal Behav 22:341–357.

Sydney-Smith J, Kiloh LG (1981). The investigation of dementia: Results in 200 consecutive admissions. Lancet i:824–827.

Tarter RE, Hegedus AM, Van Thiel DH, Schade RR, Gavaler JS, Starzl TE (1984). Nonalcoholic cirrhosis associated with neuropsychological dysfunction in the absence of overt evidence of hepatic encephalopathy. Gastroenterology 86:1421–1427.

Taylor JA (1955). A personality scale of manifest anxiety. J Abnorm Soc Psychol 48:285–290.

Terman LM, Merrill LA (1973). Stanford-Binet Intelligence Scale: 1972 Norms Edition. Boston, Houghton Mifflin.

Thomas PD, Hunt WC, Garry PJ, Hood RB, Goodwin JM, Goodwin JS (1983). Hearing acuity in a healthy elderly population: Effects on emotional, cognitive, and social status. J Gerontol 38:321–325.

Thurstone TG (1958). Manual for the SRA Primary Mental Abilities 11–17. Chicago, Science Research Associates.

Thurstone LL, Thurstone TG (1949). Examiner Manual for the SRA Primary Mental Abilities Test. Chicago, Science Research Associates.

Tulving E (1983). Elements of Episodic Memory. Oxford, Oxford University Press.

Tulving E (1987). Multiple memory systems and consciousness. Hum Neurobiol 6:67–80.

Uhlman RF, Larson EB, Koepsell TD (1986). Hearing impairment and cognitive decline in senile dementia of the Alzheimer type. J Am Geriatr Soc 34:207–210.

US Bureau of the Census (1989). Statistical Abstract of the United States: 1989. Washington, DC, US Government Printing Office.

Wallace RB, Lemke JH, Morris MC, Goodenberger M, Kohout F, Hinrichs JV (1985). Relationship of free recall memory to hypertension in the elderly. The Iowa 65+ Rural Health Study. J Chronic Dis 38:475–481.

Wechsler D (1945). A standardized memory scale for clinical use. J Psychol 19:87–95.

Wechsler D (1983). Manual for the Wechsler Adult Intelligence Scale. Revised. New York, Psychological Corporation.

Weingartner H, Grafman J, Newhouse P (1987). Toward a psychobiological taxonomy of cognitive impairments. In GG Glenner, RJ Wurtman (eds.), Advancing Frontiers in Alzheimer's Disease Research. Austin, University of Texas Press.

Weinstein BE, Amsel L (1986a). Hearing impairment and cognitive function in Alzheimer's disease: Letter to the editor. J Am Geriatr Soc 35:274–275.

Weinstein B, Amsel L (1986b). Hearing loss and senile dementia in the institutionalized elderly. Clin Gerontol 4:3–15.

Whitbourne SK (1985). The aging body: Physiological Changes and Psychological Consequences. New York, Springer-Verlag.

White N, Cunningham WR (1988). Is terminal drop specific or pervasive? J Gerontol: Psychol Sci 43:P141–P144.

Whybrow PC, Prange AJ, Treadway CR (1969). Mental changes accompanying thyroid gland dysfunction. Arch Gen Psychiatr 20:48–63.

Wilkie F, Eisdorfer C (1971). Intelligence and blood pressure in the aged. Science 172:959–962.

Wilkie FL, Eisdorfer C, Nowlin JB (1976). Memory and blood pressure in the aged. Exp Aging Res 2:3–16.

Willenbring ML (1988). Organic mental disorders associated with heavy drinking and alcohol dependence. Clin Geriatr Med 4:869–887.

Wood WG (1985). Mechanisms underlying age-related differences in response to ethanol. In E

Gottheil, KA Druley, TE Skoloda, HM Waxman (eds.), The Combined Problems of Alcoholism, Drug Addiction, and Aging. Springfield, IL, Charles C Thomas.
Winograd CH (1984). Mental status tests and the capacity for self care. J Am Geriatr Soc 32:49.
Wollf-Klein GP, Silverstone FA, Levy AP, Brod MS, Breuer J (1989). Screening for Alzheimer's disease by clock drawing. J Am Geriatr Soc 37:730–734.
Woodruff-Pak DS, Thompson RF (1988). Classical conditioning of eyeblink response in the delay paradigm in adults aged 18–83 years. Psychol Aging 3:219–229.
Yerkes RM (1921). Psychological examining in the United States Army. Mem Nat Acad Sci 15:1–877.
Yesavage JA (1984). Relaxation and memory training in 39 elderly patients. Am J Psychiatr 141:778–781.
Zelinski EM, Light LL (1988). Young and older adults' use of context in spatial memory. Psychol Aging 3:99–101.
Zelinski EM, Miura SA (1988). Effects of thematic information on script memory in young and old adults. Psychol Aging 3:292–299.
Zelinski EM, Gilewski MJ, Thompson LW (1980). Do laboratory tests relate to self-assessment of memory ability in the young and old? In LW Poon, JL Fozard, LS Cermak, D Arenberg, LW Thomspon (eds.), New Directions in Memory and Aging. Hillsdale, NJ, Erlbaum.
Ziesat HA, Logue PE, McCarty SM (1980). Psychological measurement of memory deficits in dialysis patients. Percept Motor Skills 50:311–318.
Zung WWK (1965). A self-rating depression scale. Arch Gen Psychiatr 12:63–70.

III

IMPORTANT MEASUREMENT THEMES IN THE ELDERLY

10

Assessing Physical Function in Older Populations

JACK M. GURALNIK AND ANDREA Z. LACROIX

As aging research has evolved in recent years, there has been a shift of focus from mortality and longevity to health status and quality of life. An important component of quality of life, from the perspectives of both the older individual and those responsible for his or her care, is functional independence. When disease compromises functioning to the point that older persons cannot fully care for themselves, the burden on the family and medical care system can be substantial.

Figure 10-1 illustrates the magnitude of loss of independence for the total population age 65 and older and for the age groups 65–74, 75–84, and 85 and older. With increasing age, there is a marked rise in the proportion of the population either residing in a nursing home or living at home and needing the help of another person. Among those aged 85 and older, 46 percent of men and 62 percent of women are either in a nursing home or need help at home. In the future, as life expectancy increases and unprecedented numbers of individuals live to the oldest ages, this loss of independence will have an increasing impact (Guralnik et al, 1988). Epidemiologic studies aimed at understanding the distribution, determinants, and consequences of functional loss in the older population are thus critical.

Epidemiologic research has traditionally focused on the study of specific diseases or injuries, rather than measures of functional status. The general epidemiologic approach used for traditional measures of mortality and morbidity are appropriate when employing measures of function, but a number of methodologic issues are unique to the assessment of function in epidemiologic research. This chapter will focus on the domain of physical functioning and disability. It will present a theoretical framework for assessing functioning, the process of selecting appropriate measures of physical function, general issues of functional assessment as well as specific assessment instruments, methodologic issues and challenges, and examples of the use of physical functioning in analytic research.

THE IMPACT OF DISEASE ON FUNCTIONING

A theoretical framework for describing the impact of disease on functioning is valuable for the development and evaluation of measures of function. Despite certain deficien-

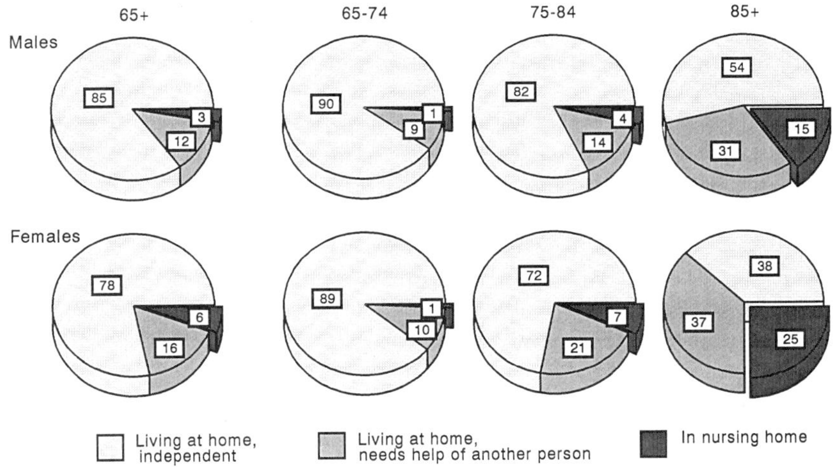

Figure 10-1 Percentage of the population that lives at home independently, at home but with the help of another person, or in a nursing home. *Source:* Schneider EL, Guralnik J (1990). The aging of America: impact on health care costs. JAMA 263:2335–2340.

cies in its practical application, the approach proposed by the World Health Organization, which defines a pathway from disease to impairment, disability, and handicap, has proven quite useful as a conceptual basis for work in this field (World Health Organization, 1980). Figure 10-2 shows this pathway and definitions of each of these classifications. Of importance in understanding this pathway is that, although some individuals follow the pathway through to a handicap, impairment does not necessarily lead to disability and disability does not necessarily lead to handicap. Furthermore, an instrument that assesses one of these domains may not provide information on another. The conceptual framework established by this approach has led to increased awareness of the importance of assessing the functional consequences of disease (Lan-

The World Health Organization Model of Impairment, Disability and Handicap

DISEASE ——> IMPAIRMENT ——> DISABILITY ——> HANDICAP

Impairment

In the context of health experience, an impairment is any loss or abnormality of psychological, physiological, or anatomical structure or function

Disability

In the context of health experience, a disability is any restriction or lack (resulting from an impairment) of ability to perform an activity in the manner or within the range considered normal for a human being

Handicap

In the context of health experience, a handicap is a disadvantage for a given individual, resulting from an impairment or a disability, that limits or prevents the fulfilment of a role that is normal (depending on age, sex, and social and cultural factors) for that individual

Figure 10-2 World Health Organization model of impairment, disability, and handicap. *Source:* World Health Organization (1980). International classification of impairments, disabilities, and handicaps. Geneva: World Health Organization.

cet editorial, 1986). It has been further proposed that this framework should serve as a basis for establishing strategies and goals for prevention in older populations (Fried and Bush, 1988).

Despite the usefulness of the WHO approach in promoting the concepts of impairment, disability, and handicap, there are a number of difficulties in operationalizing this approach. In practice, it is sometimes difficult to define clearly the distinction between the three categories. For example, the inability to grasp an object could be either an impairment or a disability. Defining this difficulty in terms of the specific muscles affected would clearly be a measure of impairment, but epidemiologic studies rarely assess a level of dysfunction that is this detailed. WHO developed a formal classification system based on the concepts of impairment, disability, and handicap (World Health Organization, 1980), which is modeled after the International Classification of Diseases (ICD). The goal of this system was to have patients classified not only according to an ICD code, but also according to an International Classification of Impairment, Disability, and Handicap (ICIDH) code. However, there has been difficulty actually putting this system into practice (Lankhorst, Hoppener, and Evert 1985; Last, 1985; Barrs and Dowell, 1985), and it has generally not received a wide degree of acceptance for this purpose (Lancet editorial, 1986).

SELECTING MEASURES OF FUNCTIONING

A wide range of instruments has been developed for the assessment of physical functioning. The specific use, the setting, and the population to be evaluated should guide the choice of assessment tools. Functional assessment plays an important role both in the clinical management of older patients and in clinical and epidemiologic research. In the clinical setting, measurement of functional status may be used to establish a baseline functional level, screen for problems undetected by the standard clinical examination, aid in diagnosis, set goals for therapy or rehabilitation, and follow a patient's course (Applegate et al, 1990). It is important to distinguish between performing functional assessments for the individual, in the clinical setting, and for a group, in the research setting, such as in an epidemiologic study (Kane and Kane, 1981). The individual assessment, as used in patient care, needs to minimize false positives and false negatives, even at the expense of ease and economy of administration and the need for a high-level professional to perform the assessment. Group measures, in the context of epidemiologic research, are often administered by multiple assessors with lower levels of professional training. These measures should have high levels of interrater reliability, should minimize dependence on professional judgment, and should be able to be administered in reasonable time, with minimal burden on the respondent.

The overall health status of the population to be evaluated should play an important role in the choice of an assessment tool or battery of tools. Many of the most commonly employed physical functioning instruments were originally developed to assess severe decrements in function, such as needing help with eating or dressing. In a nursing home population this is an entirely appropriate target for assessment. In the community-dwelling older population, however, these problems are much less common, even at the oldest ages. Although it is valuable to identify the small minority with these problems, the use of additional instruments is necessary if the older population is to be characterized across the full spectrum of functioning. Recent interest in defining healthy aging has led investigators to propose functional definitions of this state. In a study using the Framingham cohort, good function was defined as needing no help or having no difficulty in a wide variety of tasks ranging from basic activities of daily living through activities such as carrying a weight over 10 pounds and stooping, crouching, or kneeling and standing in one place for a long time (Pinsky, Leaverton, and Stokes, 1987). In a study using the Alameda County cohort, respondents were scored on these same kinds of activities as well as vigorous exercise and recreational activities, with the top quintile of scores being used to define healthy aging (Guralnik and Kaplan, 1989). If the aim of a study is to identify those with severe disability as well as those functioning at a high level, then the use of more than one assessment instrument will clearly be required.

The choice of functional measures also depends on whether they will be used to describe a population or to study the functional consequences of a specific disease or intervention. Descriptive studies of functional status play a valuable role in our understanding of the health problems and needs of the aging population. Measures of physical functioning reflect the impact of one or more diseases as well as a host of environmental infuences, and as such they can be very valuable in summarizing the health status and level of independence of older populations. Measures to describe populations should capture a wide range of dysfunction (e.g., upper-body as well as lower-body problems). In contrast to the broad instruments useful for descriptive studies, research that is analyzing specific risk factors or interventions should focus on functional assessments specific and appropriate to the problem under study. A study of the risk factors for functional decline related to arthritis must use functional measures related to joint disease. An intervention trial aimed at reducing poor functional outcomes that may result from hip fractures should employ measures that assess mobility and lower-body strength, balance, and endurance.

Finally, in selecting an instrument one must consider whether the assessment will evaluate function at one point in time only or will assess change in function. An instrument that may work well to describe the functional status of a population may not be sensitive to the kind of changes important to assess in longitudinal observational studies or intervention trials. A dichotomous measure, such as needing help walking versus not needing help walking, may not perform as well in the evaluation of change over time as an instrument that has several gradations of function. Continuous variables may have real advantage in longitudinal studies. These would include measures that are naturally continuous, such as timing someone walking a specified distance, and aggregate measures, such as those constructed from multiple questionnaire items.

GENERAL APPROACHES TO MEASURING PHYSICAL FUNCTION

The assessment of physical functioning has been employed in research and clinical settings for many years, although in recent years the use of these instruments has become much more common. In 1948 a report was published on self-assessed functioning of cancer patients receiving nitrogen mustard therapy (Karnofsky et al, 1948).

Katz and colleagues introduced a formal instrument for the assessment of activities of daily living in 1963 (Katz et al, 1963). As research efforts in gerontology have increased, so have the number of instruments to assess physical functioning (Kane and Kane, 1981).

In evaluating older persons, it is critical to recognize that physical functioning is just one of the many domains of functioning that are important to consider in evaluating overall health status and the impact of disease. Other domains include cognitive, psychological, and social function, as well as sensory function, including vision and hearing. These domains are very much interrelated, a fact that must be kept in mind when attempting to make measurements in any of these areas. To understand the complex relationships of these domains better, it would be ideal to measure each one separately. But although it is a worthwhile goal to attempt to measure one domain independently of the other domains, it is probably impossible. Any measure of physical functioning will have a cognitive component, and social functioning is strongly related to all the other domains of function. These relationships must be considered when developing and interpreting measures of physical functioning.

The most commonly used method of assessing physical functioning is through self-report. For those too physically or cognitively impaired to report on their functioning, proxies have been successfully employed, although reports from proxies with different roles and different relationships to the subject may vary from each other (Rubinstein et al, 1984). Evaluation of proxy data requires consideration of who the proxy is, the setting in which the subject is being observed, the amount of time actually spent with the subject, and the kind of questions being asked of proxies (Magaziner et al, 1988). This issue is covered in detail in another chapter in this volume. Direct observation of physical functioning may also be used as an approach to assessment. This may take the form of informal, nonstructured observation, such as a staff member reporting on the activities of a nursing home patient, or may be formal measures of physical performance administered according to a standardized protocol.

There are a number of generic, practical considerations in the choice or construction of questionnaire items used to assess functioning through self-report. For a specific clinical setting or research project, decisions about item construction must consider a number of different options:

1. A decision must be made whether to ask respondents (a) if they actually perform a specific task (such as walking half a mile) or (b) if they feel they have the capacity to perform the task. In the former approach, those who are not disabled but who choose not to do an activity may be misclassified as unable to perform the activity, whereas with the latter approach, misclassification will result among those who have not recently performed the activity being queried and who incorrectly assess their capacity to perform this activity.
2. For certain tasks, respondents may be unable to provide a satisfactory answer because they have never (or have not recently) performed the activities for reasons other than health problems. Men, for instance, may be unable to respond to questions on cooking or preparing meals, and individuals who have a housekeeper may be unable to answer questions about the ability to do heavy housework. Even for tasks done frequently in the past, respondents may be unable to provide current information on their ability to perform these activities. For

example, persons living in a house without stairs who do not otherwise encounter stairs may be unable to test their ability to climb stairs and thus may be unable to answer questions about this activity. The coding and analytic uses of these kinds of items should consider this category of response.

3. There may be a great deal of fluctuation in functioning in older populations and a decision must be made about whether to query functioning on the day of the interview or over a specified time interval. Some questionnaires ask respondents about problems in the recent past and then ask about their current state.
4. Two common methods of assessment through self-report are to ask the respondent to assess the degree of difficulty in performing a task (e.g., "a little," "some," "a lot," "can't do the task at all") or to ask the respondent if help is necessary to perform the task. A number of issues are involved in deciding on the approach that is desirable for a particular study. For some items (i.e., ability to write), it is inappropriate to ask about the need for help, and the question should focus on level of difficulty. Querying the need for help is very appropriate in clinical care settings and research on the need for health services, whereas the understanding of level of difficulty may be more appropriate for interventional studies or research in which physical functioning is serving as an indicator of health status. In general, the respondent will be more challenged to answer questions about the level of difficulty, especially when faced with several levels of response options, and this may have an impact on the reliability of using this approach. Some questionnaires combine these two approaches, first asking about level of difficulty and then inquiring about need for help among those with any difficulty.
5. In constructing a questionnaire item that asks about help in performing a task, a decision must be made about asking if help is needed or, specifically, if help is actually being received. For certain types of items, such as activities of daily living, it is also sometimes asked if help is from a person, from a device (e.g., a cane or a bar to aid getting in and out of the shower), or from both.

VALIDITY AND RELIABILITY

In selecting a physical function measure from existing scales, one should also consider what is known about the reliability and validity of the alternative measures. Similarly, the decision to modify an existing scale or to develop a new scale de novo for clinical or research purposes should be accompanied by a clear rationale for such a decision and by a thorough evaluation of the reliability and validity of the new or modified measure. This discussion will be limited to reliability and validity within the context of measuring physical function. Briefly, reliability refers to several properties reflecting the reproducibility of a measure over time, across observers, and across individual items of a multi-item scale. Validity is a property reflecting how well the scale or item measures what it was intended to measure. In longitudinal studies, clinical trials, and clinical settings where monitoring change over time is an important goal, consideration should also be given to the responsiveness of the measure to detecting change (Feinstein, Josephy, and Wells, 1986; Guyatt et al, 1989).

Reliability encompasses three types of psychometric evaluation. Interrater reliability refers to the degree of agreement in scoring a measure by multiple observers. For example, the Katz Scale of Activities of Daily Living was originally designed to be scored by trained observers who could evaluate the performance of persons in a real situation. The scale was found to have excellent agreement (≥95 percent) in scoring across trained observers (Katz et al, 1963). Interrater reliability does not apply to measures that rely on self-report, whether the data are collected by an interviewer or by self-administration. A related type of reproducibility is intrarater reliability, which is the consistency of scoring by a single observer on more than one occasion.

Test–retest reliability refers to the consistency of scores obtained using the same measure administered on more than one occasion over a short period of time. Change in physical function can vary widely in older adults and some will experience wide variation in a short time. The concept of evaluating test–retest reliability might seem at odds with the notion that a measure of physical function should be capable of distinguishing between persons with stable function and those who have meaningful improvement or deterioration. However, a good measure of physical function should be capable of demonstrating test–retest reliability among persons known to have reasonably stable function over the time interval. A measure without adequate test–retest reliability in groups with stable function will be unable to distinguish meaningful from random changes in the whole population.

The third type of reliability is internal consistency, a property reflecting item cohesion in a multi-item scale. The degree of internal consistency is measured by examining the average correlation of individual items in a scale. However, the degree of internal consistency depends both on the interitem correlations and on the total number of items; longer instruments will have greater internal consistency (Nunnally, 1978). The degree of internal consistency is greater as coefficient alpha, the measure of internal consistency, approaches 1.

Assessments of reliability have been lacking as new or modified measures of physical function have proliferated during the last several decades. In a review of 43 published scales measuring activities of daily living, Feinstein and colleagues (1986) reported that only 12 scales were accompanied by evaluations of interrater or intrarater reliability. Test–retest reliability was evaluated in only five of the 43 published reports (Feinstein et al, 1986). Internal consistency is perhaps the most frequently assessed type of reliability, perhaps because its evaluation does not require repeated data collections by the same observers of the same subjects, but simply relies on cross-sectional analysis of items in a scale. Several published reports have demonstrated a high degree of internal consistency in measures of physical function. For example, the Functional Status Questionnaire includes a scale measuring basic activities of daily living with an internal consistency of 0.79 and a scale measuring instrumental activities of daily living with an internal consistency of 0.82 (Jette et al, 1986). The Medical Outcomes Study Short-Form General Health Survey includes a six-item measure of physical function with an internal consistency of 0.86 (Stewart et al, 1988).

Four types of validity assessments can be made in evaluating measures of physical function. Content validity is established by the subjective evaluation of experts that the items included in a scale represent the domain being measured. For example, a measure of mobility would be expected to contain items pertaining to ambulation, stair climbing, and so on. The inclusion of items on continence or eating in a mobility scale might be judged to lack content validity. Criterion validity is established by comparing measurements obtained from a new instrument to measurements obtained from an external "gold standard." For measurement of physical function there are no existing gold standards. For this reason, some have dismissed criterion validity as an impossible goal to attain for any measure of physical function (Spector, 1990). However, it is possible to make comparisons to several external indicators that ought to be closely related to levels of physical function. These external indicators can be physiologic measurements, physical examination findings, or clinical judgments of disability levels. Confidence in the criterion validity of a new measure would be increased to the extent that the measure compared consistently favorably to several external indicators. Construct validity is established by stating a priori hypotheses about the relation of the physical function measure with other measures of health and function, and then providing empirical evidence that the majority of the predicted relationships exist. For example, it might be postulated that a measure of mobility would be associated with other measures of disability such as limitations in activities of daily living, restricted-activity days, and bed-limitation days, with self-reported health status and with the presence of multiple chronic diseases (co-morbidity). The ability to confirm these predictions with data would support the construct validity of the mobility measure. Finally, the predictive validity of the physical function measure can be established by relating the level of physical function to other outcomes of interest such as future risk of institutionalization or death. A brief review of the predictive capabilities of several physical function measures is presented later in this chapter. As with reliability assessments, only a minority of the existing physical function measures have been subjected to rigorous evaluation of their validity. In Feinstein and colleagues' (1986) review of 43 indexes of activities of daily living, only 10 of 43 scales had published any data concerning comparisons between the proposed new measure and existing scales or different versions of the same scale, or between the proposed measure and clinical assessments of function.

It has been well documented that change in physical function is large in older adult populations and occurs in both the direction of improvement in function and deterioration (Branch et al, 1984; Manton, 1988). A variety of possible explanations can account for change in physical function, including the progression of disease, development of new disease, response to treatment or intervention, changes in the environment such as the availability or lack of aids or prosthetic devices, nonstandard conditions of measurement, response to measurement such as learning effects, differences in observers, and statistical artifacts such as regression to the mean (van Belle et al, 1990). The investigator or clinician must distinguish meaningful change in function from that which is due to random variation or noise (van Belle et al, 1990).

The concepts of reliability and validity can also be applied to measurement of change of function, although their application to measures of change is somewhat distinct from single (one-time) measurements of function. The reliability of a change score has been defined as "a measure of how well the individuals in a group can be ranked on the basis of the observed change scores" (van Belle et al, 1990, page 591). Therefore, the reliability of change scores is a property of scales that applies to groups rather than to individuals. Van Belle and colleagues (1990) note that the reliability of change scores is a function of the group's variability in true change, the residual variability or noise about the true change within individuals, and the number and spacing of the observations upon which the change scores are based.

The validity of change scores concerns the degree to which the measured change reflects change in the actual dimension of interest. Responsiveness to change refers to the ability of the scale to detect meaningful differences in function over time, even if the changes are of a small magnitude (Guyatt et al, 1989). Both concepts are critical aspects of the ability of physical function measures to determine which subjects have improved and which have worsened. Deyo and Centor (1986) have proposed the use of receiver operating characteristic (ROC) curves to compare alternative scales used to measure change against various external criteria. This approach provides data for evaluating both the validity of change and responsiveness to change of various physical function measures.

INSTRUMENTS FOR ASSESSING FUNCTIONING

A wide range of instruments has been developed for use in assessing physical functioning in aging populations. The reader is referred to several excellent reference works that list many of these instruments (Branch and Meyers, 1987; Kane and Kane, 1981; Mangen and Peterson, 1984). Because of the large number of instruments and approaches used in the assessment of physical functioning, it is helpful to develop a general classification scheme for these measures. An understanding of the categories of instruments within the domain of physical functioning is helpful in the selection of instruments to be applied in a clinical or research situation. Five general categories of instruments will be discussed (Table 10-1).

The most commonly assessed measures of functioning are self-care activities, usually known as activities of daily living (ADLs). These measures were originally developed to assess older individuals in long-term care or rehabilitation settings, and reflect a substantial degree of disability. They have now been widely utilized in representative community-dwelling populations, and although the prevalence of difficulty or the need for help in these populations is low, these items do serve well in identifying the most severely disabled individuals. For most uses of ADLs there are five basic activities that are always assessed. These include, in order of decreasing prevalence of disability: bathing, dressing, transferring from bed to chair, using the toilet, and eating. The original ADL scale introduced by Katz and colleagues also included continence (Katz et al, 1963). Although continence is an important area of assessment in older populations, it is generally not included in population estimates of ADL impairment, as incontinence has many forms and may be present in persons who are otherwise in very good health. Walking has also been incorporated as an ADL measure (Branch et al, 1984), which may be appropriate as a component of self-care when it queries walking a short distance, such as across a room. The prevalence of disabilities in ADLs has been assessed in several U.S. national surveys (Table 10-2). Overall, these surveys found

Table 10-1 General Categories of Instruments Used to Assess Physical Functioning

1. Self-care: activities of daily living
2. Maintenance of independence in the community: instrumental activities of daily living
3. Other measures of usual functioning
4. Physical activity/exercise/recreation
5. Performance measures of functioning

Table 10-2 Estimates of Disabilities in Activities of Daily Living in Four National Surveys of Persons Aged 65 and Older US Noninstitutionalized Population as Measured by Percent Receiving the Help of Another Person

ADL	1982 National long-term care survey	1984 National long-term care survey	1984 Supplement on aging	1987 National medical expenditure survey
One or more ADLs	7.8	7.8	5.0	8.1
Bathing	6.3	6.3	4.6	6.9
Dressing	4.2	4.0	2.9	4.4
Transferring	4.2	4.0	2.6	3.5
Toileting	3.4	3.3	2.4	2.4
Eating	2.5	2.3	0.7	[a]

Source: Wiener and Hanley (1989).
[a]Cell size too small for reliable estimate.

that between 5.0 percent and 8.1 percent of people age 65 years and older needed help from another person in performing one or more ADLs. Most surveys have found a steeply increasing prevalence of ADL disability with age and a somewhat higher prevalence of disability in women compared with men of the same age group.

The instrumental activities of daily living (IADLs) are activities that are necessary for independent living in the community but are more difficult and complex than the personal self-care domain represented by ADLs. Lawton and Brody (1969) first described a scale with a number of these activities, including shopping, food preparation, housekeeping, doing laundry, using transportation, taking medications, handling finances, and using the telephone. In Figure 10-3, data from the Supplement on Aging to the National Health Interview Survey are used to demonstrate dependence in IADLs (Fulton et al, 1989). The percentage of the U.S. population age 65 and older having difficulty or being unable to perform a specific activity because of a health problem is shown, according to age group and sex, for preparing meals, shopping for personal items, and doing light housework.

The IADLs, by their nature, incorporate more than just the physical domain of functioning and may be difficult to interpret as direct measures of physical functioning and disability. In particular, cognitive functioning plays an important role in the ability to perform these tasks, although it should be noted that cognitive impairment may play a role in ADL disability as well. Motivation, especially as influenced by depression, can have a large influence on the performance of IADL tasks. Opportunities to perform these activities will be important not only in influencing respondents' ability to answer questions about them but also in maintaining the ability to perform them. Persons residing in a nursing home rarely get the opportunity to practice some of the IADLs and may actually lose the ability to perform tasks they were capable of performing before they entered the nursing home (Kane and Kane, 1981). Interpreting IADL responses can also be quite difficult. Reporting difficulty in shopping can mean many things, depending on geographic location, availability of transportation, and type of shopping being done. Nevertheless, the IADLs can serve a valuable role as indicators of need for help to perform tasks that are necessary if the individual is to continue to reside in the community.

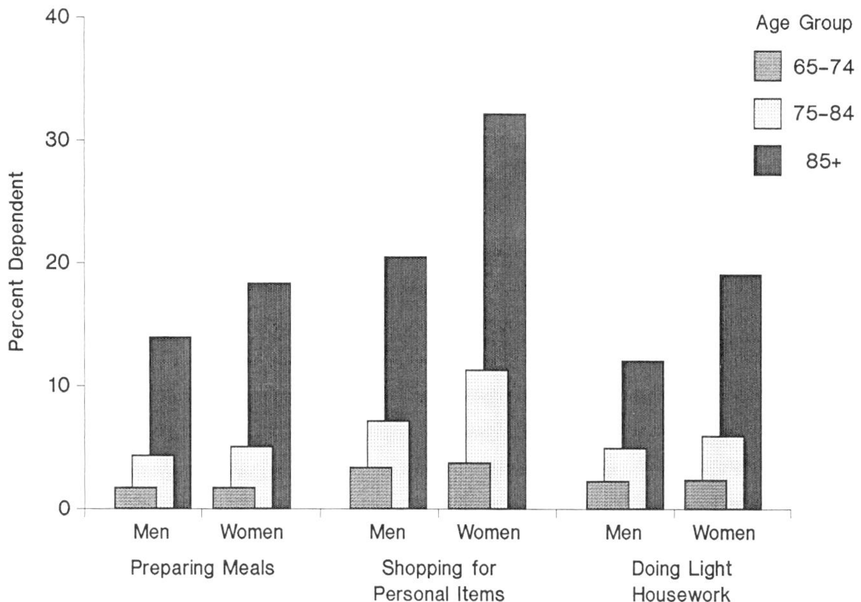

Figure 10-3 Percentage of population dependent in three instrumental activities of daily living (United States, 1984). (Dependence is defined as having difficulty or being unable to perform a specific activity by oneself because of a health problem.) *Source:* Fulton JP, Katz S, Jack SS, Hendershot GE (1989). Physical functioning of the aged (United States, 1984). National Center for Health Statistics. Vital Health Stat, Series 10, No. 167. DHHS Publication No. (PHS) 89-1595, Hyattsville, MD, March 1989.

A number of other activities in addition to ADLS and IADLs have been used to assess physical functioning in older populations. Although this is a miscellaneous class, its items may be characterized as being less complex than the IADLs, or even the ADLs, although they may actually be more vigorous. These are in general questions that assess a particular function of the human body, rather than a task that has multiple components. These functions are in the categories of mobility, range of motion, strength, and endurance.

Examples of these kinds of items are found in the Supplement on Aging, the Framingham Disability Study (Jette and Branch, 1981), and the Established Populations for the Epidemiologic Study of the Elderly (EPESE), sponsored by the National Institute on Aging (Cornoni-Huntley et al, 1986). They all used modifications of scales developed by Rosow and Breslau (1966) and by Nagi (1976). The Rosow-Breslau scale employed in these studies includes two mobility items, walking up and down stairs to the second floor and walking a half mile, and heavy housework. Figure 10-4 shows the percentage of the population unable to perform the mobility items without help for the EPESE populations in East Boston, Massachusetts; New Haven, Connecticut; and two rural counties in Iowa. The Nagi scale contains items assessing a heterogeneous group of tasks, including lifting arms above the shoulders, handling small objects, lifting weights over 10 pounds, moving large objects, and stooping, crouching, or kneel-

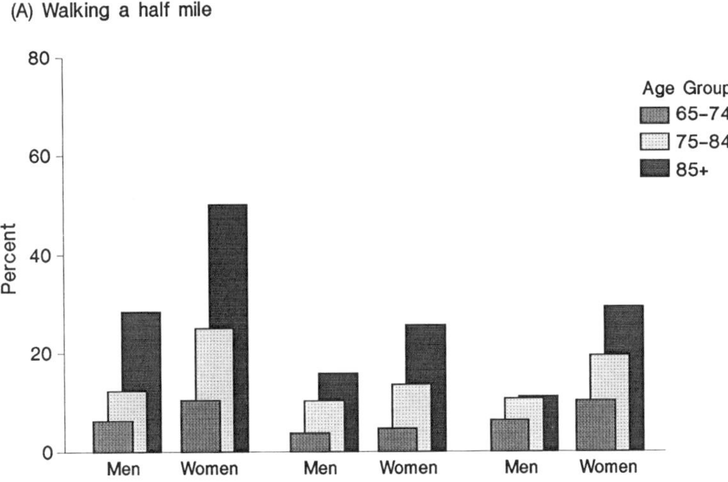

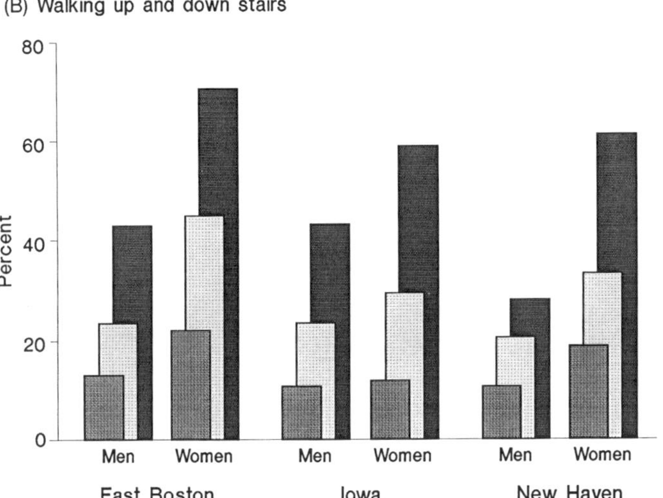

Figure 10-4 Percentage of population needing help or unable to (a) walk a half mile and (b) climb up and down stairs to the second floor. *Source:* Cornoni-Huntley J, Brock DB, Ostfeld A, Taylor JO, Wallace RB, eds. (1986). Established Populations for Epidemiologic Studies of the Elderly, Resource data book. National Institutes of Health, NIH Pub. No. 86-2443, 1986.

ing. Figure 10-5 shows the prevalence of those having difficulty with or unable to perform stooping, crouching, or kneeling and pushing or pulling a large object such as a living room chair. Need for help or difficulty in both the Rosow-Breslau mobility items (see Figure 10-4) and the Nagi items (see Figure 10-5) is more prevalent than it is for ADLs and IADLs.

In addition to ADLs, IADLs, and other measures of usual functioning, physical activity, exercise, and vigorous recreational activities may serve as a measure of phys-

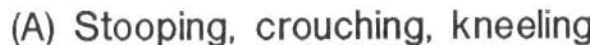

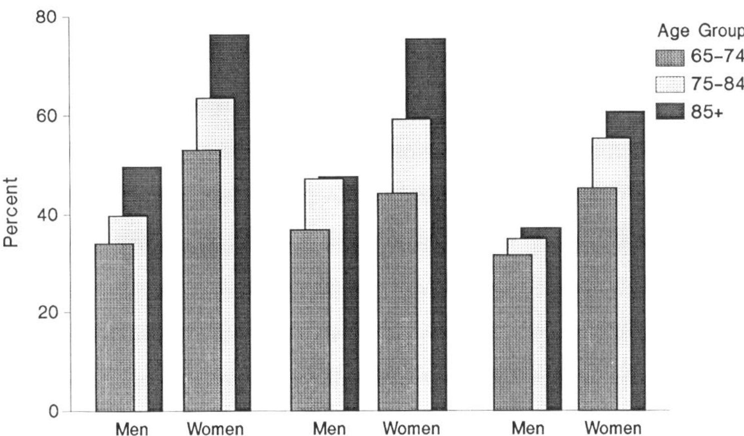

(B) Pulling or pushing large objects

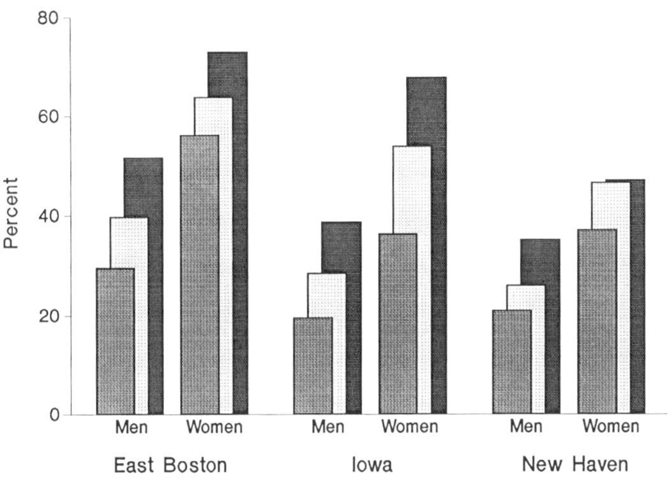

Figure 10-5 Percentage of population having difficulty or unable to perform (a) stooping, crouching, or kneeling and (b) pushing or pulling a large object, such as a living room chair. *Source:* Cornoni-Huntley J, Brock DB, Ostfeld A, Taylor JO, Wallace RB, eds. (1986). Established Populations for Epidemiologic Studies of the Elderly, Resource data book. National Institutes of Health, NIH Pub. No. 86-2443, 1986.

ical functioning in older populations. In community-dwelling populations of older adults, ADLs, IADLs, and other measures of usual function may do little to characterize a substantial portion of the population that is functioning at higher levels (Guralnik, 1987). Assessment of physical activity in this segment of the older population with no serious disability may be of value in placing them along the continuum of the full spectrum of physical functioning. The Iowa site of the EPESE study queried the following activities: gardening or doing yardwork in season; taking walks; jogging, bike riding, swimming, or other vigorous exercise; and hunting, fishing, camping, or boating in season. These kinds of activities may be thought of as discretionary, as they do not have to be performed for the individual to remain independently living in the community. As such, they may not be valid indicators of health status in those who are very healthy but simply choose not to engage in such activities. However, they do indicate high levels of functioning in those who do perform them, and assessment of these kinds of activities can give insight into the effects of physical activity on numerous diseases and conditions of aging (Washburn and Montoye, 1986). A number of existing instruments have been used to assess physical activity in epidemiologic studies (Washburn and Montoye, 1986), although there may be problems with their use in older populations (Washburn et al, 1990).

The final general category of physical functioning instruments listed in Table 10-2 is performance measures of functioning. Although clinical specialties such as physical therapy, neurology, and rheumatology have long relied on the assessment of patient performance, the standardized assessment of physical performance has not been used extensively in clinical research or epidemiologic studies (Guralnik et al, 1989a). A performance measure of physical functioning may be defined as an assessment instrument in which an individual is asked to perform a specific task and is evaluated in an objective, standardized manner using predetermined criteria. For some measures these criteria may define whether the task was successfully completed, whereas for others the assessment may include the counting of repetitions or timing of the activity. This category relates to a technique used to measure functioning rather than the kind of functioning being measured. The general approach is analogous to that used in other domains of functioning in which the function may be assessed both by asking the respondent questions about the level of functioning and by assessing performance in the domain through a standardized examination. For example, cognitive functioning is assessed by asking the respondent or family member about such areas as difficulty with memory and problem solving skills and is also assessed directly by having the respondent demonstrate performance in these areas.

Performance measures can be used to assess a wide range of functioning, including self-care activities (Kuriansky and Gurland, 1976); basic physical maneuvers, such as rising from a chair (Jette and Branch, 1985); gait and balance (Tinetti, 1986); and vigorous exercise, such as rapid walking (McGavin et al, 1978). There has been a minimal amount of methodological work comparing performance measures to self-report measures. There are, however, a number of theoretical advantages, as well as disadvantages, to using objective performance measures (Table 10-3). Further work will be necessary to define the appropriate application of performance measures in geriatric practice and research, but it is likely that both self-report and performance measures will serve complimentary roles in the assessment of physical functioning.

SUMMARY MEASURES OF FUNCTIONING

Epidemiologists have a great deal of experience in analyzing data in which variables represent a single piece of information. Examples of common end points in analytic studies are "dead" versus "alive" and "incident disease" versus "free of disease." Independent variables may be continuous (blood pressure, cholesterol) or categorical

Table 10-3 Theoretical Advantages and Disadvantages of Performance Versus Self-report Measures of Physical Functioning

Advantages:
- Face validity clear for task being performed
- Better reproducibility
- Greater sensitivity to change
- Usual activity versus maximal capacity not an issue
- Influenced less by poor cognitive functioning
- Influenced less by culture, language, and education

Disadvantages:
- More time-consuming
- Adequate space and special equipment needed
- Special training of examiners required
- Modifications necessary for home surveys
- Potential injuries
- Simple tests may not reflect performance on complex tasks or adaptation to environment in daily life

Source: Guralnik et al (1989).

(smoking status). In assessing functional status, however, a single questionnaire item is generally not adequate to capture the range of problems that older people may have with functioning, and it is necessary to combine information relating to a number of activities to gain a comprehensive picture. A simple way of summarizing multiple items that has been used extensively in gerontologic research is exemplified in the way ADLs are often reported. Persons are classified as to needing help in one or more of a list of ADLs versus not needing help with any of the ADLs. This approach is valuable, but more comprehensive scaling is necessary if functional status is to be classified along a continuum instead of simply dichotomized into disabled versus not disabled.

Researchers from the Rand Corporation spent considerable effort in developing aggregate measures of functioning for studies in which they were evaluating the impact on health of several methods of financing health care (Stewart, Ware, and Brook, 1981). They summarized the advantages of aggregating multiple items into a single measure as follows:

1. Using aggregate measures, functional status can be summarized meaningfully using one or a few scores.
2. Reliability of the aggregate measure is higher than that for individual items.
3. For those with some missing data, adjustments can be made to assign them a score on an aggregate measure.
4. In testing hypotheses in analytic studies, an aggregate score results in greater precision.

The development of useful aggregate scales demands a great deal of methodologic work, and many scales of physical functioning have not been fully evaluated (Spector, 1990). There are several necessary steps for both the development and evaluation of scales (Kirshner and Guyatt, 1985). To create a scale, a pool of items must be selected, the number of items must then be reduced so that each item provides nonredundant information, and a scoring system must be applied to the remaining items. The scale must then be evaluated for reliability, validity, and responsiveness, or sensitivity, to change.

The aggregation of multiple items into a single scale or index may be accomplished through a number of techniques, which have generally been developed and refined by those working in the social sciences, where scale construction is common. The two most commonly used types of scales are the summated and the cumulative scales (Selltiz et al, 1976). In the summated scale, also often called an index, individual items are scored and then summed to arrive at an aggregate score. Before adding items, certain summated scales apply weights, obtained through various analytic techniques, to each item. Cumulative scaling, also called Guttman scaling (Guttman, 1944), is appropriate when the items being assessed are hierarchical, such as when they can be ranked in some order related to level of difficulty. The scores that subjects receive place them in an exact location on the scale. When subjects endorse an item with a certain level of difficulty, it can be assumed in a cumulative scale that they would endorse all easier items. This is the main feature that distinguishes cumulative scales from summated scales, in which identical total scores can be obtained through multiple patterns of response.

An example of a modified summated scale of physical functioning is the Health Assessment Questionnaire Disability Index, developed to assess the impact of arthritis on functional status (Fries et al, 1982). The scale includes eight different domains: dressing and grooming, hygiene, arising, eating, walking, conducting IADL-type activities, reaching, and gripping. Each domain includes two or three items, with each item scored as a 0 (no difficulty), 1 (some difficulty), 2 (much difficulty), or 3 (unable to do). The score for the domain is the individual's poorest score in that domain. The scores for the eight domains are summated and then averaged, so the total score ranges from 0 to 3.

An example of a cumulative or Guttman scale of functioning is the scale employed by Pinsky and colleagues to analyze data from the Framingham Disability Study (Pinsky et al, 1985; Pinsky et al, 1987). They found a strong hierarchical pattern for three sets of questionnaire items—the ADLs, Rosow-Breslau items, and Nagi items. In this cumulative scale, 0 indicates no disability in any of the three subscales, 1 indicates disability in Nagi items only, 2 indicates disability in Nagi and Rosow-Breslau items, and 3 indicates disability in all three subscales. In their study only 28 out of 1138 study participants either did not fit this hierarchical pattern for the three subscales or had missing data in all three subscales and were dropped from the analysis. In applying this cumulative scale in another population, it was found that a higher proportion of individuals did not fit the hierarchical pattern, and an alternative scoring system had to be devised to summarize functional level for these participants in order to include them in the analyses (Berkman et al, 1986). Using other data, a hierarchical relationship between ADLs and IADLs has also been found, and a three-level scale has been proposed using these subscales (Spector et al, 1987).

Aggregate scales of functioning have a number of advantages as summary measures, but the burden of proof as to the validity and reliability of these scales is on those who employ them. Some argue that an aggregate scale hides too many details and that items in many aggregate scales represent different domains or constructs and therefore should not be combined (Feinstein et al, 1986). In a study of the association of knee osteoarthritis with physical disability in older persons it was found that the use of an aggregate index of physical functioning led to an underestimate of the impact of arthritis on disability when compared to the impact of arthritis on specific tasks such as stair climbing, walking a mile, and housekeeping (Guccione et al, 1990). Analyzing the large amount of information that may be collected on physical functioning often does necessitate aggregation of variables at some level, but appropriate caution should be exercised in creation of scales and indexes.

THE ASSOCIATION OF DISEASE AND DISABILITY

Much of the work on physical functioning and disability in older populations has been done without consideration of the specific disease causing the disability. This approach is not inappropriate, as there is much to be learned about the distribution and impact of disability itself, but ultimately a comprehensive understanding of disability requires that functional impairment be linked with the underlying diseases that are its cause. For example, efforts at prevention of disability will be focused in most cases on specific diseases that cause disability rather than being generic interventions for disability. Research has been done on the impact on disability of single diseases, such as stroke and arthritis, in patients who have these diseases (Cunningham and Kelsey, 1984; Wade and Hewer, 1987). However, only a limited amount of research has been done that addresses the relative impact of many different diseases in representative populations.

Using data from the Supplement on Aging, Verbrugge found that in cross-sectional analyses cerebrovascular disease and hip fracture had the largest impact on disability, with visual impairment, osteoporosis, and atherosclerosis next in level of importance (Verbrugge et al, 1989). Other diseases, such as arthritis, had less impact on individual disability, but because they were prevalent they had a large impact on the total population burden of disability. Similar results were found in a small cross-sectional study of persons 74–95 years old, in which stroke had by far the largest impact on individual disability among a list of 11 important chronic conditions (Ford et al, 1988). In this study, arthritis and rheumatism accounted for 34 percent of the total burden of disability in the study sample, with stroke, visual impairment, heart trouble, and dementia together accounting for 50 percent of the burden of disability. The Framingham Disability Study prospectively evaluated the impact of stroke on disability and found it to be statistically significant in both men and women, but of much greater magnitude in men (Jette et al, 1988). In both sexes angina pectoris, arthritis, other neurologic conditions, and back problems were also found to be predictive of disability. Congestive heart failure and cancer were predictive of disability in women, and respiratory problems were predictive in men. The preceding studies make important contributions to our understanding of the diseases associated with disability, but much work remains to be done in this area. In particular, the examination of a cohort of older disabled persons to determine the concurrent disease or diseases that are actually causing their disability has not yet been accomplished.

The impact of multiple chronic diseases on disability is also an important area for study in the older population, in whom co-morbidity, or co-existing multiple conditions, is common. A study using data from the Supplement on Aging evaluated the association of disability in ADLs with number of conditions, using a list of nine com-

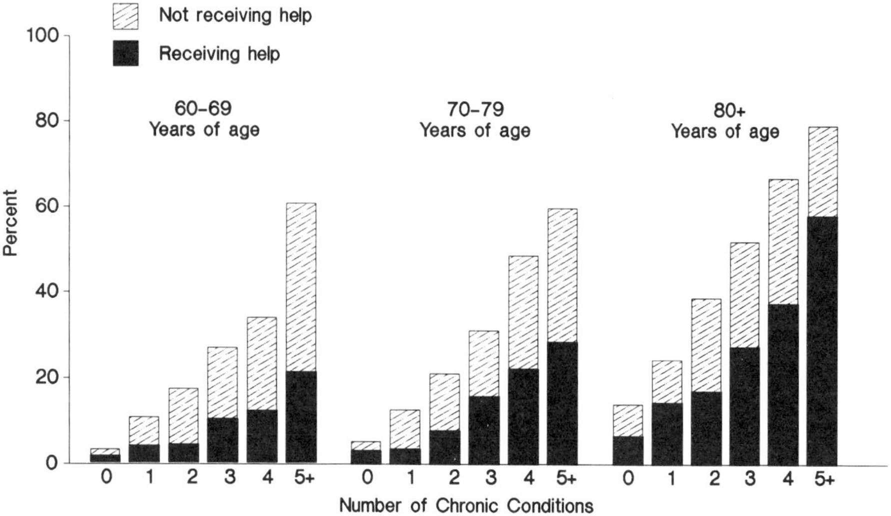

Figure 10-6 Prevalence of women 60 years of age and over having difficulty in one or more activities of daily living by number of chronic conditions and age group. *Source:* Guralnik JM, LaCroix AZ, Everett DF, Kovar MG (1989). Aging in the eighties: the prevalence of co-morbidity and its association with disability. Advance data from vital and health statistics; No. 170. Hyattsville, MD: National Center for Health Statistics.

mon chronic conditions assessed in the study (Guralnik et al, 1989b). In age groups 60–69, 70–79, and 80 and older, there was a stepwise increase in the prevalence of disability with an increasing number of chronic conditions. Figure 10-6 shows these results for women. Results are similar for men. This study simply used the total number of conditions. The next step in understanding the impact of co-morbidity is to evaluate the impact of specific pairs of conditions, with the hypothesis that the pairing of certain conditions will have a synergistic effect on disability compared to what would be expected from the effects of each condition alone (Verbrugge et al, 1989).

FUNCTIONAL STATUS MEASURES IN ANALYTIC EPIDEMIOLOGIC STUDIES

The two broad categories of epidemiologic studies are descriptive epidemiology and analytic epidemiology. Data previously shown in this chapter for prevalence rates of several different measures of disability (Table 10-2, Figures 10-1, 10-3–10-6) are examples of how descriptive epidemiology is applied in aging research. These data provide a picture of the magnitude of disability in various domains and give information on the distribution of disability in the older population according to age group and sex. Analytic epidemiology evaluates determinants of disease, testing specific hypotheses about risk factors for disease and factors related to high and low rates of disease. Although functional status and disability are not specifically diseases, the basic approaches of analytic epidemiology can be applied in research employing measures of physical functioning. Studies have been done in which physical functioning has served both as an independent variable, predicting a number of important outcomes, and as a dependent, or outcome, variable. Several examples of the use of measures of physical functioning in analytic research will be given.

Physical function measures have been found to be strong predictors of a number of important outcomes in older populations. Those with physical disability are at substantially increased risk of death compared to those free of disability. This has been found to be true in community-dwelling older persons (Branch, 1980; Koyano et al, 1986; Warren and Knight, 1982) as well as in institutions, where those disabled are more likely to die than those who are nondisabled (Donaldson et al, 1980). Among those disabled, there is also a strong mortality gradient according to the degree of disability. Two-year follow-up data from the National Long Term Care Survey showed mortality rates rising from 15.2 percent in those with IADL disability only to 20.7 percent in those with disability in one or two ADLs, 24.0 percent in those with three or four ADLs, and 37.2 percent in those with five or six ADLs (Manton, 1988). In addition to mortality, poor physical functioning is predictive of institutionalization (Branch and Jette, 1982; Greenberg and Ginn, 1979) and further declines in functioning (Branch et al, 1984). Studies of factors related to falls have also found physical functioning to be an important independent predictor of this outcome. Performance measures of functioning were found to be highly predictive of falls both within an institution (Tinetti et al, 1986) and in the community (Nevitt et al, 1989; Tinetti et al, 1988).

Because poor physical functioning is a strong predictor of adverse outcomes and because it is also an important marker for older persons' quality of life, there is much to be gained from understanding factors related to the development of poor functional status. Epidemiologic research into this potentially fruitful area has only just begun but is certain to increase in the coming years. Studies that have used functional status as the outcome of interest have taken two general approaches, evaluating factors related to functional level in the overall population and studying factors associated with functioning for those with specific clinical conditions. Using the first approach, investigators have evaluated predictors of poor functioning, such as the development of ADL and IADL disability (Keil et al, 1989; Palmore et al, 1985), and have studied predictors of maintaining high levels of functioning (Guralnik and Kaplan, 1989; Harris et al, 1989; Mor et al, 1989; Pinsky et al, 1987). Examples of the second approach, in which functional outcome is evaluated in relation to specific conditions or interventions, include the use of functional status measures to evaluate the impact of cataract surgery (Elam et al, 1988), recovery from hip fracture (Magaziner et al, 1990), and the value of comprehensive geriatric assessment (Applegate et al, 1990).

CONCLUSION

Measures of physical functioning play an important role in aging research. A large amount of experience has accumulated in this field, and, in general, appropriately chosen measures of physical functioning should now be included as both baseline and outcome variables in population-based epidemiologic studies and clinical trials that involve older populations. Despite the extensive use of measures of physical functioning, a large amount of methodologic and substantive work remains to be done in this field. Areas in which future contributions would be highly beneficial include reliability and validity assessment, scale construction, application of performance measures, the association of specific diseases with impaired functioning, and the assessment of high levels of functioning.

REFERENCES

Applegate WB, Blass JP, Wiliams TF (1990). Instruments for the functional assessment of older patients. N Engl J Med 322:1207–1214.

Applegate WB, Miller ST, Graney MJ, et al (1990). A randomized, controlled trial of a geriatric assessment unit in a community rehabilitation hospital. N Engl J Med 322:1527–2578.

Barrs I, Dowell AM (1985). Trial use of ICIDH, October 1983. Int Rehabil Med 7:67–70.

Berkman LF, Berkman CS, Kasl S, et al (1986). Depressive symptoms in relation to physical health and functioning in the elderly. Am J Epidemiol 124:372–388.

Branch LG (1980). Functional abilities of the elderly: An update on the Massachusetts Health Care Panel Study. In Haynes SG, Feinleib M, eds. Second Conference on the Epidemiology of Aging. Bethesda, MD, U.S. DHHS, NIH Pub. No. 80-969.

Branch LG, Jette AM (1982). A prospective study of long-term care institutionalization among the aged. Am J Public Health 72:1373–1379.

Branch LG, Katz S, Kniepmann K, et al. (1984) A prospective study of functional status among community elders. Am J Public Health 74:266–268.

Branch LG, Meyers AR (1987). Assessing physical function in the elderly. Clin Geriatr Med 3:29–51.

Cornoni-Huntley J, Brock DB, Ostfeld A, Taylor JO, Wallace RB, eds (1986). Established Populations for Epidemiologic Studies of the Elderly, Resource Data Book. National Institutes of Health, NIH Pub. No. 86-2443.

Cunningham LS, Kelsey JL (1984). Epidemiololgy of musculoskeletal impairments and associated disability. Am J Public Health 74:574–579.

Deyo RA, Centor RM (1986). Assessing the responsiveness of functional scales to clinical change: An analogy to diagnostic test performance. J Chronic Dis 39:897–906.

Donaldson LJ, Clayton DG, Clarke M (1980). The elderly in residential care: Mortality in relation to functional capacity. J Epidemiol Comm Health 34:96–101.

Elam JT, Graney MJ, Applegate WB, et al (1988). Functional outcome one year following cataract surgery in elderly persons. J Gerontol Med Sci 43:M122–M126.

Feinstein AR, Josephy BR, Wells CK (1986). Scientific and clinical problems in indexes of functional disability. Ann Intern Med 105:413–420.

Ford AB, Folmar SJ, Salmon RB, et al (1988). Health and function in the old and very old. J Am Geriatr Soc 36:187–197.

Fried LP, Bush TL (1988). Morbidity as a focus of preventive health care in the elderly. Epidemiol Rev 10:48–64.

Fries JF, Spitz PW, Young DY (1982). The dimensions of health outcomes: The health assessment questionnaire, disability and pain scales. J Rheumatol 9:789–793.

Fulton JP, Katz S, Jack SS, et al (1989). Physical functioning of the aged: United States, 1984. National Center for Health Statistics, Vital Health Statistics Ser. 10, No. 167. DHHS Pub. No. (PHS) 89-1595, Hyattsville, MD, March.

Greenberg JN, Ginn A (1979). A multivariate analysis of the predictors of long-term care placement. Home Health Care Serv Quart 1:75–99.

Guccione AA, Felson DT, Anderson JJ (1990). Defining arthritis and measuring functional status in elders: Methodological issues in the study of disease and physical disability. Am J Public Health 80:945–949.

Guralnik JM (1987). Capturing the full range of functioning in older populations. In National Center for Health Statistics, Proceedings of the 1987 Conference on Records and Statistics: Data for an Aging Population. DHHS Pub. No. (PHS) 88-1214. Hyattsville, MD, 236–240.

Guralnik JM, Branch LG, Cummings SR, et al (1989a). Physical performance measures in aging research. J Gerontol Med Sci 44:M141–M146.

Guralnik JM, Kaplan GA (1989). Predictors of healthy aging: Prospective evidence from the Alameda County Study. Am J Public Health 79:703–708.

Guralnik JM, LaCroix AZ, Everett DF, et al (1989b). Aging in the eighties: The prevalence of co-morbidity and its association with disability. Advance data from vital and health statistics, No. 170. Hyattsville, MD, National Center for Health Statistics.

Guralnik JM, Yanagishita M, Schneider EL (1988). Projecting the older population of the United States: Lessons from the past and prospects for the future. Milbank Mem Fund Q 66:283–308.

Guttman L (1944). A basis for scaling qualitative data. Am Soc Rev 9:139–150.

Guyatt GH, Deyo RA, Charlson M, Levine MN, Mitchell A (1989). Responsiveness and validity in health status measurement: A clarification. J Clin Epidemiol 42:403–408.

Harris T, Kovar MG, Suzman R, et al (1989). Longitudinal study of physical ability in the oldest-old. Am J Public Health 79:698–702.

Jette AM, Allyson RD, Cleary PD, et al (1986). The Functional Status Questionnaire: Reliability and validity when used in primary care. J Gen Intern Med 1:143–149.

Jette AM, Branch LG (1981). The Framingham disability study: II. Physical disability among the aging. Am J Public Health 71:211–216.

Jette AM, Branch LG (1985). Impairment and disability in the aged. J Chronic Dis 38:59–65.

Jette AM, Pinsky JL, Branch LG, et al (1988). The Framingham Disability Study: Physical disability among community-dwelling survivors of stroke. J Clin Epidemiol 41:719–726.

Kane RA, Kane RL (1981). Assessing the Elderly: A Practical Guide to Measurement. Lexington, MA, Lexington Books.

Karnofsky DA, Abelmann WH, Craver LF, et al (1948). The use of nitrogen mustards in the palliative treatment of carcinoma. Cancer 1:634–656.

Katz SC, Ford AB, Moskowitz RW, et al (1963). Studies of illness in the aged. The index of ADL: A standardized measure of biological and psychosocial function. JAMA 185:914–919.

Keil JE, Gazes PC, Sutherland SE, et al (1989). Predictors of physical disability in elderly blacks and whites of the Charleston Heart Study. J Clin Epidemiol 42:521–529.

Kirshner B, Guyatt G (1985). A methodological framework for assessing health indices. J Chronic Dis 38:27–36.

Koyano W, Shibata H, Haga H, et al (1986). Prevalence and outcome of low ADL and incontinence among the elderly: Five years follow-up in a Japanese urban community. Arch Gerontol Geriatr 5:197–206.

Kuriansky J, Gurland B (1976). The performance test of activities of daily living. Int J Aging Human Devel 7:343–352.

Lancet (1986). Assessment of disability (editorial). Lancet 1:591–592.

Lankhorst GJ, Hoppener MGWC, Evert van der Kaaij J (1985). Preliminary experiences with WHO's ICIDH; a user's report. Int Rehabil Med 7:70–72.

Last PM (1985). First experiences with ICIDH in Australia's largest nursing home. Int Rehabil Med 7:63–66.

Lawton MP, Brody EM (1969). Assessment of older people: Self-maintaining and instrumental activities of daily living. Gerontologist 9:179–186.

Magaziner J, Simonsick EM, Kasner TM, et al (1988). Patient–proxy response comparability on measures of patient health and functional status. J Clin Epidemiol 41:1065–1074.

Magaziner J, Simonsick EM, Kashner TM, et al (1990). Predictors of functional recovery one year following hospital discharge for hip fracture: a prospective study. J Gerontol Med Sci 45:M101–M107.

Mangen DJ, Peterson WA (eds) (1982; 1984). Research Instruments in Social Gerontology. Minneapolis, University of Minnesota, 3 vols.

Manton KG (1988). A longitudinal study of functional change and mortality in the United States. J Gerontol (Soc Sci) 43:S153–S161.

McGavin CR, Artvinli M, Naoe H, et al (1978). Dyspnea, disability, and distance walked: Comparison of estimates of exercise performance in respiratory disease. Br Med J 2:241–243.

Mor V, Murphy J, Masterson-Allen S, Wiley C, et al (1989). Risk of functional decline among well elders. J Clin Epidemiol 42:895–904.

Nagi SZ (1976). An epidemiology of disability among adults in the United States. Milbank Mem Fund Quart 6:493–508.

Nevitt MC, Cummings SR, Kidd S, et al (1989). Risk factors for recurrent nonsyncopal falls: A prospective study. J Am Med Assoc 261:2663–2668.

Nunnally JC (1978). Psychometric Theory. New York, McGraw-Hill.

Palmore EB, Nowlin JB, Wang HS (1985). Predictors of function among the old-old: A 10 year follow-up. J Gerontol 40:244–250.

Pinsky JL, Branch LG, Jette AM, et al (1985). Framingham Disability Study: Relationship of disability to cardiovascular risk factors among persons free of diagnosed cardiovascular disease. Am J Epidemiol 122:644–656.

Pinsky JL, Leaverton PE, Stokes J III (1987). Predictors of good function: The Framingham Study. J Chronic Dis 40:159S–167S.

Rosow I, Breslau N (1966). A Guttman health scale for the aged. J Gerontol 21:556–559.

Rubinstein LZ, Schairer C, Wieland GD, et al (1984). Systematic biases in functional status assessment of elderly adults: Effects of different data sources. J Gerontol 39:686–691.

Selltiz C, Wrightsman LS, Cook SW (1976). Research methods in Social Relations. New York, Holt, Rinehart and Winston.

Spector WD (1990). Functional disability scales. In Spiker B (ed), Quality of Life Assessments in Clinical Trials. New York, Raven Press, pp. 115–129.

Spector WD, Katz S, Murphy JB, et al (1987). The hierarchical relationship between activities of daily living and instrumental activities of daily living. J Chronic Dis 40:481–489.

Stewart AL, Hays RD, Ware JE (1988). The MOS Short-form General Health Survey: Reliability and validity in a patient population. Med Care 26:724–732.

Stewart AL, Ware JE Jr, Brook RH (1981). Advances in the measurement of functional status: construction of aggregate indexes. Med Care 19:473–488.

Tinetti ME (1986). Performance-oriented assessment of mobility problems in elderly patients. J Am Geriatr Soc 34:119–126.

Tinetti ME, Speechley M, Ginter SF (1988). Risk factors for falls among elderly persons living in the community. N Engl J Med 319:1701–1707.

Tinetti ME, Williams, TF, Mayewski R (1986). Fall risk index for elderly patients based on number of chronic disabilities. Am J Med 80:429–434.

van Belle G, Uhlmann RF, Hughes JP, Larson EB (1990). Reliability of estimates of changes in mental status test performance in senile dementia of the Alzheimer type. J Clin Epidemiol 43:589–595.

Verbrugge LM, Lepkowski JM, Imanaka Y (1989). Comorbidity and its impact on disability. Milbank Mem Fund Quart 67:450–484.

Wade DT, Hewer RL (1987). Functional abilities after stroke: measurement, natural history and prognosis. J Neurol Neurosurg Psych 50:177–182.

Warren MD, Knight R (1982). Mortality in relation to the functional capacities of people with disabilities living at home. J Epidemiol Comm Health 36:220–223.

Washburn RA, Jette AM, Janney CA (1990). Using age-neutral physical activity questionnaires in research with the elderly. J Aging Health 2:341–356.

Washburn RA, Montoye HJ (1986). The assessment of physical activity by questionnaire. Am J Epidemiol 123:563–576.

Weiner JM, Hanley RJ (1989). Measuring the activities of daily living among the elderly: A guide to national surveys. The International Forum on Aging-Related Statistics and the Brookings Institution, 1989.

World Health Organization (1980). International Classification of Impairments, Disabilities, and Handicaps. Geneva, World Health Organization.

11
Epidemiologic Methods for the Study of Health Service Use by Older People

LAURENCE G. BRANCH

The epidemiologic methods outlined in previous chapters are powerful tools for quantifying the distributions and determinants of death, disease, and disability among defined populations. Let us now consider expansions of the traditional methods of clinical epidemiology, to explaining the distribution and determinants of other outcomes important in the public's health.

EXPANDING THE OUTCOMES

Disease and its consequences are not the only concerns of those attempting to organize, deliver, and finance health services to populations in need. The same methods used to study the distribution and determinants of specific diseases and the consequences of these diseases can be applied to the distribution and determinants of the *use* of individual personal health care services, such as acute hospitals, institutional long-term care facilities, community long-term care services, physician services, other ambulatory care services, ambulatory surgeries, and a host of other types of health care utilization. Epidemiologic methods have also been used in attempts to quantify a *population's needs* in certain areas, as well as to understand the configurations of manpower and services required to *supply the health services* necessary to meet those population needs.

The Major Complexity in Expanding the Outcome

Traditional clinical epidemiology has a major advantage that the expansion of epidemiologic methods to health services research does not share. This advantage should be appreciated. The traditional outcome of clinical epidemiologic research, whether it be mortality or morbidity (in the conservative definition of a disease, not a consequence of disease such as disability), is a clear dichotomy that is either present or absent. In addition to the characteristic of having a clear dichotomy, the presence of the outcome is immutable and therefore unidirectional in nearly all circumstances. That is, once a person dies, the person remains dead. As another example, once a person is diagnosed as having coronary heart disease or a myocardial infarction, the individual would always be classified as having CHD or having had an MI. Again, there is no need to consider mutable transitions or bidirectional change.

Categorizing health service use does not share this characteristic of dichotomous classification from absent to present, nor the characteristic of immutability (i.e., once present, always present). Consider the example of hospitalization. Because an individual can be hospitalized for a variety of reasons and could be hospitalized multiple times for a single reason, the application of an epidemiologic model to understanding hospital utilization often uses a "multichotomous," or continuous, dependent variable. A dichotomous dependent variable is simply too crude (although some investigators have correctly used the dichotomous variable of never having used hospital care versus having used hospital care one or more times during the period of study).

In addition to multichotomous, or continuous, dependent variables in health services research, some health services research incorporates *mutable* multichotomous dependent variables. These mutable outcomes present more complex challenges to the analytic design. Let us consider the example of active life expectancy as operationally defined by Katz and his colleagues (1983). In this example, the outcome is dichotomous [i.e., active life (operationally defined as living in the community *and* being independent in specific activities of daily living) versus dependence (operationally defined as living in the community *and* being dependent in one or more activities of daily living, *or* living in a nursing home, *or* expiring)]. With this dichotomous dependent variable, classifications are mutable. That is, an individual could have been independent in ADLs at one point in time, dependent in ADLs at a second point in time, and returned to independence in ADL at a third point in time. Therefore, the transitional probabilities are both mutable and bidirectional. The traditional life table approach of calculating probabilities assumes a dichotomous outcome that is *both* immutable and unidirectional. Mutability of the outcome violates the assumption, and different analytical models are necessary.

Multistate increment–decrement models adapted from methodologies developed by statisticians in the Bureau of Labor Statistics to calculate work life estimates have been adapted and applied to the calculation of active life expectancy among older people (Branch et al, 1991; Rogers et al, 1989). The Bureau of Labor Statistics statisticians faced an analogous situation in which individuals enter and exit the labor force multiple times throughout their lives. Adaptation of these techniques in a life table logic is complex but has become an important methodological expansion of traditional clinical epidemiologic methods that enables health service researchers to understand the quantitative relationships among more complex variables.

A Minor Complexity in Expanding the Outcome

The application of epidemiologic methods to health services research very often involves a reliance on self-reported information for some critical variables. Although it is possible to go to administrative records to document the use of specific services, the use of services is often estimated by self-reported responses to questionnaires. The reliability and validity of self-reported information is an important topic in its own right. Some traditional epidemiologists assume that administrative records represent a gold standard against which the accuracy of self-reported information should be judged. However, extensive methodologic research over three decades has indicated that the gold standard does not exist in the context of health service utilization. Administrative records are not completely accurate in all circumstances and reflect trends in billing procedures and quality assurance mechanisms over time. That is, when administrative records are used for billing purposes, it becomes more likely that errors of undetected additional services might occur, rather than errors of omission in which delivered services are omitted from the administrative record. This makes intuitive sense. If you are a provider who submitted changes for a delivered service, you would notice and correct an error of omission if no reimbursement or a reduced reimbursement was sent. However, if an increased or an extra reimbursement was sent, a provider might be less diligent in correcting that error. Therefore, in these circumstances an error in the administrative record is more likely to be detected when it is an omission rather than an extraneous addition. This differential in the possibility of more overcounts in the administrative record than undercounts leads to an overestimate of utilization. Consider another example when the administrative record is not used for billing purposes but is used for quality assurance purposes. In these circumstances it is more likely that an error in the administrative record would be detected when it is an erroneous addition rather than an omission; hence, an underestimate is more likely. Again, if you are a provider who has been requested to render a QA review based on an erroneous addition in the administrative record, you will take steps to correct the record. However, comparable diligence would not be expected in correcting erroneous omissions. So the incentives for correcting errors are uneven.

Similarly, methodologic research has demonstrated that self-reported information is not completely accurate either. There are problems of memory and problems of telescoping (i.e., a respondent knowing the event occurred but assuming it occurred more recently than it did) among well-intended respondents, as well as the obvious problems of inaccuracy among those who intentionally might want to deceive for some reason.

In summary, the source of data for health services research can be problematic. Administrative records that were established for one purpose do not necessarily reflect the gold standard for another purpose. Self-reported information has its own set of concerns for reliability and validity.

The National Center for Health Services Research (the forerunner of the current Agency for Health Care Policy and Research) and the National Center for Health Statistics have sponsored a series of conferences during the last 15 years on health services research methods (NCHSR, 1977; NCHSR, 1979; NCHSR, 1989). These publications provide important discussions of these and related topics. Survey research is a professional discipline in its own right. The epidemiologist or health service researcher is well advised to incorporate survey research expertise on the research team.

The Importance of Defined Populations

The value of real estate has often been described as a function of three factors—location, location, and location. Similarly, the value of epidemiologic methods can be expressed by three key characteristics—defined populations, defined populations, and defined populations. The defined population becomes the denominator in the calculation of rates, be they prevalence rates, incidence rates, or odds ratios (simply two rates considered simultaneously). An exclusive focus on the number of people who have the characteristic of interest (e.g., those who have a specific disease, those who use institutional long-term care, those who receive hospice services, those in adult day treatment programs) is simply incomplete. Knowing who has what disease or who receives what service is just the first part of the scientific inquiry (and obviously an important part, particularly if you are the person with the disease or the individual with responsibility for care or intervention). But the ability to compare and contrast these with the larger defined population is the basis of the power and utility of epidemiologic methods.

The literature has some examples of investigations whose utility could have been enhanced considerably if the defined population of interest had been kept firmly in mind. For example, the National Center for Health Statistics does periodic surveys of institutionalized long-term care patients. These periodic National Nursing Home Surveys have great utility. The members of the defined population for the cross-sectional survey are the current nursing home residents on the given day the sample is selected. This means the defined population is *not* the people who enter long-term care (that would be an admission cohort of nursing home residents) and the defined population is *not* the people at risk of receiving long-term care (that would require longitudinal data from a population not currently receiving long-term care). Trying to clarify certain features of an admission cohort or identifying risk factors for long-term care are worthwhile scientific efforts, but the initial defined population must exist and be appropriate for the epidemiologic analysis.

The ability to define a population is necessary but not sufficient for the scientific base. The defined population should *not* be a self-selected group whose basis of selection might have any influence on the outcome variable of interest. For example, an investigator would not select a population of HMO enrollees to study the utilization of preventive health care services. The competing hypothesis that those who self-select into an HMO might simultaneously have a value that predisposes them to preventive health care use simply is too compelling to logically discard. Hence, the ability to define a population is necessary, but an *appropriately* defined population is sufficient.

Epidemiologic Designs and Health Services Outcomes

With the development of more sophisticated multiple regression techniques, it is increasingly rare to encounter a purely descriptive epidemiologic study, either in clinical epidemiology or in epidemiologic methods applied to health services utilization. The multivariate models make it very easy to undertake an analytic study with appropriate comparison groups. The comparison groups may be defined by the presence or absence of a specific variable or the degree to which a characteristic presumed to be related to the outcome is present in the sample. Conceptually, many of the independent variables in a regression analysis may be considered as exposures.

Most epidemiologic health services research studies can be classified into one of two major types: observational–nonintervention studies or experimental–intervention studies.

Observational Studies

Concerning observational–nonintervention studies, both cross-sectional and longitudinal designs are common. The literature prior to 1980 was dominated by the nonintervention cross-sectional design, or the one-time survey approach if you will. A variety of methodological issues demand attention, even with the one-time cross-sectional survey. Limitations to the generalizability of a survey have multiple sources: sampling errors, sample nonresponse, interviewer errors, coding errors, data entry and data processing errors, as well as analyst errors. (See Fowler, *Survey Research Methods,* 1984, or Andersen et al, *Total Survey Error,* 1979, for more comprehensive treatments of the issues influencing the limits of generalizability of survey research data to the population of interest.)

The major problem with cross-sectional designs, even those from a defined population and employing multivariate regression techniques, is that neither causation nor a temporal sequence can be established. An example from the long-term care literature will serve to illustrate. In 1979, the National Center for Health Statistics published data from the 1977 Survey of Nursing Home Residents and compared characteristics of nursing home residents with characteristics of people age 65 and over living in the community, as reported in the National Health Interview Survey. Among other characteristics that distinguished nursing home residents from the comparison group was that the nursing home residents had a greater percentage of women. In part as a consequence of this study and as a consequence of other studies with additional methodological limitations, the long-term care conventional wisdom assumed for many years that women were at increased risk of nursing home placement compared to males. There are two problems with this interpretation that require clarification. The first stems from a limitation of cross-sectional studies—namely, they cannot identify risk factors because the temporal sequence is confounded. Cross-sectional studies may identify correlates, but the concept of a risk factor implies that the presence of a factor renders the individual at increased risk for a specific *subsequent* outcome, other things being equal. Longitudinal studies can identify risk factors; cross-sectional studies can identify correlates.

The second problem with that interpretation is that multivariate models are necessary to implement the caveat of "other things being equal." Obviously, it is essential to clarify which factor among several correlates is most predominantly associated wih the outcome of interest. In much of the long-term care research before 1980, multivariate statistical controls were not employed. When age is not controlled, it appears as if women are at greater risk for long-term care. However, the correlations between age and sex at the end of the lifespan are quite high, because women's life expectancy is greater than that of men. Appropriate controlled multivariate analyses subsequently demonstrated that advancing age was the predominant risk factor for nursing home placement controlling for other factors, not being female.

The observational longitudinal design comes in two varieties and has many advantages. The first is the prospective longitudinal design, and the second is the retrospective longitudinal design. Examples of each are forthcoming, but the reader is forewarned that there are a group of analyses that engender quite heated dialogue over their classification as either retrospective or prospective. Let us consider the simpler cases first, however. A team of investigators wishes to clarify the risk factors for the use of a variety of health services (e.g., hospitalization days, physican visits, dental visits, home care, ambulatory care, and institutional long-term care). They enroll a defined population (e.g., a statewide probability sample of all people aged 65 and over living in the communities) and prospectively monitor subsequent utilization. The potential risk factors are measured prior to outcome ascertainment. The analytic objectives are defined at the beginning, and the data are collected subsequently. This is an example of a prospective longitudinal observational (nonintervention) study.

Another team of investigators wishes to clarify the role of posthospital physical therapy on rehospitalization rates among women aged 75 or older who have had a hip replacement. They have access to the hospital records of all hospitalized patients during the prior three full calendar years from all hospitals in a defined geographic area. From these records, they can select all cases who meet their inclusion criteria (i.e., female, aged 75 or older, and hospitalized for a hip replacement) during the first two calendar years of the record, thereby allowing at least 12 months for the outcome of rehospitalization to occur. The records indicate whether and how much physical therapy was provided following first discharge (the critical independent variable). This is an example of a retrospective longitudinal study. The investigators have access to administrative data that have already been collected for an entirely different purpose, but they are amenable to the clarification of their hypothesis.

Consider a third example. After the first team of investigators has completed its prospective longitudinal study of the risk factors of various health service utilizations, a new investigator requests using the data for another analysis. For the new investigator, is this a prospective longitudinal design or a retrospective longitudinal design? There are differences of opinions here.

Analytic Models in Observational Longitudinal Designs. The observational design usually does not have a major independent variable that is the lynch pin for hypothesis testing that occurs in the RCT (the randomized clinical trial, a specific form of the prospective intervention study). Consequently, the investigators must be careful not to succumb inadvertently (or advertently, for that matter; but that is a different topic) to a form of "data-dredging" or a "fishing expedition." These phrases refer to procedures that take advantage of the Type I error—namely, that for every 20 statistical tests conducted using the traditional 0.05 level of confidence, one will erroneously indicate statistical significance where none exists. If one has a whole computer full of data and begins simply looking for statistical associations, 100 tests should produce five "significant" associations that really are not.

To counteract this potential problem, analytic paradigms are useful. Andersen and Aday have proposed a behavioral model of health services utilization (Andersen et al, 1979) that has guided many quantitative studies of health care use. Their model conceptualizes utilization behavior as a consequence of characteristics of the health delivery system and of characteristics of the population at risk. The population at risk, in turn, is characterized as having predisposing, enabling, and need characteristics. Predisposing variables are mutable or immutable characteristics that exist prior to the onset of illness. Mutable variables are those that health policy or related efforts (e.g., health care attitudes) can alter; immutable variables are unchangeable, or at least they cannot be changed by the health policy system (e.g., level of formal education). The enabling component describes the "means" individuals have available to them for use of services. This component includes resources specific to the individual (e.g., insurance coverage) and attributes of the community in which the individual lives (e.g., rural–urban). The need component refers to illness level, which is the most immediate cause of utilization. Need for care can be either that perceived by the individual (e.g., symptoms) or as evaluated by members of the delivery system (e.g., physican assessment of the severity of conditions reported).

Although the model has been used extensively, some have noted that its utility for clarifying health services use has been limited, at least from the perspective of the amount of variance in utilization explained. However, it is worth noting that most analysts have not employed a test of the full model; instead, they have used the model for organizing a subset of variables that their particular study can bring to bear on the topic.

Intervention Studies

Intervention studies, by definition, usually have prospective designs. (A "naturally occurring experiment" might come along about once a decade.) The RCT, when properly executed, is the design that enables an investigator to address the causation of the observed effect. [From one technical perspective, a statistical association demonstrated by a correlational test (such as a regression analysis) should be refered to as "an affect of x on y," whereas a statistical association demonstrated in the context of an RCT can appropriately be referred to as "an effect of x on y."] In the simplest of RCTs, the unit of analysis is the individual, and randomization occurs at the level of the individual as well. The ability of the investigator to assign participants randomly to conditions is the sine qua non of the experimental design referred to as the RCT (Campbell and Stanley, 1963).

The Veterans Administration is trying to adapt the logic of RCTs for randomized health services interventions as well. Just as new clinical interventions are subjected to testing by means of the experimental design of an RCT to determine their effectiveness in a causal model, so also, the VA reasons, can the effectiveness of different organization, delivery, and financing systems be subjected to randomized intervention trials. Of course the element of randomization and the unit of analysis in the traditional RCT is the individual, whereas the element of randomization for a randomized health services trial needs to be a delivery system. For example, the VA is considering a randomized health services trial in which some VA medical centers would be randomly assigned to receive a new configuration of hospital-based home care that would include an experimental care coordination and cost capitation component, and other VA medical centers would continue to participate with traditional hospital-based home care programs. Obviously, randomized trials of health services configurations create additional challenges for calculation of design effects and appropriate sample sizes. Nevertheless, the logic of the RCTs can be applied to randomized trials of health services interventions as well.

Case Example: The Massachusetts Health Care Panel Study.[1] The Massachusetts Health Care Panel Study (MHCPS) is an example of a prospective longitudinal study

[1]This description of the MHCPS was taken from Branch LG, Applications of epidemiological research in aging to planning and policy: The Massachusetts Health Care Panel Study. In: Brody JA, Maddox GL (eds), *Epidemiology and Aging: An International Perspective,* Springer Publishing Co., New York, 1988, pp. 177–188.

of a defined population that has provided data to clarify predictors of subsequent health service utilization and to estimate the needs of the defined population for long-term care.

Before discussing these epidemiologic applications, however, it is helpful to describe the methodology of the original panel study.

The Participants. The MHCPS began in 1974–1975 with a statewide survey of noninstitutionalized people aged 65 years and older living in the communities of Massachusetts. The original sample was identified by a stratified statewide area probability sample of housing units. After stratifying by the eight health planning regions of Massachusetts and by three levels of density (central city, other urban, other place), a systematic selection process was applied. Approximately 400 enumeration districts were to be identified, based on probability proportionate to the 1970 census count of the number of people aged 65 or over in each enumeration district. In fact, 403 enumeration districts were systematically selected, each with the likelihood of containing approximately six to seven older people.

From these 403 enumeration districts, 8,614 addresses were generated by listers who identified every possible housing unit within the boundaries of the enumeration district by a series of site visits. Of these, 803 were vacant and 127 were not dwelling units, leaving 7,684 occupied housing units to screen for eligible respondents, that is, those aged 65 or over at the time of initial household contact. Interviewers were then sent to these occupied housing units to screen each household for the age, sex, and relationship of every member of the household. This screening information was provided by any responsible adult in the household.

All noninstitutionalized people aged 65 years or older at the time of the household screening were eligible for participation in this panel study. Predicated on the assumption that older people occupied the relatively few housing units for which no contact was ever made at the same rate at which older people occupied the housing units for which contact was made, 79 percent of all of the age-eligible people participated in the initial wave of this project.

The screening and interviewing took place from November 1974 through February 1975, and the process is referred to as the 1975 baseline interview (or Year 0 or Wave I interview). There were 1,625 community respondents in this first wave. By definition, there were no nursing home respondents or decedents at this baseline interview.

The panel has been interviewed three more times after the baseline interview. Table 11-1 presents a summary of the field dates, number and age of respondents, and participation rates for the four waves of interviews. Over three-quarters (76 percent) of those who responded to the baseline interview either continued to participate in the panel study by giving interviews in 1985 or continued to participate until their death.

The Questionnaire. A structured questionnaire whose administration time averaged from 45 to 60 minutes was administered by trained lay interviewers at each wave of the panel study. The core questionnaire secured the following information: sociodemographic characteristics, self-reported health status, physical health status (including walker or wheelchair use as indicators of limitation in moving about one's environment), emotional health status, health services utilization (including acute hospital

Table 11-1 Summary of Field Results for the Massachusetts Health Care Panel Study

	Wave I (year 0, 1975, baseline)	Wave II (year 1.25, 1976)	Wave III (year 6, 1980)	Wave IV (year 10, 1985)
Field dates	11/74–2/75	2/76–5/76	10/80–12/80	1/85–3/85
Community respondents	1625	1317	825	541
Nursing home respondents	INAP	27	61	62
Decedents	INAP	102	316	270
Lost to follow-up	INAP	179	142[a]	44
Participation rate	79%	89%	89%	95%
Age	65+	66+	71+	75+

[a]Of these, 28 became reeligible at wave IV; 22 had died, three were in nursing homes, and three were interviewed.

use, nursing home use, physician contact, dental contact, and other special services), social service knowledge and use, social activities, income and expenditure information, areas of needs assessment (transportation, personal care, housekeeping, social opportunities, emergency assistance, grocery shopping, and food preparation), and housing arrangements. An adapted Functional Health Scale (Rosow & Breslau, 1966) and a modified Activities of Daily Living Scale (Katz et al., 1970) were also administered.

In addition to these core items, each questionnaire contained some supplemental information that was not reassessed at each interview. The baseline questionnaire, for example, contained additional items on housing and neighborhood satisfaction. The Year 1.25 questionnaire contained supplemental information on dietary habits, cigarette and alcohol consumption, and additional items on morale. The Year 6 questionnaire contained extensive information on potential informal support networks available to the respondents; further information on self-reported physical abilities in other domains; and an innovation in functional assessment for the personal interview mode that required performance testing of the respondents for certain range of motion (upper extremity and lower extremity) activities, adapted from Keitel (Eberl et al., 1976). The Year 10 questionnaire contained additional information on medical history, cognitive function, financial assets, and out-of-pocket expenditures.

As is often the case with population sample surveys, limited time for interviewing precluded the common psychometric strategy of using multiple items or multiple approaches to measure the same concept. The multiple-measure approach undeniably facilitates the ascertainment of reliability and validity. The MHCPS questionnaires, however, have tried to incorporate the best single items to assess single concepts.

Assessing Population Needs. In 1974, the Massachusetts Commissioner of Public Health was considering the realities associated with the possible large-scale deinstitutionalization of many middle-aged and older adults from state mental health facilities and nursing homes. To support an eventual state policy of deinstitutionalization, the Commissioner of Public Health requested three simultaneous studies. The first was a survey of the level-of-care needs of people currently in mental institutions and nursing homes in order to determine how many of the current residents could in fact be deinstitutionalized if support services were available in the communities. The second study was an analysis of the costs required to provide a comparable service, such as a meal or assistance in dressing, from various settings (e.g., institutional settings, community settings, or home-based settings). Third, a needs assessment survey among the non-institutionalized elders was commissioned to determine what percentage of those currently in the communities would likely be placed in institutions if beds became available, as well as what percentage of the noninstitutionalized elderly would need community and home-based support services if such services were made available to support the deinstitutionalized population.

The MHCPS began as the third commissioned study, a statewide needs assessment required for the initial step of estimating the size and characteristics of the community-living elders with presumptive risk of needing long-term-care support (either institutional or home-based). Bear in mind two things about this 1974 needs assessment. First, it was an initial step in establishing a statewide network of home care services as an alternative for those with long-term-care needs. Therefore, individuals who requested information about services could only be referred to the local council on aging; the complementary purpose of case finding for an existing service system did not exist. Second, the needs assessment was planned prior to the 1975 passage of Title XX of the Social Security Act, which provided federal support for planning and partial federal support for implementing state social support programs. In predating Title XX, the initial needs assessment could not build upon a consensus among professionals concerning such elementary issues as what domains are important in a needs assessment.

Needs Assessment. The estimate of the size of the population with presumptive risk of need for specific home-based support services was necessary in order to plan the configuration of services to be provided and to allocate sufficient funds to meet the needs. A task force of approximately 25 clinicians working in various state agencies was convened to develop consensus on the areas for needs assessment and on the information necessary to place individuals into one of four of the following categories:

Need met—No apparent problem
Need met—Apparent problem
Uncertain—Apparent problem
Need unmet—Current problem

The areas for needs assessment agreed upon in 1974 were:

Transportation
Grocery shopping
Food preparation
Housekeeping
Personal care
Social activities

In each of these needs assessment domains, the clinicians agreed they would require both objective information and subjective evaluations from individuals in order to categorize them. By objective information they meant finding out specifically who does the task in the household, the frequency with which it is accomplished, and so forth. For subjective information, the clinicians agreed they needed estimates of the individual's satisfaction with the frequency with which a task is completed and, if dissatisfied, reasons for dissatisfaction. For each domain, approximately seven to ten elements of information were agreed upon by the task force of clinicians as necessary to classify an individual into one of the four categories. Furthermore, they agreed that only a subset of the information was necessary to identify an individual in the most independent category of "Need met—No apparent problem." These were the individuals who reported they accomplished the specific activities themselves, as frequently as they desired, and in the way they wished.

The distinction between the first two groups (both with needs met, but a difference between no apparent problem and an apparent problem) revolved around the issue of who in fact was accomplishing the task at present; and, if it was not the respondent, how easily it would be for the respondent either to do the task him- or herself or to find someone else to do it if the original person were unavailable. In the parlance of the day, the role and stability of the informal support network were taken into consideration in making this distinction.

After pretesting the original needs assessment items, administering a revised version to all the respondents of the first wave, and conducting a validation substudy during the first wave in which a second set of clinicians interviewed a subsample of the respondents, we implemented the final revision of the needs assessment items on the second wave of interviews. A copy of the final revisions of the scoring procedures for each of the needs assessment areas is available from the author. The final scoring procedures were converted to a computer algorithm.

With the second wave of the MHCPS, clinicians and policy makers alike agreed that accurate estimates of presumptive risk for long-term care support were available. By that time, the Massachusetts Department of Elder Affairs had responsibility for implementing a statewide network of Home Care Corporations.

For the purposes of implementation, the Commonwealth was divided into 27 planning and service areas. The first two Home Care Corporations had been established in 1973. By July 1977, each of the 27 areas was covered by its own Home Care Corporation. During 1976 and 1977, state officials asked Department of Elder Affairs' planners to project the maximum size of the home care network based on the expected number of clients. During 1977 and 1978, the Home Care Corporations were maturing into coordinated service agencies.

During 1975 and 1976, the first two waves of the statewide needs assessments were analyzed and reanalyzed to produce an estimate of the total size and characteristics of the noninstitutionalized population with presumptive risk of needing long-term care support. A summary index of presumptive risk was developed, identifying the size of the target group at approximately 5–7 percent of the noninstitutionalized population aged 65 and older in Massachusetts (Branch, 1980).

During the period from 1975 to 1980, the funding for the Massachusetts network of Home Care Corporations changed from near total reliance on Title XX funding to total reliance of state funds. The level of services authorized by case managers steadily increased until it reached approximately 5.5–6.0 percent of the noninstitutionalized population aged 65 or over. (In 1982 and 1983, there were approximately 40,000 clients in the home care network, representing approximately 5.5 percent of the 727,000 people aged 65 or over enumerated in the 1980 federal census.)

Predictors of the Use of Health Services. The MHCPS was one of the first prospective longitudinal studies to identify true risk factors for nursing home placement (Branch and Jette, 1982). Kane and Kane (1987) subsequently reviewed much of the published literature on antecedents or risk factors for institutional placement, and summarized their findings in Figure 11-1. Notice that of the nine studies that examined gender as a risk factor for institutional placement, only two observed any statistical association. The risk factors for institutional placement are advancing age, race (being white), living alone, lack of social supports, certain diagnostic conditions (including incontinence and dementia), physical disabilities (e.g., problems with activities of daily living, problems with instrumental activities of daily living, using ambulatory aids, or being confined to a bed), cognitive disabilities, and increased contact as outpatient or inpatient.

The importance of the risk factors identified for institutional placement by traditional epidemiological methods in health services research is not overwhelming. The percent of variance explained by most of the studies is less than 20 percent. This means of course that 80 percent of the factors leading to institutional placement are not identified. Two reasons seem to explain this phenomenon. First, many of the prospective studies do not include an appropriate list of medical conditions for inclusion in the predictive models. There are many reasons for this omission, including difficulty in obtaining reliable and valid self-reported information of medical diagnoses and substantial logistic difficulties in obtaining office-based information on diagnoses and conditions. The second is that the interval between ascertainment of the risk factor at

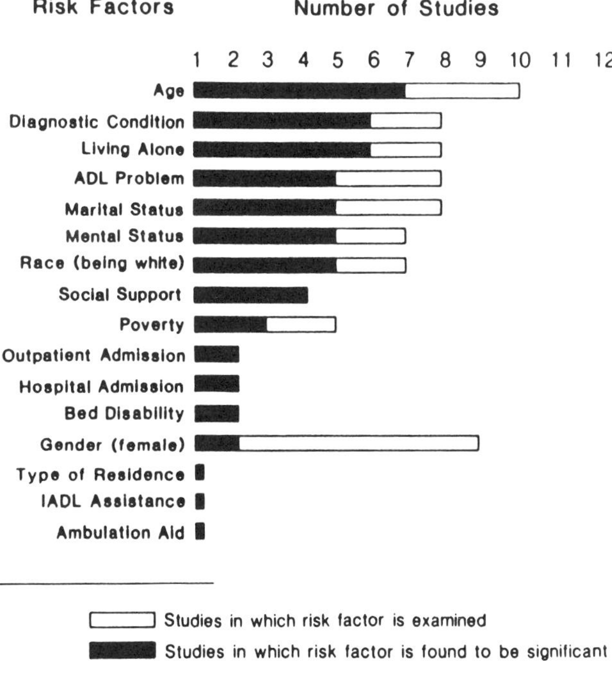

Figure 11-1 Commonality of risk factors for entering a nursing home among 12 studies. (*Source:* Kane and Kane, 1987).

baseline and the outcome might be excessively long. There is some anecdotal evidence to suggest that the decision to seek long-term care through an institution is made quite rapidly and as a result of a changing set of precipitating stimuli. To the extent that the outcome is triggered by these fast-acting and proximate events, traditional methodologies for risk factor ascertainment of chronic conditions will be insufficient.

The MHCPS was also used to identify risk factors associated with the utilization of other health services (Branch et al., 1981; Evashwick et al., 1984). The risk factors identified at baseline were able to explain 27 percent of the variance in physician visits during the subsequent 15 months, 23 percent of the use of home care, 15 percent of the number of days hospitalized and the number of dental visits, but only five percent of ambulatory care (Branch et al., 1981). In general, predisposing characteristics explained less than two percent of the variance in all services except dental services (where it explained 10 percent of the variance). Enabling characteristics explained over 10 percent of the variance for both physician visits and dental visits, but less than five percent for the other types of health service use. Need characteristics as measured in this kind of epidemiologic prospective study accounted for the major portion of the variance in hospital days, physician visits, and home care, but relatively little in ambulatory care and dental visits. Indicators of specific oral health service needs were not addressed in the baseline instrument, so it is not surprising that the study failed to identify need characteristics.

Conclusion. Epidemiologic methods can be applied to understanding many health issues beyond the determinants and distribution of diseases and mortality. The methods can be applied to many public health outcomes, including the ascertainment of population needs and risk factors for health service use. However, the expansion of the epidemiologic methods to those other applications will necessitate additional methodological advances, including statistical methods for dealing with multichotomous or continuous dependent variables, and outcomes that are mutable.

REFERENCES

Andersen R, Kasper J, Frankel MR, and associates (1979). Total Survey Error. San Francisco, Jossey-Bass.

Branch LG (1980). Vulnerable elders. Gerontological Society Monographs, No. 6, pp. 1–48.

Branch LG, Guralnik JM, Foley DJ, Kohout FJ, Wetle TT, Ostfeld A, Katz S (1991). Active life expectancy for 10,000 Caucasian men and women in three communities. J Ger: Med Sci. 46(4):M145–150.

Branch LG, Jette AM, Evashwick CJ, Polansky M, Rowe G, Diehr P (1981). Toward understanding elders' health service utilization. J Community Health 7(2):80–92.

Branch LG, Jette AM (1982). A prospective study of long-term care institutionalization among the aged. Am J Public Health 72(12):1373–1379.

Campbell DT, Stanley JC (1966). Experimental and Quasi-Experimental Designs for Research. Chicago, Rand McNally.

Eberl DR, Rahlfs FV, Schleyer RI, Wolf R (1976). Repeatability and objectivity of various measurements in rheumatoid arthritis: A comparative study. Arthritis Rheum 19(6):1278–1286.

Evashwick C, Rowe G, Diehr P, Branch LG (1984). Factors explaining the use of health care services by the elderly. Health Serv Res 19(3):357–382.

Fowler FJ (1984). Survey Research Methods. Beverly Hills, CA, Sage Publications.

Kane RA, Kane RL (1987). Long-Term Care: Principles, Programs and Policies. New York, Springer, p. 31.

Katz S, Branch LG, Branson MH, Papsidero JA, Beck JC, Greer DS (1983). Active life expectancy. New Engl J Med 309(20):1218–1224.

Katz S, Downs T, Cash H, Grotz R (1970). Progress in development of the index of ADL. Gerontologist 10:20–30.

National Center for Health Services Research (1975). Advances in Health Survey Research Methods: Proceedings of a National Invitational Conference. DHEW Publication No. (HRA) 77–3154.

National Center for Health Services Research (1977). Health Survey Research Methods, Second Biennial Conference. DHEW Publication No. (PHS) 79–3207.

National Center for Health Services Research (1989). Health Survey Research Methods (Floyd J. Fowler, Jr. Editor). DHHS Publication No. (PHS) 89–3447.

Rogers RG, Rogers A, Belanger A (1989). Active life among the elderly in the United States: Multistate life-table estimates and population projections. Milbank Mem Fund Q 67(3–4):370–411.

Rosow I, Breslau N (1966). A Guttman scale for the aged. J Gerontol 21:556–559.

12

Social Networks and Social Support Among the Elderly: Assessment Issues

LISA F. BERKMAN, THOMAS E. OXMAN,
AND TERESA E. SEEMAN

Social networks and the support they can provide may be important to the elderly for a number of reasons. In this chapter we review basic concepts of social network structure, support and subjective assessments of adequacy of support or strain, how they are associated with one another in a population-based elderly cohort, and available instruments to measure these constructs. We conclude with a brief discussion of future directions for research in this area. The reader is referred to several other recent reviews for an in-depth discussion of the relationships between health status and social networks and support (Berkman, 1988; Broadhead et al, 1983 Cohen and Syme, 1985; House et al, 1988;).

The idea that social relationships influence health and well-being is not new. For at least 100 years scientists have noted that isolation, bereavement, and lack of social integration are related to increased mortality risk. Most studies to date, contrary to what one might think, have *not* shown that older people are more vulnerable to the losses that may occur in their social network. Older people in many studies have very similar mortality risks associated with social isolation when compared to middle-aged cohorts, although their *risk of exposure* (i.e., risk of experiencing such isolation) may be greater. In reviewing evidence on these issues, we shall pay particular attention to two questions that permeate the literature. The first question asks "Are specific aspects of network structure or support conceptually or empirically interchangeable or distinct?" The second question asks, "If they are distinct, do they have specific impacts on health and functioning?"

CONCEPTS AND THEORIES OF SOCIAL NETWORK AND SUPPORT: THE MULTIDIMENSIONAL NATURE OF SOCIAL RELATIONSHIPS

To understand the specific role that networks and support play in influencing health and functioning and to plan effective interventions it is important to outline the multidimensional nature of social relationships. Three major dimensions of social relationships are (1) their structure (e.g., size and composition of the social network), (2) their content (e.g., the availability, type, amount, and source of social support provided by members of the network), and (3) the subjectively perceived adequacy of support provided, or, conversely, the amount of conflict and strain produced by members of the individual's network. As Cohen (1988) has noted, it is likely that aspects of network structure and the support or conflict produced by network members will have specific disease influences. Their impact will depend on characteristics of the individual's disease status, the specific pathophysiologic or behavioral pathways linking a specific characteristic of the network or support to a clinically relevant disease outcome, and the length of time or stability of exposure. For instance, the sudden loss of emotional support due to the death of a close friend may have a critical impact on the health of a very vulnerable and frail older person and a much weaker impact on a healthy and vigorous older person. Alternatively, an adult who lives a life of 10, 20, or 30 years of social isolation may develop diseases that in themselves take a long time to develop (e.g., atherosclerosis). In this latter instance, it is unlikely that a relatively short-term exposure could substantially contribute to a long-term disease process. For instance, Cohen and Matthews (1987) have reported that satisfaction with support or perceived availability would not be likely predictors of atherosclerosis because they tend to be relatively unstable or variable over time. Finally, as a third example of the potential specificity of network effects on outcomes, the type of support that prevents an older person from being admitted to a nursing home may be very different, involving the mobilization of support for very tangible and instrumental purposes (help with shopping, transportation, activities of daily living) from the kind of support needed in preventing depressive episodes.

In addition, to date, most investigators have focused on one or another of these dimensions of network structure or support and proposed either main (direct) or buffering effects. Buffering is usually meant to identify an effect of support only in the presence of another stressor (e.g., job loss, bereavement, major illness). Main effects are direct or have an independent effect on health outcomes. We propose that since, by their very nature, social relationships are multidimensional, it is possible that some aspects, for instance, of support will only influence outcomes in the presence of other stressful experiences, whereas stable measures of network structure and size will exert direct effects on health outcomes. Only through careful assessment strategies will we discover the degree to which characteristics of networks and support exert either direct or buffering effects and are specific with regard to health outcomes.

The Structure of Social Ties

Much of the work uncovering the structure of social ties grew from social science research in the area of social network analysis (Fischer, 1982). Social networks classically were seen as the web of social ties surrounding an individual, and measures were constructed that characterized the links tying people together. Typical structural measures of ties are size (number of network members), frequency of contact, geographic proximity, percent of network comprised of kin, durability (how long members were known to one another), reciprocity, homogeneity (how similar network members are to one another), and density (how many network members know one another). Most of these measures focus on actual behaviors (e.g., "How often do you see any relatives?" "How many of your friends know one another?") rather than hypothetical situations (e.g., "If you needed a ride, who would you call on?").

Most prospective community-based studies in which social ties predict subsequent increased mortality risk have relied on this theoretical base, although it is important to note that most of the summary indices used in these studies do not tap many specific network measures. Rather, they often lump several dimensions of network structure together to form a more global measure (i.e., often measured by items on marital status, number of close friends and relatives, participation in church and group activities). Even with these summary measures, studies in Alameda County (Berkman and Syme, 1979; Seeman et al, 1987), Tecumseh, Michigan (House, et al, 1982), North Carolina (Blazer, 1982), and several recent studies in Scandinavia (Kaplan et al, 1988; Orth-Gomer and Johnson, 1987; Welin et al, 1985) have all found lack of social ties to be related to long-term mortality risk, often between 10 and 20 years after baseline assessments.

An advantage of this approach is that these measures often rely on common behaviors and activities. They are relatively objective, stable, and only weakly related to indices of social desirability. Also, they appear to tap the degree to which people are very isolated (at one end of the scale) or very integrated (at the upper end of the scale) within their network and communities. These measures of social network structure often show direct or main effects on mortality risk. House (1987) reports these effects are often additive rather than showing a threshold effect. Such an additive effect suggests that it is not extreme isolation alone that accounts for increased risk.

The disadvantage of these measures is that they are so global that they give little indication of what elements of networks are protective to health and well-being. They give little insight into the actual character of social relationships and little basis on which to plan interventions. Nonetheless, these instruments are among the most powerful and consistent predictors of important health outcomes. If they in fact tap the extent to which people are integrated into their respective communities through active contacts with friends and relatives and participation in religious and voluntary activities, interventions aimed at maintaining older people's involvement in their respective communities may be of critical importance to the health of the elderly.

The Functions of Social Networks: The Provision of Support

The second important component of social relationships is the availability and amount of specific kinds of social support received or provided, that is, the types of resources that flow through social networks. Although network measures characterize the structure of ties, they reveal little about whether such ties are actually supportive. A major question in this field is to understand the conditions under which networks provide support (Wellman, 1985). Barrera and colleagues (1983, 1986) in extensive reviews describe numerous types of support functions. However, subsequent empirical research (Barrera and Ainlay, 1983; Caldwell and Reinhart, 1988) suggests that three types of functions capture the majority of types of social support. The first is emotional support, the availability or presence of someone to talk to about personal matters and express comfort and concern for one's well-being. The second is often called instrumental or tangible support—having someone available to help with tasks, provide transportation, help with groceries, and so on. The third is informational or guidance oriented—help with information, giving directions, or suggesting action. Aspects of support that are important to measure include current availability as well as availability under hypothetical conditions, and source (i.e., who provides support). At this time, for example, we have very little descriptive information on exactly *who* provides support to older individuals, whether a single individual or many are likely to provide various kinds of support. There is also little evidence identifying whether it matters in terms of disease risk who provides support.

A major advantage of assessing support is its focus on the functions of social ties. Theoretically, social networks are important because they function in certain ways and provide the individual with support and information. They contribute to the individual's feelings about themselves and the world around them. In terms of interventions, it may be possible to mobilize network members to provide specific kinds of support, which may in turn promote health and optimal levels of functioning. It is also likely that specific kinds of support will be related to specific outcomes. For example, the availability of instrumental support may enable an older person to remain living at home rather than enter a nursing home. Availability of emotional support, however, may play a stronger role in recovery from illness by reducing anxiety and encouraging the older person to become active in social roles. The link between the kind of support and specific outcomes depends on our hypotheses concerning the pathogenesis of a particular disease or decline and the process by which a particular kind of support inhibits that process or promotes recovery.

A major disadvantage of focusing solely on the nature of support is that its availability may be highly correlated with the actual need for help with that particular function. For instance, an older person at home with major difficulties in activities of daily living will need substantial instrumental support. A less impaired older person may report little help with daily tasks because he or she has no current need for help. Even hypothetical (what if. . .?) questions may not accurately represent the healthy person's structure or current, but untapped, available support. Thus, we have a situation where functional disability may cause the individual to mobilize levels of support rather than social support influencing a health outcome. We will return to this issue in the next section.

Perceived Adequacy of Social Support

The third major component of social relationship measures is the perceived adequacy of social support. In contrast to the number of providers of support or types of support, the perceived adequacy of support usually focuses on the recipient's subjective assessment that the support available, or received, would or did, enhance his or her well-being (Barrera et al, 1981). There is evidence that at least some of the benefit of social support is cognitively mediated (Antonucci, 1985; Barrera, 1981; Cohen et al, 1985), influencing health via the perception and cognitive understanding of its presence. Furthermore, some evidence suggests that not all apparently supportive acts are perceived as supportive (Wortman and Lehman, 1985).

Equally important with respect to perceived adequacy of support is the more recent attention given to negative aspects of social relationships—not all networks provide support, and recently it has been hypothesized that not all aspects of support are health promoting. For instance, support that increases the older person's feelings of low self-esteem, lack of competence, or autonomy and dependence may be potentially damaging (Barrera, 1986; McFarlane et al, 1984; Pagel et al, 1987; Parmelee, 1983; Rook, 1984).

Furthermore, especially for older people, social relationships may be stressful at the same time they are long-standing and emotionally close as individuals in the older person's network become frail or ill and have growing needs for care. One of the major hypotheses proposed for explaining the frequently reported weaker network effects among women is that women do not lack networks but are often the providers rather than the receivers of support (Kessler and MacLeod, 1985). Older people, especially older women, may be providing support to even more frail network members. This suggests the importance of assessing reciprocity in relationships, perhaps over the life course, and certainly the effects of both giving and receiving. Thus, it is of potential importance, especially for the older person, to assess the perceived adequacy of support and the strain from the amount of support the older person provides to other members of his or her network. Such perceptions of adequacy and strain broadly conceived may be very important additions to measures of network structure and support function of networks.

A disadvantage of assessing perceived adequacy by itself is that a person's mental state, coping style, and degree of illness may exert profound influences on perceived adequacy measures (Cutrona, 1986; Sarason et al, 1983). For instance, older people who are depressed or very ill may report that support is available but inadequate to meet their needs because they perceive their needs to be so great or resources to be so limited. Thus, these measures reflect not only who in the network is available to provide support but also the older person's actual level of need and perceived level of need.

Social Ties, Support, and Perceived Adequacy of Support Among the Elderly

Instruments

Although many "first-generation" studies of social ties and health status consisted of secondary analyses of existing data where only crude measures of social ties were available (e.g., generally global measures of social integration), a host of more sophisticated "second-generation" studies now exist in which rigorous attempts have been made to conceptualize and measure the multidimensional nature of networks and support. Studies from investigators using data from the Duke Epidemiology Catchment Area Study and from the Older Americans Resources and Services Community Survey (Blazer, 1982), investigators using data from the University of Michigan, Institute for Survey Research survey of Social Networks in Adult Life and Americans Changing Lives (House, 1987; Depner and Ingersoll-Dayton, 1988) and investigators from Yale using the Establishment of Populations for the Epidemiologic Study of the Elderly (EPESE) (Seeman and Berkman, 1988) have advanced our understanding of specific aspects of social networks and support among the elderly in critical ways. Other investigators have developed similar multidimensional instruments designed for adults of all ages. It is important that survey instruments and results related to them be based on studies in which the samples come from well-defined populations and in which participation rates are high. Studies of volunteers are particularly likely to be biased and give a distorted perspective of network composition and support characteristics. Furthermore, findings based on cohorts of college studies may not be relevant for older populations, since the network configurations, types of support, and relevant health outcomes of these young well-educated groups are often very different from those of older populations.

In Table 12-1 we have selected some important research instruments and highlighted the strengths and areas of concentration of each. For a more detailed description of these instruments the reader is referred to our earlier paper (Oxman and Berkman, 1990).

The Social Network Questionnaire from the Yale Health and Aging Project was developed for the National Institute on Aging's EPESE and has thus been used in a large elderly community-dwelling population. It includes assessments of structural components of networks (size, density, geographic proximity, percentage kin-based, and number of visual and nonvisual contacts) as well as the availability, sources, and perceived adequacy of emotional, instrumental, and financial support (Seeman and Berkman, 1988).

The Survey Research Center at the University of Michigan has conducted several surveys of older adults (Antonucci, 1985; Israel and Antonucci, 1987; Kahn and Antonucci, 1980). Assessments of network ties and support were derived from an initial list of social network members that respondents are asked to provide, indicating their degree of emotional closeness to each individual named. Using this list measures density, frequency, proximity, and reciprocity of both emotional and tangible support are averaged across close network members. In addition, each close network member is rated for the frequency of emotional and tangible aid support. The reported measures have shown a consistent relationship to psychological well-being in three different samples.

The Duke Social Support Index (DSSI) is a thirty-five-item scale utilized in the Piedmont Health Survey and the Epidemiologic Catchment Area Program (ECA) (Landerman, George, Campbell, in press). To determine the parameters of social support in a community population, the DSSI was designed to be desegregated into individual components, including a four-item network scale, a four-item interaction scale, and a confidant question, each with known mean values from the Piedmont Health Survey.

The Social Health Battery is an 11-item measure of both access and use of social resources (Donald and Ware, 1984). It was developed for the Health Insurance Experiment and thus administered to a large sample of 4603 individuals. It was designed to focus on the more objective measures of available social ties and frequency of contact with them.

The Social Support Questionnaire developed by Schaefer, Coyne, and Lazarus (1981) covers both actual support and perceived adequacy. Respondents are asked to respond to hypothetical situations. Dimensions of support are related to emotional support, guidance, and tangible support.

The Interview Schedule for Social Interaction (ISSI) of Henderson et al (1980, 1981) was designed to delineate how social relationships protect against psychiatric disorders under adversity. Both Henderson et al (1980) and Sarason et al (1983) were guided by Weiss' conception (1974) of six benefits from relationships: attachment, integration, caring for others, self-reassurance, reliable alliance, and available help.

Table 12-1 Comparison of Features of Twelve Social Relationship Measures

	Yale–New Haven SNQ	Duke social support index	Social networks in adult life	Rand social health battery	Social support questionnaire (Schaefer)	Interview schedule for social interaction	Social relationship scale	Inventory of socially supportive behaviors	Interpersonal support evaluation list	Social support questionnaire (Sarason)	Multi-dimensional scale of perceived social support	Perceived social support questionnaire
Description:												
Number of items	49	35	8[a]	11	19	53	6[a]	40	40	27*	12	40
Administration	Interview	Interview	Interview	Self-report	Interview	Interview	Interview assisted	Self-report	Self-report	Self-report	Self-report	Self-report
Social network structure and composition:												
Size of available members	X	X	X	X			X			X		
Frequency of actual contacts	Weekly and monthly	Weekly	Week, month, year	Monthly		Past year	Variable period					
Geographic proximity	X	X	X									
Composition (friend, children, relatives)	X						X			X		

Presence of confidante	X	X							X	
Reciprocity	X		X	X		X	X			
Type and amount of support function:										
Emotional	Available		Average number of members			Available and variable time		Past month available		
Tangible guidance	Available	Ever	Average number		Available			Past month available		Available	Available
Perceived adequacy of social support:										
Adequacy by composition	Past year						Variable period			
Adequacy by type of support	Past year				Past month and ever	Variable period		Available		
Adequacy by problem										
Total adequacy		Available					Variable period	Available	Available	Available
Negative aspects						X	X	X	X	

[a]Asked of each identified network number.

Only the first two of these benefits could be distinguished by Henderson and colleagues in their development of the interview. Reliability and validity have been established for scores based on the 53 items assessing the availability and perceived adequacy for social attachment and social integration.

The Social Relationship Scale (McFarlane et al, 1980, 1983, 1984) was developed to measure the effects of social relationships on illness responses in each of six areas in which a subject may have experienced life changes. Respondents are asked to identify each person they talked to about a problem, the type of relationship, the helpfulness of the discussion, and the reciprocity with each person.

The Inventory of Socially Supportive Behaviors is a 40-item self-report inventory of activities for assessing types of support (Barrera and Ainlay, 1983; Barrera et al, 1981; Caldwell and Reinhardt, 1988). Three types of social support are covered: emotional, tangible aid, and guidance. Although initially developed on college students, Krause (1987) applied a modified form of the instrument to a community cohort of elderly. Another support instrument developed by Cohen et al (1985), The Interpersonal Support Evaluation List, emphasizes both standard aspects of support and the subject's perceptions that these support functions would be available if needed. The ISEL has been used for a variety of purposes in different populations and has adequate reliability.

The Social Support Questionnaire of Sarason et al (1983) is a 27-item scale. It asks respondents to list up to nine potential providers of support for each of 27 different hypothetical or commonly occurring types of support situations. A six-point overall satisfaction scale from very satisfied to very dissatisfied is asked for each situation, rather than each individual, providing support. The SSQ has not been tested in the elderly and some of the support situations may be less relevant to an older population.

The Multidimensional Scale of Perceived Social Support was designed to be a quick, easily administered, self-report inventory of perceived adequacy of social support (Zimet et al, 1988). It includes 12 items that divide into three groups (family, friends, and significant others). However, it also has a total score and can be used as an overall measure of perceived adequacy. The validity and test–retest reliability have been adequately demonstrated. Disadvantages include that it focuses more on subjective evaluation of providers than on the support function provided. Another instrument to assess perceived adequacy of support was developed by Procidano and Heller (1983), designed to measure the degree to which a person perceives his needs for support are met by friends and family. It consists of two 20-item scales.

Associations Between Dimensions of Networks and Support: Findings from the New Haven EPESE

One important issue is the extent to which measures of social networks and support are so highly correlated with one another that they are essentially tapping the same phenomena even though they are theoretically distinct. We examined this issue in detail using data from the New Haven site of the EPESE program (Seeman and Berkman, 1988). The study is based on a probability sample of 2806 noninstitutionalized men and women aged 65 and older living in New Haven, Connecticut, in 1982. These NIA-funded studies in Iowa, East Boston, and Durham, North Carolina, have a core series of network items. However, several sites have unique and additional measures of dimensions of networks and support. The New Haven study had as one of its major focuses a study of social networks and support among the elderly. We are particularly interested in two related questions (Seeman and Berkman, 1988):

1. Are there aspects of network structure that lend themselves to the maximal provision of support?
2. Are there certain people or specific kinds of relationships that are crucial to the provision of particular kinds of support?

Table 12-2 illustrates the association between a network measure of number of monthly face-to-face contacts between the respondent and his or her friends, children, and other relatives and the proportion reporting the availability of instrumental and emotional support. Although there is a clear positive association between the number of face-to-face contacts and the availability of support, 60 percent of those reporting no face-to-face contacts with either children, close friends, or relatives still report that instrumental and emotional support are available. These two measures, although related, clearly illustrate the point that the measures are not measuring the same phenomena. It is possible, for instance, that people rely on others for support who are not "counted" as close friends or relatives.

Also revealing are regression analyses of the relationships between aspects of social networks (size, geographic proximity, and direct, face-to-face contact) and availability of emotional and instrumental support. Table 12-3 shows again that network size is related to both types of support. However, closer inspection reveals that it is only geographically proximate and face-to-face contacts that provide instrumental support. This distinction between more distant and unseen ties and closer ties seems logical, since instrumental support implies direct, tangible assistance, a type of assistance likely to require the supporter's presence. Thus, geographic proximity may be important in determining those network members capable of helping an increasingly frail older person to maintain himself or herself in terms of living at home. Both proximal and nonproximal ties are significantly related to availability of emotional support (although geographically proximate ties have the stronger association). When comparing face-to-face contacts with the number of nonvisual contacts by mail or phone, only face-to-face contacts show strong and significant associations with the perceived adequacy of instrumental and emotional support.

Table 12-2 Availability of Support by Total Number of Monthly Face-to-Face Contacts with Children, Close Friends, and Relatives (New Haven EPESE baseline data, 1982, $N = 2806$)

	Proportion reporting availability of support	
Face-to-face contacts	Instrumental support	Emotional support
0	65.6[a]	62.2
1–2	87.6	72.5
3–5	91.6	84.1
6–10	94.1	87.9
11+	97.2	90.9

[a]Percentage of "contacts" category reporting that type of support is available.

Table 12-3 Availability of Instrumental and Emotional Support and Network Structure[a] (New Haven EPESE baseline data, 1982, $N = 2806$)

		Instrumental support (no = 0; yes = 1)			Emotional support (no = 0; yes = 1)		
Model	Variables	B^b	X_2	P-value	B^b	X_2	P-value
1	Network size	0.06	39.93	0.0000	0.07	36.16	0.0000
2	Number of proximal ties	0.03	22.17	0.0000	0.04	15.30	0.0002
	Number of nonproximal ties	0.009	1.16	0.3	0.02	4.69	0.03
3	Number of direct face-to-face contacts	0.05	23.40	0.0000	0.07	20.19	0.0000
	Number of indirect nonvisual contacts	0.008	0.61	0.4	0.004	0.19	0.6

[a]Results presented are each adjusted for age, sex, race, and income.
[b]Regression coefficient.

The New Haven EPESE program explored who provides support to the older person and the extent to which that support is seen as adequate. For instance, having a spouse is unrelated to perceived adequacy of support. On the other hand, having a confidant (whether a spouse or someone else) is related to adequacy of both instrumental and emotional support. Children, friends, and extended family contributed to the perception of adequate instrumental support, but children are *not* the major sources of emotional support. Ties with close friends and relatives show stronger associations with such support. This sort of differentiation in terms of who the older person views as likely to provide adequate support and the difference between measures of networks and availability of support suggest that these features of social relationships are not interchangeable. Each may have unique health effects and be influenced by quite different processes, both psychosocial and biomedical. These data also indicate that intuitively important sources of support commonly assessed by living arrangements (with whom the older person lives) and the presence of children (particularly daughters who live nearby) may not tap the rich resources for support that many older people feel are available to them.

When we examine the cross-sectional association between measures of networks and support and health variables such as functional status, quite interesting patterns emerge, suggesting the different associations between functional status, networks, and support. Table 12-4 shows mean scores on an index of functional ability and measures of visual, face-to-face ties, number of contacts by mail or phone, and two measures of support: number of sources of support and perceived adequacy. The measure of functional ability is a Guttman scale comprised of three subscales of activities of daily living and higher-order physical functioning, including bending, reaching, walking half a mile, moving furniture, lifting groceries, and so on. The scale goes from 1 to 4, with higher scores signifying increasing disability. Numbers of face-to-face contacts are inversely related to level of disability [i.e., those with the most contacts have the least

Table 12-4 Functional Ability and Network Structure (New Haven EPESE baseline data, 1982, $N = 2806$)

	Functional ability (mean scores)[a]	N
Visual ties (no. of contacts)		
0	2.75	178
1–2	2.84	628
3–5	2.59	810
6–10	2.40	712
11+	2.18	405
		($\chi^2 = 67.2$; $p = .0000$)
Nonvisual contacts (no. of contacts)		
0	2.55	139
1–2	2.52	453
3–5	2.53	761
6–10	2.64	830
11+	2.38	546
		($\chi^2 = 7.92$; $p = .11$)
Instrumental support (no. of sources)		
0	2.28	274
1	2.67	1325
2+	2.69	704
		($\chi^2 = 10.7$; $p = .005$)
Adequacy		
Need a lot more	3.43	73
Need some more	3.27	128
Need a little more	3.27	201
Adequate	2.50	1896
		($\chi^2 = 68.7$; $p = .0000$)
Emotional support (no. of sources)		
0	2.42	361
1	2.54	1537
2+	2.65	348
		($\chi^2 = 1.4$; $p =$ NS)
Adequacy		
Need a lot more	3.14	68
Need some more	2.87	124
Need a little more	2.86	137
Adequate	2.46	1889
		($\chi^2 = 27.2$; $p = .0000$)

disability ($p = .001$)]. Contacts made by phone or mail show basically no relationship with physical functioning. The number of sources of people who provide support is *positively* associated with impairment (i.e., elderly who report more sources of support have more disability). The differences are greater and statistically significant for instrumental support, but the trends are in the same direction for emotional support. Finally, older men and women who report they need "a lot more" emotional *or* instrumental support have the highest scores on the disability scale.

There are several ways to interpret these data, and since they are cross-sectional, no definitive interpretation is possible. Although it is possible that different aspects of support lead to disability, it seems more likely that these associations reflect the impact

Table 12-5 Reciprocity with Children by Age (New Haven EPESE baseline data, 1982, $N = 2806$)

	65–69	70–74	75–79	80–84	85+
Proportion of things respondent does for children[a]	.57	.51	.45	.39	.34
Proportion of things children do for respondent[b]	.55	.55	.58	.59	.67
Relative difference (children help vs. you help) [proportion children do for respondent, proportion respondent does for children]	−.02	.05	.13	.21	.33

[a]List of possible things done includes (1) give gifts, (2) help with money, (3) help when ill, (4) help around house, and (5) help with child care.

[b]List of possible things done includes (1) give gifts, (2) help with money, (3) help when ill, (4) help around house, (5) run errands or provide transportation, (6) prepare meals.

that functional disability has on the ability of the older person to maintain active visits with friends and relatives and its lack of impact on contacts maintained by phone or letters. Increasing disability may also lead the older person to have increased need for social support and the mobilization of several sources of support. Thus, the number of sources of support is related not only to the background network structure but to need for support. The opposite association between the number of face-to-face contacts and the number of sources of support with functional disability points to the very real danger of equating measures of support with those of network size.

Patterns of reciprocity of support between older men and women and their adult children also change as older persons age. Using data from the New Haven EPESE, we have shown that men and women over the age of 75 do fewer things for their children than their children do for them. Between the ages of 65 and 75, both the elderly and their adult children provide about the same amount of support to each other. Table 12-5 shows the proportion of tasks older people do for their children, the proportion of tasks children do for their parents, and the relative difference for different age groups of "parents." Under the age of 75, there is no relative difference in proportions; however, by age 85, children have increased the proportion of tasks they help their elderly parents with from 55 percent to 67 percent. Even more dramatically, the older parents have decreased support from 57 percent of tasks to 34 percent.

There are gender and ethnic differences in the provision of support as well as age (or potentially cohort) differences. More elderly women than men and more blacks than whites are likely to receive support from their adult children. Similar findings with regard to gender differences are also reported by Depner and Ingersoll-Dayton (1988).

CONCLUSIONS

To conclude, we have shown that social networks and support are theoretically and empirically multidimensional constructs measuring various aspects of social relationships. Although there are a wide variety of research instruments available to assess aspects of network structure and support, most instruments focus on a limited number of dimensions. Furthermore, not all of these instruments were developed for use in elderly populations. Instruments developed for other populations must be carefully scrutinized for their appropriateness in older populations where the majority of people are not employed full time and where children are likely to be neither young nor dependent.

Perhaps most important to investigators wishing to select instruments to predict health or medical care outcomes in the elderly is the need to specify a priori those dimensions or characteristics of networks and support they hypothesize to lead to critical health outcomes. The selection of measures should be guided by how the investigator suspects the social "phenomenon" will be behaviorally or biologically linked to the outcome of interest. Although there is not yet much evidence to guide this process, the investigator will do well to work out the potential pathways or mechanisms. As stated earlier, if, for instance, the provision of instrumental support by a geographically proximate network member is most likely to enable the frail older person to remain living at home, network and support questions can be selected accordingly. These items may well be very different from aspects of network structure that are related to the development of atherosclerosis or from those aspects of support that are related to recovery from myocardial infarction or hip fractures.

Finally, it is important to understand that many conditions influence networks and support, and they are likely to do so in relatively specific ways. For instance, functional disability is likely to restrict an older person's network in terms of size but expand the number of sources of support. Patterns of reciprocity between older people and their adult children or even between spouses are likely to be influenced by current levels of frailty and need. Although we have not discussed environmental determinants of networks and support, much work needs to be done to uncover the ways in which the physical environment (e.g., housing characteristics, transportation, urban versus rural environments) and the social environment and structure (socioeconomic status, patterns of migration and mobility, and work conditions) either enable or inhibit the development of stable networks capable of functioning effectively.

ACKNOWLEDGMENTS

This work has been supported by NIH Grant No. N01-AG-0-2105 (Dr. Berkman), John D. and Catherine T. MacArthur Foundation Network on Successful Aging (Drs. Berkman and Seeman), and NIMH Grant No. MH00687 (Dr. Oxman).

Parts of this chapter have been adapted from Oxman and Berkman, "Assessment of Social Relationships in Elderly Patients," *International Journal of Psychiatry in Medicine* 20(1):65–84, 1990 and Seeman and Berkman, "Structural Characteristics of Social Networks and their Relationship with Social Support in the Elderly: Who Provides Support," *Social Science and Medicine*, 26:737–749, 1988.

REFERENCES

Antonucci TC (1985). Social support: Theoretical advances, recent findings and pressing issues. In Social Support: Theory, Research and Applications, IG Sarason and BR Sarason (eds.). The Hague, Martinus Nijhoff, pp. 21–37.

Barrera M (1981). Social support in the adjustment of pregnant adolescents: Assessment issues. In Social Networks and Social Support, BH Gottlieb (ed.), Beverly Hills, CA, Sage, pp. 69–96.
Barrera M (1986). Distinctions between social support concepts, measures, and models. Am J Community Psychol 14:413–445.
Barrera M, Ainlay SL (1983). The structure of social support: A conceptual and empirical analysis. J Community Psychol 11:133–143.
Barrera M, Sandler IN, Ramsay TB (1981). Preliminary development of a scale of social support: Studies on college students. Am J Community Psychol 9:435–443.
Berkman LF (1988). The changing and heterogeneous nature of aging and longevity: A social and biomedical perspective. Ann Rev Gerontol Geriatr 8:37–68.
Berkman LF, Syme SL (1979). Social networks, host resistance, and mortality: A nine-year follow-up study of Alameda County residents. Am J Epidemiol 109:186–204.
Blazer DG (1982). Social support and mortality in an elderly community population. Am J Epidemiol 115:684–694.
Broadhead WE, Kaplan BH, James SA, Wagner EH, Schoengach VJ, Grinson R, Heyden S, Tibblin G, Gehlbach SH (1983). The epidemiologic evidence for a relationship between social support and health. Am J Epidemiol 117:521–537.
Caldwell RA, Reinhart MA (1988). The relationship of personality to individual differences in the use of type and source of social support. J Soc Clin Psychol 6:140–146.
Cohen C, Teresi J, Holmes D (1985). Social networks, stress, and physical health: A longitudinal study of an inner-city elderly population. J Gerontol 40:478–486.
Cohen S (1988). Psychosocial models of the role of social support in the etiology of physical disease. Health Psychol 7(3):269–297.
Cohen S, Marmelstein R, Kamarch T, Hoberman HM (1985). Measuring the functional components of social support. In Social Support: Theory, Research and Applications, IG Sarason and BR Sarason (eds.), Dordrecht, Martinus Nijhoff.
Cohen S, Matthews KA (1987). Editorial: Social support, type A behavior and coronary artery disease. Psychosom Med 44:325–330.
Cohen S, Syme SL (1985). Social Support and Health, New York, Academic Press.
Cutrona CE (1986). Objective determinants of perceived social support. J Pers Soc Psychol 50:349–355.
Depner C, Ingersoll-Dayton B (1988). Supportive relationships in later life. Psychol Aging 3(4):348–357.
Donald CA, Ware JE Jr (1984). The measurement of social support. Res Community Mental Health, 4, 334–335.
Fischer CS (1982). To Dwell Among Friends; Personal Networks in Town and City. Chicago, University of Chicago Press.
Henderson S, Byrne DG, Duncan-Jones P (1981). Neurosis and the Social Environment. Sydney, Academic Press.
Henderson S, Duncan-Jones P, Byrne DG, Scott R. (1980). Measuring social relationships: The interview schedule for social interaction. Psycholog Med 10:723–734.
House JS (1987). Social support and social structure. Soc Forum 2(1):135–146.
House J, Robbins C, Metzner H (1982). The association of social relationships and activities with mortality: Prospective evidence from the Tecumseh community health study. Am J Epidemiol 116:123–140.
House JS, Umberson B, Landis KR (1988). Structural processes of social support. Ann Sociol 14:293–318.
Israel BA, Antonucci TC (1987). Social network characteristics and psychological well-being: A replication and extension. Health Educ Quart 14:461–481.

Kahn RL, Antonucci TC (1980). Convoys over the life course: Attachment, roles, and social support. Life-Span Devel Behav 3:253–285.

Kaplan GA, Salonen JT, Cohen RD, Brand RJ, Syme SL, Puska P (1988). Social connections and mortality from all causes and from cardiovascular disease: Prospective evidence from eastern Finland. Am J Epidemiol 128:370–380.

Kessler RC, McLeod JD (1985). Social support and mental health in community samples. In Social Support and Health, S Cohen and SL Syme (eds.). New York, Academic Press, pp. 219–240.

Krause N (1987). Satisfaction with social support and self-rated health in older adults. Gerontologist 27:301–308.

Landerman R, George LK, Campbell RT, et al (in press). Social support, stress and depression: Alternative models of the stress buffering process. Am J Community Psychol.

McFarlane AH, Neale KA, Norman GR, Roy RG, Streiner DL (1980). Methodological issues in developing a scale to measure social support. Schizophrenia Bull 7:90–100.

McFarlane A, Norman GR, Steiner DL, Roy RG (1983). The process of social stress: Stable, reciprocal, and mediating relationships. J Health Soc Behav 24:160–173.

McFarlane AH, Norman GR, Streiner DL, Roy RG (1984). Characteristics and correlates of effective and ineffective social supports. J Psychosom Res 28:501–510.

Orth-Gomer K, Johnson JV (1987). Social network interaction and mortality: A six-year follow-up study of a random sample of the Swedish population. J. Chronic Dis 40:949–957.

Oxman TE, Berkman LF (1990). Assessment of social relationships in elderly patients. Int J Psychiatr Med 20(1):65–84.

Pagel MD, Erdly WW, Becker J (1987). Social networks: We get by with (and in spite of) a little help from our friends. J Pers Soc Psychol 53:793–804.

Parmelee PA (1983). Spouse versus other family caregivers: Psychological impact on impaired aged. Am J Community Psychol 11:337–349.

Procidano M, Heller K (1983). Measures of perceived social support from friends and from family: Three validation studies. Am J Community Psychol 11:1–24.

Rock KS (1984). The negative side of social interaction: Impact on psychological well-being. J Pers Soc Psychol 46:1097–1108.

Sarason IG, Levine HM, Basham RB, Sarason BR (1983). Assessing social support: The social support questionnaire. J Pers Soc Psychol 44:127–139.

Schaefer C, Coyne JC, Lazarus RS (1981). The health-related functions of social support. J Behav Med 4:381–406.

Seeman TE, Berkman LF (1988). Structural characteristics of social networks and their relationship with social support in the elderly: Who provides support. Social Sci Med 26(7):737–749.

Seeman TE, Kaplan GA, Knudsen L, Cohen R, Guralnik J (1987). Social network ties and mortality among the elderly in the Alameda County study. Am J Epidemiol 126:714–723.

Stoller EP (1985). Exchange patterns in the informal support networks of the elderly: The impact of reciprocity on morale. J Marriage Fam 47:335–342.

Weiss RS (1974). The provisions of social relationships. In Doing unto Others, Z Rubin (ed.). Englewood Cliffs, NJ, Prentice-Hall, pp. 17–26.

Welin L, Tibblin G, Svardsudd K, Tibblin B, Ander-Peciva S, Larsson B, Wilhelmsen L (1985). Prospective study of social influenccs on mortality: The study of men born in 1913 and 1923. Lancet 1:915–918.

Wellman B (1985). From social support to social network. In Social Support, Theory, Research, and Applications, Sarason IG, Sarason BR (eds.). The Hague, Martinus Nijhoff, pp. 205–222.

Wortman C, Lehman D (1985). Reactions to victims of life crises: Support attempts fail. In Social Support: Theory, Research, and Applications. Sarason IG, Sarason BR (eds.). Dordrecht, Martinus Nijhoff, pp. 463–489.

Zimet GD, Dahlem NW, Zimet SG, Farley GK (1988). The multidimensional scale of perceived social support. J Pers Assess 52:30–41.

13

Psychiatric Epidemiology in Elderly Populations

DAN L. TWEED, DAN G. BLAZER,
AND JAMES A. CIARLO

The epidemiologic study of psychiatric disorders in elderly populations is a challenging endeavor. In this chapter we will explore the tools that are available for such studies and the various factors that make such studies particularly difficult. We begin by examining recent developments within psychiatry itself that influence the manner in which epidemiologic research is conducted.

The last several decades have seen major changes in psychiatry, including important developments in psychopharmacology and the ascendancy of biologic models of psychopathology (Klerman, 1986, 1989). With these changes have come (1) a resurgence in interest in psychiatric nosology and the classification of psychiatrically morbid conditions and (2) a specific concern for improving the reliability of the diagnostic process (Goodwin and Guze, 1989; Klerman, 1986). As a consequence of these changes, three developments have occurred that have shaped the nature of contemporary epidemiologic research in psychiatry.

1. Development of explicit diagnostic criteria. First, the strong emphasis on increasing the reliability of the diagnostic process has led to several systematic attempts at generating explicit criteria for making diagnostic decisions that would be widely acceptable in both the clinical and research communities. Without such criteria meaningful psychiatric epidemiologic research among the elderly cannot proceed.

The most successful of the earlier attempts were the Feighner Criteria (Feighner, et al, 1972) and the related Research Diagnostic Criteria (RDC) (Spitzer et al, 1978). The most influential event, however, was the publication of the Diagnostic and Statistical Manual of Mental Disorders, 3rd edition (DSM-III)—the official statement of diagnostic nomenclature of the American Psychiatric Association (1980). Unlike earlier DSM editions, DSM-III emphasized the careful delineation of criteria for assessing the presence of clinically important psychiatric syndromes. Also unlike earlier versions, it avoided etiologic stances in the specification of these criteria. In a field notorious for competing etiologic theories (Millon, 1986), this "agnostic" approach was an essential precondition for the widespread adoption of the DSM-III nomenclature.

2. Development of structured diagnostic interviews. The second major development was in the areas of instrumentation and measurement—tools for the empirical identification of cases essential for psychiatric epidemiologic research. Until recently, psychiatric epidemiologists have relied either on (a) clinical records in institutional settings (with little or no standardization in reporting protocols) or on (b) simple screening scales, symptom indices, or global scales intended to measure *levels* of psychological impairment rather than to determine the presence or absence of clinically significant syndromes. Clinical records, although useful for certain types of epidemiologic investigation, were of little use in studying community populations. Hence, epidemiologists worked with symptom indices and/or impairment scales. Instruments such as the Center for Epidemiologic Studies—Depression Scale (CES-D) (Sawyer-Radloff and Locke, 1986), the Langner 22-item screening scale (Langner, 1986), and the General Well-Being Schedule (GWB) (Dupuy, 1973) are examples of these earlier, prediagnostic instruments.

Such symptom indices and screening scales continue to play an important role in epidemiologic research by allowing us to quantify the level of impairment or psychopathology in populations. At the same time they have posed problems for the psychiatric epidemiologist concerned with estimating the prevalence of specific psychiatric disorders. First, many of these scales provided only global measures of impairment and provided little information regarding specific psychiatric disorders. Second, even when scales for assessment within specific domains have been developed (e.g., the CES-D for depression), questions remain regarding the level of impairment that must be observed to record the presence of a disorder. Arbitrary cutting points are often adopted. In the study of the elderly, or any population, the use of such arbitrary cutting points was not optimal and reflected the "gap" between clinical psychiatry and epidemiology (Klerman, 1985).

The developments in psychiatric nosology leading up to the publication of the DSM-III, however, made feasible the development of structured diagnostic instruments—instruments designed to yield diagnostic information. One of the most successful initial attempts at developing a diagnostic interview instrument was the Schedule for Affective Disorders and Schizophrenia (SADS), which was based upon the RDC criteria and provided for the collection of the data necessary to make RDC diagnoses. Currently, three versions of the SADS are available: (1) the regular version, focusing upon current psychiatric status (SADS); (2) the lifetime version (SADS-L), deemed to be most appropriate for community samples where current morbidity is low; and (3) a version for measuring change (SADS-C) (Endicott and Spitzer, 1978; Williams et al, 1989).

The first attempt to use the SADS (the SADS-L variant) in a large-scale community epidemiologic study was in New Haven, Connecticut (Weissman and Myers, 1978). Using nonpsychiatric mental health professionals as interviewers, more than 500 people were interviewed. Over 15 percent of the sampled individuals qualified for one or more of 19 specific RDC-based diagnoses. More than any other study, the New Haven study demonstrated that the resurgence of interest in psychiatric diagnoses could lead to advances in psychiatric epidemiology. At last it was possible to collect data in community samples and generate prevalence estimates for specific disorders.

3. Development of the epidemiologic catchment area program and DSM-III/DIS. These developments laid the foundations for the National Institute of Mental Health's Epidemiologic Catchment Area (ECA) program (Regier et al, 1985)—a series of five large-scale epidemiologic surveys conducted between 1980 and 1984 designed to generate diagnosis-specific prevalence and incidence data. The instrument adopted for use in the ECA program was the Diagnostic Interview Schedule (DIS) (Robins et al, 1981). It was chosen over instruments like the SADS-L for two reasons. First, it was a direct implementation of the DSM-III diagnostic system rather than an implementation of either the RDC or Feighner criteria (though it is possible to score the DIS using these criteria as well). Using the American Psychiatric Associations's official diagnostic criteria was naturally desirable.

Equally desirable was the fact that the DIS interview could be conducted by intensively trained lay interviewers rather than by clinicians—as was necessary for the SADS. For community surveys this was highly cost effective and made large-sample studies feasible. However, the use of lay interviewers has raised issues of credibility regarding the DIS, and the controversy concerning the value of lay versus clinically trained interviewers continues (Klerman, 1985).

As noted, five survey sites were included in the ECA program—New Haven, Baltimore, St. Louis, Los Angeles, and the Raleigh–Durham area of North Carolina. A total sample of 18,571 psychiatric interviews was conducted, with each site contributing between 3004 and 5034 subjects. Included in this sample were 5702 persons aged 65 years or older (Regier et al, 1988). The ECA data base is the repository of much of what we now know about the burden of psychiatric morbidity (as described in the official nomenclature) within the elderly population.

In the remainder of this chapter we accomplish two things. First, we present the basic findings from the ECA program as they pertain to the burden of psychiatric morbidity in the elderly population. Second, we use the ECA findings as a spring board to raise pertinent questions regarding the conduct of epidemiologic research in general, and with regard to elderly populations in particular.

ECA FINDINGS

The main findings from the ECA appeared in a special issue of the Archives of General Psychiatry in October of 1984. Lifetime and six-month prevalence data were presented for three of the five sites. One-month prevalence data were presented for all five sites in November of 1988 (Regier et al, 1988). The latter data, based upon rates standardized to age, sex, and race distribution of the 1980 noninstitutionalized population of the United States, are reported here because of the completeness of the data and the fact that the one-month data avoid some methodologic issues that will be discussed latter.

Table 13-1 presents the age-specific one-month prevalence rates for disorders assessed at all five sites. The data are aggregated across the five sites. The patterns are striking. In nearly every case, the prevalence of psychiatric impairment is lower in the elderly age group (aged 65 or older) than in any other age group. Moreover, this pattern was found across sites and for both males and females.

The Initial Response

The ECA findings surprised many investigators for three reasons. First, the ECA age-prevalence pattern was inconsistent with previous studies that indicated that (1) the

Table 13-1 Standardized One-Month Prevalence Rates of DIS/DSM-III Disorders for All ECA Sites Combined (percent)[a]

	Age category			
Diagnostic category	18–24	25–44	45–64	65+
Any DIS disorder	16.9 (1.0)	17.3 (0.6)	13.3 (0.7)	12.3 (0.6)
Alcohol abuse–dependence	4.1 (0.6)	3.6 (0.3)	2.1 (0.3)	0.9 (0.2)
Drug abuse–dependence	3.5 (0.5)	1.5 (0.2)	0.1 (0.0)	0.0 (0.0)
Schizophrenic disorder	0.7 (0.2)	0.9 (0.1)	0.4 (0.1)	0.1 (0.0)
Schizophreniform disorders	0.1 (0.1)	0.1 (0.1)	0.0 (0.0)	0.0 (0.0)
Manic episode	0.6 (0.2)	0.6 (0.1)	0.2 (0.1)	0.0 (0.0)
Major depressive episode	2.2 (0.4)	3.0 (0.3)	2.0 (0.3)	0.7 (0.1)
Dysthymic disorder	2.0 (0.4)	4.0 (0.3)	3.8 (0.3)	1.8 (0.2)
Phobic disorder	6.4 (0.6)	6.9 (0.4)	6.0 (0.4)	4.8 (0.3)
Panic disorder	0.4 (0.2)	0.7 (0.1)	0.6 (0.2)	0.1 (0.2)
Obsessive–compulsive	1.8 (0.4)	1.6 (0.2)	0.9 (0.2)	0.8 (0.2)
Somatization disorder	0.1 (0.0)	0.1 (0.0)	0.1 (0.0)	0.1 (0.0)
Antisocial personality	0.9 (0.3)	0.8 (0.1)	0.1 (0.1)	0.0 (0.0)

Source: Regier et al (1988).

[a]The rates presented are standardized to the age, sex, and race distribution of the 1980 noninstitutionalized population of the United States aged 18 years and over. Standard errors are presented in parentheses.

lowest rates were among the youngest age groups (Dohrenwend and Dohrenwend, 1969) and (2) that the elderly had relatively high rates of psychopathology (Blazer and Houpt, 1979; Edgerton et al, 1970; Mortimer et al, 1983; Schwab et al, 1974; Warheit, 1976; Zung, 1967).

Second, working within the social causation framework that dominated pre-ECA epidemiology, the ECA findings were counterintuitive. The elderly in our society are known to have a high risk of exposure to a number of risk factors for psychopathology including;

- Loss of social roles (parental, occupational, etc.)
- Death of significant others
- Increased illness, declining health, and risk of age-related trauma (e.g., falls and burns)
- Loss of autonomy

Increased likelihood of isolation
Decrements to income
Declines in cognitive functioning

The knowledge that the elderly are relatively disadvantaged with respect to factors such as these made "pre-ECA" findings seem theoretically plausible. As Klerman (1988, p. 6) noted, the "expected increase of depression with aging has intuitive 'face validity'." The ECA findings, on the other hand, appeared theoretically dissonant and enigmatic.

Third, studies employing other indices of mental well-being have reported findings that are inconsistent with the ECA findings. For example, suicide remains more prevalent among the elderly than at other stages of the life cycle—and continues to increase (Blazer et al, 1987b; Leenaars, 1989). Though the increased prevalence of suicide in the elderly has historically been explained almost exclusively by a dramatic increase among white males, there is evidence that future cohorts of the oldest old in general, and nonwhite elderly males in particular, may suffer increased prevalence from suicide (Manton et al, 1987). Such mortality from suicide reflects a psychiatric burden among the elderly that is not reflected in the ECA results.

Patterns of psychotropic drug use constitute another factor that does not coincide with ECA findings. Though persons 65 years of age and over constitute 12 percent of the total population, 15 percent of the antianxiety drug use occurs in this population. One study (Sussman, 1988) suggests that the rate of regular anxiolytic use among the elderly is approximately five times that seen in the general population. Again, as can be seen in Table 13-1, this is simply not reflected in the ECA results.

Yet the ECA findings of an inverse relationship between psychiatric disorder and age, independent of disorder, age, and location, seems incontrovertible. The samples were large and were scientifically drawn random samples of the household population. The age-prevalence pattern held, regardless of disorder, for every study site and for both males and females. In addition, the DIS was the state-of-art reflection of the current psychiatric nosology as embodied in the DSM-III. In spite of the surprise and skepticism, the ECA findings were persuasive.

Based on the ECA findings, the evidence seemed clear—the prevalence, and hence the burden, of psychiatric morbidity was lower in the elderly population than for any other age group. Apparently, psychiatric morbidity is not a major public health problem among the elderly. Perhaps age provides even some protection against psychiatric illness.

For the remainder of this chapter we want to evaluate whether such conclusions are warranted or whether epidemiologists (as methodologists) need to consider some of the questions the ECA data raise and the limitations inherent in the ECA design that might make it necessary to hedge on drawing such conclusions.

QUESTIONS OF NOSOLOGIC ADEQUACY

By admission and design, DSM-III is a provisional system that reflects the somewhat uneasy current consensus regarding the structure of psychopathology. As Spitzer (APA, 1980, p. 12) notes in the introduction to DSM-III and reiterates in the introduction to the 1987 revision, DSM-III-R, the current nomenclature is "only one still frame in the ongoing process of attempting to understand mental disorders." As a system for conducting epidemiologic research in elderly populations, the DSM-III has two limitations.

First, the DSM-III makes little reference to variation in the structure of psychiatric morbidity as might be manifested at later stages of the life cycle. In particular, there is little specification regarding the manner in which symptomatology associated with specific disorders may vary with age, and no attempt is made to identify disorders unique to various stages of the adult life cycle. For example, is late-life depression comparable to depression experienced at earlier stages of life? Is the symptomatic expression the same? Research has begun to address questions such as these (Blazer et al, 1987a; Blazer et al, 1987c), but much remains to be done. The DSM-III does provide, however, the basic tools to launch systematic investigations into the comparative nature of psychiatric morbidity as it affects different age groups—as long as researchers are mindful of its provisional nature and the strong need for nosologic investigation along developmental lines.

Second, there appears to be a justifiable concern for the adequacy of DSM-III as a tool for describing extant forms of psychopathology as found in nonclinical, community populations. One significant finding in this regard is the surplus symptomatology found in various applications of the DIS and related structured diagnostic interviews. By surplus symptomatology we mean that the survey data reveal a large number of individuals who display clear pathology—with implications for significant impairment—but whose pathology is not well described within existing DSM-III diagnostic categories. Focusing on the depressive domain alone, for example, Blazer, Hughes, and George (1987c) determined that 27 percent of community-dwelling elderly suffered depressive symptoms, whereas only 0.8 percent qualified for a diagnosis of major depression. Similar findings hold for other diagnostic domains. Simply put, there is a gap between the range of symptomatology seen in community studies and our ability to diagnose.

What does this excess symptomatology mean? Some of it, of course, could simply represent nonpathologic symptomatology (e.g., reactive dysphoria). Another significant portion may reflect either prodromal or residual symptomatology indicative of incipient disorder or conditions of incomplete remission. Yet there is also the possibility that this undiagnosable psychopathology reflects residual forms of clinically important psychiatric morbidity with yet uncatalogued syndromal forms. In such cases the current nomenclature, in its provisional format, fails to account for significant morbidity. The extent to which this is true requires that additional efforts be made to analyze and understand this excess symptomatology.

That a nomenclature based upon accumulated exposure to psychopathology in *clinical settings* would not work well in *community populations* is not totally surprising. There have been historical precedents in psychiatry. For example, when psychiatry was mainly practiced by administrative physicians within the confines of insane asylums, the nomenclature that developed was principally useful in describing the severely and chronically ill. As psychiatry moved into the confines of general hospitals and other institutional settings, the existing nomenclature was not found to be particularly useful. Again, during World War II, as psychiatrists became involved in military service, they found that the existing nomenclature was of limited use.

> A wide variety of patients seen by military psychiatrists not only differed substantially from those typically admitted to public mental hospitals, but could not be assigned a label in accord with the *Standard*'s nomenclature. Not only was there no provision for the diversity of psychological disturbances that arose in combat, an understandable deficiency, but a surprisingly wide array of neurotic, personality and psychosomatic disorders could either not be categorized at all or were grouped under such broadly undifferentiated classes as to be virtually useless [Millon, 1986, p. 32]. [Note: the reference to the *"Standard"* pertains to the psychiatric section of the *Standard Classified Nomenclature of Disease* as it existed prior to World War II.]

The community study, then, represents the next point of adaptation in the evolution of psychiatric nosology. Such studies represent both a challenge and an opportunity for empirical investigations into the existence of yet poorly understood forms of psychiatric morbidity. The question for the psychiatric epidemiologist is the extent to which this diagnostic uncertainty is correlated with age, and the extent to which excess symptomatology reflects nontrivial conditions affecting the psychiatric burden of the elderly.

QUESTIONS OF SELECTION AND DESIGN

How do we interpret the persistent inverse correlation between age and prevalence as presented in Table 13.1? Why are the elderly consistently characterized by the lowest prevalence of psychiatric morbidity? The interpretation of such findings, particularly in the context of a cross-sectional design, is always tricky.

Selection Factors

Selective Mortality

First, it is reasonable to assume that differential mortality is at work in the observed relationship (Robins et al, 1984). We know that the respondents aged 65 and over at the time of the interview are not a random sample of those born 65 years prior to the interview. Persons most prone to mental disorders are less likely to survive into old age. For certain types of psychiatric disorder this selection "bias" operates in a readily understandable manner. Individuals with antisocial personality disorders, for example, are prone to act in ways that increase their risk of violent death. Substance abusers are at higher risk of accidental death and mortality because of medical complications arising from their addictive behavior. But research also suggests that there is a link between psychiatric illness and mortality due to natural causes (Tsuang and Simpson, 1985). For example, links have been posited between anxiety and coronary heart disease (Paffenbarger et al, 1966), and depression and cancer (Shekelle et al, 1981). A recent 16-year prospective study (Murphy et al, 1987) reports that respondents with depressive or anxiety disorders at the baseline interview had experienced 1.5 times the number of deaths expected on the basis of rates for a large reference population.

In general, these reports have suggested a link between emotional disturbance, compromised resistance to disease, and subsequent death. The resultant selection will leave persons having a lower risk of mental illness. This will necessarily affect cross-sectional designs, such as those on which the ECA prevalence rates are based. They can also affect longitudinal studies, however, as age-cohorts lose members to death over the course of the study. The Duke experience with elderly respondents in a multiwave longitudinal design suggests an annual loss to mortality of more than 5 percent, increasing with successive waves of the study.

Selective Institutionalization

Second, it is also reasonable to assume that differential rates of institutionalization account for the lower rates of the elderly in the community. As Figure 13-1 indicates, the rate of institutionalization of the elderly has been steadily increasing over the last several decades. Moreover, the risk of institutionalization increases with age. Hing (1987) found that about 1 percent of persons aged 65–74 were institutionalized. Among those 85 years of age and over, 22 percent resided in institutional settings (Smyer, 1989).

It is likely that the mentally ill elderly are being disproportionately selected out of the noninstitutional population (and surveys of that population) by our society's tendency to protect them from their frailty by placing them in protected, custodial settings, such as intermediate-care medical treatment settings and long-term nursing home environments. This prospect is supported by recent studies. Koenig et al (1988), using DSM-III diagnostic categories, estimated the rate of depressive disorders in 130 consecutively admitted male patients 70 years of age and older to a Veteran's Administration Medical Center. Major depression was found in 11.5 percent of these patients, which is considerably above that found in community studies. Another 23 percent suffered significant depressive symptoms not captured by the DSM-III nomen-

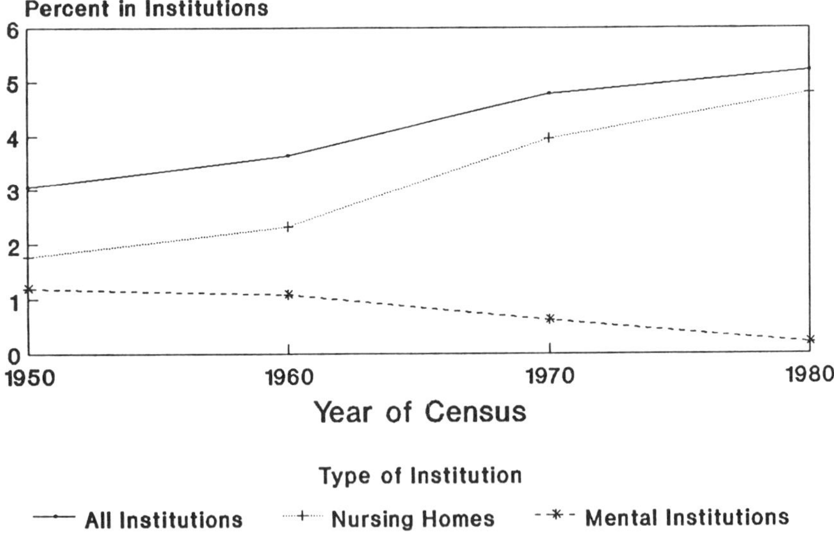

Figure 13-1 Percent of persons aged 65 and over in long-term care institutions: 1950–1980. (*Source:* US Bureau of the Census).

clature. Parmalee, Katz, and Lawton (1989) estimated the prevalence of major depression in a nursing home population to be 12.4 percent. An additional 30.5 percent of the sample had undiagnosed but clinically significant depressive symptoms. Newman et al (1989), with a random sample of 828 residents of nursing homes, found that 21.1 percent of the elderly had a primary psychiatric diagnosis, whereas 83.9 percent had moderate to intense psychosocial problems not reflected in formal diagnoses. Again, these figures are well above those of the ECA community surveys.

Each of these studies illustrates two things. First, a balanced picture of the mental health of elderly populations cannot be obtained in community surveys alone. Institutionalization of the elderly will operate to bias prevalence estimates downward if only community samples are included. Nursing home environments have become increasingly important in this regard, as Figure 13-1 indicates. In 1950, 58 percent of the institutionalized elderly resided in nursing homes. By 1980 this figure had risen to over 92 percent.

Second, these studies illustrate another troublesome feature of studying psychiatric morbidity in elderly populations—the problem of co-morbidity (Feinstein, 1970). In medical settings, for example, the elderly are typified by a host of physical ailments and organic pathology. In arriving at a psychiatric diagnosis, care must be taken to ensure that symptoms attributable to psychiatric causes (such symptoms as anxiety) are not, in fact, of organic origin. Nowhere is this more obvious than in cases involving organic brain disorders. In the nursing home study, Parmalee, Katz, and Lawton (1989) found that nearly half of the respondents diagnosed with major depression also had significant cognitive deficits. The problem arises because (1) it is known that depression symptoms can arise secondary to dementia and (2) depression can create cognitive deficits in the absence of organic causes (depressive epsudodementia). Hence, care must be taken in assigning diagnoses based upon a single interview. It has been suggested that pseudodementia can be detected by inconsistencies in cognitive test performance, but such inconsistencies are only determinable by repeated testing (Alexopoulos et al, 1988). Most community surveys are not designed to do this, although it would not be entirely out of the question, given a base rate of severe cognitive impairment of under 5 percent in the community-based elderly population (Regier et al, 1988).

It appears to be beyond the capacity of symptom-based, self-report instruments, such as the DIS or SADS, to make such differential diagnoses. Hence, epidemiologists concerned with such phenomena need to report patterns of co-morbidity carefully until satisfactory techniques for generating diagnostic hierarchies can be devised.

Other Selection Factors

It has been suggested that the inverse relationship between age and the prevalence of psychiatric conditions could be a function of factors that tend to select the morbid elderly out of the population prior to household sampling.

Other factors are also important in this regard, such as homelessness. Since community survey techniques are generally predicated upon assumptions regarding a stable place of residence, the older homeless simply do not get included—even though recent studies have shown them to have high rates of schizophrenia–schizophreniform disorder (7.8 percent), manic depressive illness (6.1 percent), major depression (13.3 percent), alcohol abuse–dependence (76.3 percent), and other substance abuse–dependence (17.9 percent). Although the elderly are not overly represented in the homeless population, the failure to include the homeless elderly can distort the overall picture of the psychiatric burden of the elderly. Yet the difficulties of drawing probability samples of these individuals for estimation purposes are enormous and provide a major challenge for the epidemiologist.

A final factor to be considered—respondent shielding—operates somewhat differently. Shielding occurs whenever an eligible respondent is located in a household, but household representatives disallow the possibility of an interview for the "protection" of the respondent. Three groups are most likely to be shielded from interviews: children, the elderly, and the ill or disabled. There is, of course, an overlap between the latter two populations.

When illness or disability is the issue, it is often possible to obtain a "proxy" interview. In this case the person who best knows the target respondent is interviewed to obtain symptom reports. The value of such data is highly suspect since it is based upon the assumption that psychiatric symptoms are either apparent or reported to the proxy respondent. The fact is that proxy respondents are generally unable to answer many key questions, and interviews are usually incomplete. In the Colorado Social Health Survey, a statewide survey of 4745 noninstitutionalized adults (Ciarlo et al, 1986), a total of 44 proxy interviews were collected. The average age of the target respondents was over 70 years old, as compared to an average age of 44 for the nonproxy sample.

One additional selection factor is nonresponse. Older persons with a given psychiatric condition may be less willing to participate in household surveys, or are less accessible. Also, mentally disabled respondents may be shielded by other household members. Shielding can also occur for less beneficent reasons. Shielding cases of elder abuse is of specific concern here. The incidence of this social problem in the general population, however, is difficult to estimate. The cost to the abused elderly in terms of mental and emotional anguish and related psychopathology must be extremely high.

Design Factors

Age Versus Cohort Effects

The interpretation of data from community samples of older adults in cross-sectional studies must take place within the context of period and cohort effects. Relative differences in the prevalence of symptoms or disorders across the life cycle may be incorrectly interpreted as deriving from age differences when cohort and period effects actually predominate. This problem was well illustrated in a large epidemiologic study initially fielded in 1954 in which subjects were reinterviewed in 1974 [i.e., the Midtown Manhattan Study (Srole and Fischer, 1986)]. In the 1954 survey of 1660 individuals between the ages of 20 and 59, the investigators found a symptom distribution that suggested older persons (between 50 and 59 years of age) suffered more frequent mental health impairment (22 percent) than younger persons (7 percent among the 20–29-year age group). The subjects were reinterviewed in 1974 and the same relative distribution was found; that is, among subjects 70–79 years of age, 18 percent suffered mental health impairment, whereas only 8 percent of the subjects 40–49 years of age suffered mental health impairment. When the cohorts were compared at the two points in time (the 50–59-year-olds in 1954 were the 70–79-years olds in 1974), there was no clear increase in mental health impairment with age. The cohort into which individuals were born was therefore a more important factor in determining the relative burden of symptoms than the age of the subject. Evidence of period effects was also observed.

It has been suggested that the similar cohort–period effect is at work within the ECA depression data—with the inverse relationship between age and depression prevalence due to a dramatic increase in the rate of depression among adolescents and young adults (Klerman, 1988; Klerman et al, 1985). A study of a sample of 1323 elderly respondents by Haug, Belgrave, and Gratton (1984) sought to test the hypothesis that mental health declines with age. The study found that, contrary to expectation, observed psychopathology was more likely to remain stable or improve over time, but the one-year interval seems too short to draw conclusions about age effects. Nevertheless, the wisdom of assuming the observed ECA relationship represents an age effect can be reasonably questioned.

QUESTIONS OF VALIDITY

Thus far we have looked at a number of factors that should make us pause before we draw conclusions about the nature of the relationship betwen age and the prevalence of psychiatric morbidity. We have not yet questioned the validity of the data underlying the observed relationship, however. Yet there is reason to be cautious when evaluating such data. Before attempting to explain the age–prevalence relationship, it is prudent to eliminate (or at least be aware of) other methodological factors that could bias the observed pattern in an artifactual manner.

In the remainder of this chapter we shall review several characteristics of the elderly respondent that can make the use of self-report, autobiographical symptom data problematic. We discuss the implications of these characteristics for the ECA age-specific rate data and illustrate the kinds of problems that can arise using data from the DIS-based Colorado Social Health Survey.

Response Styles

Psychologists and educators concerned with testing for individual differences have long been aware that responses to questionnaires and interviews are often determined by factors other than the constructs the component questions were designed to measure. Factors such as the respondent's intelligence and education, speed of item presentation, item complexity, and so on, can often structure the response in directions not intended. A class of such factors that are particularly pertinent here are "response styles." Nunnally (1967, p. 593) defines a response style as "(1) a reliable source of variance in individual differences which (2) is an artifactual product of measurement methods and (3) is at least partially independent of the trait which the measurement methods are intended to measure." Such response styles become important when they are correlated with a variable of central concern, such as age.

Socially Desirable Responses

Ross and Mirowsky (1984) have suggested that the tendency to give desirable responses and/or acquiescent responses may affect reported symptomatology among the elderly and lead to biased psychiatric assessments. Obtaining an indirect measure of the propensity to give socially desirable responses, these researchers found that the negative relationship between age and psychological distress (as observed in their sample) was largely accounted for by the positive correlation between age and this response style (Ross and Mirowsky, 1984, p. 196). Although more work needs to be done in this area, epidemiologists need to be aware of this potential bias and work to mitigate those conditions that might encourage such response patterns.

Reticence to Report Mood States

Related to the tendency to give socially desirable responses is the clinically observed reticence to report feeling states among the elderly (*APA,* 1980, p. 212; 1987, p. 220). Such reticence is particularly troublesome with regard to depression, where the respondent has to report a significant period of depressed mood (dysphoria or anhedonia) as a precondition for a diagnosis. Hence, if the elderly are reluctant to admit to depressed mood, they will not be given a diagnosis and the prevalence of major depression will be underestimated.

Problems with Recall and Memory

Research has demonstrated that there are strong memory decay functions operative in survey respondents in general. For example, Bradburn, Rips, and Shevell (1987, p. 158) report that a recent study of recall for personal events "found that 20% of critical details—selected at the time of occurrence to be 'certainly' remembered if the events were recognized—were irretrievable after 1 year; 60% were irretrievable after 5 years." Similar findings have been observed in studies involving respondents to longitudinal mental health surveys (Andreasen et al, 1981; Aneshensel et al, 1987; Bromet et al, 1986; Kendell, 1988). Commenting on the study by Bromet et al, Kendel notes that when the "Schedule for Affective Disorders (SADS) was administered to a community sample on two occasions 18 months apart more than half of the episodes of major depression reported on the first occasion were no longer reported, or not reported in sufficient detail to fulfill major depressive criteria, on the second occasion" (p. 375).

When the respondent is elderly the problem of recall may be exacerbated by age-related declines in general cognitive functioning and related problems in the encoding, storage, or retrieval of biographical information. There is considerable evidence that performance on memory tasks declines with age (Weinert, 1983). It is important to know why this decline occurs. Some, for example, have suggested that there is a simple decrease in mental capacity. Others have argued that the decrements arise from changes in the efficiency with which information is stored and recalled—the system becomes less efficient and slows down. Finally, others have postulated that feelings and knowledge about the ability to perform memory tasks can affect our performance on such tasks. Bandura (1989), for example, has demonstrated that perceptions regarding self-efficacy on memory tasks can predict performance on such tasks. The elderly tend to lack confidence about their ability to remember events and systematically tend to underestimate their actual performance (Weinert et al, 1983).

It is important to know whether and how these declines affect interview data. Herzog and Dielman (1985) checked on the veracity of factual reports by age group and found no reliable differences. However, the accuracy of information recalled is a different question from whether the recall process itself is impaired. Aneshensel et al (1987) analyzed patterns of discrepant symptom reports between baseline and follow-up interviews using the SADS instrument. Within the context of a multivariate model, they found that age was not a significant factor in the explanation of such discrepancies. To the extent that these discrepant reports are a function of problems with recall, this would suggest that age-related recall biases do not exist.

There is evidence within the ECA, however, that age-related deficits in recall may be creating problems and may be biasing prevalence estimates. This was suggested by Robins et al (1984) after their analysis of age patterns in the lifetime prevalence rates. Within the DIS, lifetime rates are based upon an assessment of "symptoms ever experienced" and are particularly prone to biases due to age-related problems with recall. The lifetime prevalence rates were found to parallel the one-month prevalence rates presented earlier, with the highest rates being found in the younger age groups and the lowest rates being found among the elderly. Unless there was an overwhelming cohort effect, it made little sense that the elderly (who had the greatest cumulative exposure to risk) had the lowest rates.

It would seem, however, that the effects of age-related problems with recall would be minimized when estimating one-month prevalence rates such as those presented in Table 13-1. Therefore, even if the lifetime rates are biased, the one-month rates would not be. Yet an analysis of the diagnostic algorithm used to arrive at a DIS/DSM-III diagnosis of major depression implies that effects are entirely possible, and—at least in the DIS-based Colorado Social Health Survey (Ciarlo et al, 1986) data—do appear to be operative.

This effect works in the following way. Within the DIS depression section, the interviewer begins by establishing whether the respondent has *ever* experienced the requisite period of dysphoric mood and/or anhedonia. Next, the interviewer reviews a list of 16 specific symptoms that often characterize major depression. These symptoms are organized into nine symptom domains. The interviewer then establishes if there was *ever* a time when the respondent had both a depressed mood and *some* of the associated symptoms. This kind of episode is called a "spell." If the respondent replies "yes," then the interviewer inquires as to the last time the respondent had such a "spell" and the timing and symptomatology associated with the "worst" spell ever experienced. Based upon this information the respondent will receive a one-month diagnosis if (1) they had experienced a "spell" within the month prior to the interview and (2) during the "worst" spell they had experienced symptoms within at least four of the nine symptom domains.

The problem with the DIS diagnostic algorithm is that it assesses the recency of the diagnosis at the spell level rather than at the symptom level (Von Korff and Anthony, 1982). Hence, even though the algorithm requires that the respondent experienced a spell during the past month, it does not require this spell to be fully diagnosable. For example, it is quite possible for an individual to qualify for a one-month diagnosis with a spell that involved symptoms in only one of the associated symptom domains. Lifetime symptoms, then (occurring more than one month prior to the interview), can count toward a diagnosis and lead to an inappropriate diagnosis. For such respondents the data would suggest that the "spell" was not a full-blown depressive syndrome. The result would be a false positive case of major depression.

If age-related differences in recall are operative, we would expect such false positives to be least likely to occur among the elderly, since they are the least likely to recall and report past symptomatology that might contribute to a misdiagnosis. Tweed, Ciarlo, and Blazer (in progress) were able to determine if such age-related effects were present using the modified version of the DIS employed in the Colorado Social Health Survey (CSHS). Within the Colorado version of the DIS, questions regarding recency information were incorporated at both the symptom and the spell level for several disorders, including major depression. Using these symptom-level recencies, it is possible to upgrade the depression diagnostic algorithm so that the spell necessarily involves the requisite number of symptoms within the one-month constraint. Hence, the revised algorithm ought to minimize effect of false positives. It is useful then to compare the age-specific prevalence rates for major depressive episodes and to study the pattern of false positives suggested by this comparison. This is accomplished in Table 13-2. The first column presents the rates of depression within four age groupings. Using the Colorado data, the pattern resembles that found in the ECA sites with the highest rates among the younger age groups and the lowest rates among the elderly. The chi square value suggests that the prevalence rates differ significantly among the age groups. (Note that the data in Table 13-2 are based upon unweighted sample data and should not be used for drawing inferences about the prevalence of major depression in the general Colorado population).

Table 13-2 Effect of Choice of Diagnostic Algorithm on the Estimated Prevalence of Depression (by age group)[a]

	Estimated prevalence			
Age group	Original[b] algorithm (%)	Revised[c] algorithm (%)	False[d] positive rate (%)	No. of cases
18–24	2.9	1.5	50.0	616
25–44	2.6	1.0	62.5	2165
45–64	1.4	0.6	56.3	1153
65 plus	1.3	1.1	11.1	796
Chi-square	10.1	3.3	9.57	
P-value	.02	.34	.02	

[a]Data taken from the Colorado Social Health Survey.

[b]In the original algorithm respondents get a one-month diagnosis if they have *ever* had a diagnosable "worst" spell and their most recent spell occurred within the month prior to the interview. The most recent spell need not be diagnosable.

[c]The revised algorithm requires that within the past month, the respondent must have experienced dysphoric mood plus at least four other symptoms—as per DSM-III-R guidelines.

[d]This is the percentage of cases identified under the original algorithm who failed to meet criteria under the revised algorithm.

The second column gives the results of the revised algorithm and tells a very different story. First, the shape of the relationship has changed and the elderly no longer have the lowest rates of depression. Moreover, the associated chi square is nonsignificant, suggesting that the data are consistent with the hypothesis that the prevalence of depression is uniform across age groups. Hence, the nonintuitive inverse relationship, which previously required explanation, is no longer apparent. The relationship, instead, appears to be a function of the choice of diagnostic algorithm.

The next-to-last column of Table 13-2 tells the important story. Reported are the estimated rates of false-positive diagnoses under the old diagnostic algorithm. This rate varies from an average of around 55 percent for the three youngest age groups to slightly more than 11 percent for the elderly. This pattern is consistent with the presence of an age-related recall effect.

Lessons Learned

The preceding analysis suggests two important lessons. First, indirectly at least, the effects of recall do appear to be operative in the CSHS data and are probably operative in the ECA data as well. Only a reanalysis of the data at those ECA sites that collected symptom-level recency data will verify this inference. The Duke, Baltimore, and Los Angeles ECAs collected symptom-level recency data and permit this type of reanalysis.

It is true that response-style factors could also be operative in the preceding CSHS results. It is unlikely that social desirability plays a significant role in the preceding findings, however, and should be operating to mitigate the effects of differences in recall. In fact, one would assume that if social desirability were a factor, it would be easier to admit to past "undesirable" conditions than to present ones. (It is, for instance, easier to admit to past illicit drug use than to current use.) If such effects are present they are more likely to affect the reports of current symptoms. As a consequence current rates may be underestimated. Unfortunately, there is no direct way of estimating the size of such effects.

Second, when we speak of the validity of structured diagnostic interviews, we need to think at multiple levels. For example, we can be concerned with the validity of particular items meant to assess specific symptom domains. Almost exclusively, the validation work reported on the DIS has been at the diagnosis level (Anthony et al, 1985; Helzer et al, 1985; Robins, 1985; Robins et al, 1982). Yet the diagnosis is only as good as the data on which it is based. We can work to improve the process by which symptoms are assessed so as to maximize validity. Much symptom-level validation needs to done with respect to the DIS.

Independent of the validity of the symptom data, we also need to think about validity at the level of the diagnostic process—the validity of the process by which we move from symptom data to inferences regarding the presence of a disorder. The diagnostic validation work that has been done thus far has taken the current diagnostic algorithms as given and simply looked for agreement between modes of diagnosis (DIS-based versus clinician-based, for example). Yet misspecification at the diagnostic level can lead to serious problems of internal validity even if the symptom data are perfectly valid. We have seen how such problems may interact with the characteristics of the elderly respondent to lead to inappropriate conclusions regarding the age–prevalence relationship.

PSYCHIATRIC MORBIDITY IN ELDERLY POPULATIONS: ANOTHER LOOK

As noted at the outset of this chapter, the ECA data are the repository of much of what we know about the psychiatric morbidity in elderly populations. Yet it is clear that inadequate nosology, selection factors, and diagnostic validity issues have introduced noise into the information this data base has provided us. By revising the diagnostic algorithms for a reanalysis of the existing data base we may be able to eliminate some of that noise.

The data presented here, for example, would suggest that the rates of depression in the elderly population are at least as great as those for the rest of the population—contrary to the initial inferences based upon the original diagnostic algorithm. When consideration is given to the potential biases introduced by institutional selection, response styles, and so on, the rates of psychiatric morbidity may well be much higher among the elderly. Only future research can determine this.

THE FUTURE

Instrumentation

It is clear that epidemiologists have much to do if we are to have a better understanding of the psychiatric burden of the elderly and the impact of aging on mental health. At the outset, work needs to be done in terms of instrumentation for assessing psychiatric morbidity in elderly populations. We feel that much can be done with existing instruments, such as the DIS and SADS. These instruments have much to recommend them, but more validation studies should be performed at the symptom assessment and diagnostic levels, with a special regard for how these processes can interact with characteristics of the elderly to give biased information.

There is also much that can be done (given current instrumentation) to make them better suited to the elderly. Simply modifying the speed of presentation may mitigate some of the apparent effects of recall on symptom recall among the elderly. Studies have shown that the effects of age on memory are minimized when more time is provided to perform memory tasks. Hence, interviewers need to be aware of this need and to provide ample time for elderly respondents.

The debate over lay interviewers versus clinical interviewers may also be more critical among the elderly than among the rest of the adult population, given the clinically observed reticence to report emotional status. Clinical training may be necessary when there is reason to suspect self-reports.

Nosology and Nomenclature

At the same time it is difficult to talk about improving instrumentation without a prior concern for advancing psychiatric nosology. As Robins (1989) has made clear, there is a fundamental duality between nosology and instrumentation. Instrumentation will only be as good as the nosology it embodies.

Epidemiologists have an important role to play in the evolution of psychiatric nosology through research. Kendell (1989) recently described the need to validate our diagnostic categories, suggesting that we may have been caught up in a drive for reliable diagnosis without an attendant concern for validity. Meehl (1986) has made similar observations and suggests a need to consider current diagnostic entities as "open concepts" so as to maximize the potential impact of ongoing research.

Nowhere is this more clear than in the study of psychopathology in community populations. As noted earlier, we are seeing a broad range of symptomatology in these studies that is not well described in the current DSM-III literature. Could this reflect uncatalogued forms of psychiatric morbidity? There are historical precedents that lead us to believe so. Yet postulation of new morbid conditions needs to proceed slowly, with a deep regard for validation and understanding of the lines of continuity between new morbid variants and currently understood entities.

The technology for exploring this surplus symptomatology—for uncovering recurrent and meaningful syndromes—is still developing. Techniques such as cluster analysis and Q-techniques have been applied in the past. The problem, however, is that such techniques tend to find structure when it may not be present, and the "structure" found may be more products of sampling and unreliable variance than of true latent entities. Thus, if one specifies a 10-cluster solution, that is what will be produced, regardless of the underlying structure of the data. Clearly, we need to develop taxonomic strategies that guard against such occurrences.

Recently developed techniques, such as Grade of Membership (GOM), show promise as tools for nosologic research (Woodbury and Manton, 1982). Based upon the theory of fuzzy sets rather than crisp sets, this technique allows the exploration of complex data sets in meaningful ways. At this time the prospects for understanding psychopathology through GOM look exciting (Blazer et al, 1988; Blazer et al, 1989; Swartz et al, 1986). Yet such excitement needs to be tempered by the recognition of the subsequent need for clinical and field validation.

Studies in Institutionalized Populations

Given the increasing role of nursing homes and other institutional settings in the elderly population, more basic epidemiologic research needs to be conducted in these settings. In this way we can get a more balanced perspective of the burden of mental illness among the elderly. Longitudinal studies must clearly be prepared to follow elderly populations into these settings and confront the kinds of challenges they provide for psychiatric research. Problems of co-morbidity are particularly important here.

Longitudinal Studies

The impact of aging as a risk factor for psychiatric morbidity can only be understood through prospective, longitudinal designs. Only such studies provide any hope of sorting out age effects from the cohort and period effects with which they nearly always are confounded. Cross-sectional studies, although useful in suggesting new questions and hypotheses, are of limited utility in disentangling such effects. Yet longitudinal studies must be devised carefully. Initial cohorts must be assembled carefully, so as to minimize selection effects. The impact of cohort losses to mortality and other conditions must be assessed. Undoubtedly the statistical tools used to sort out these effects in longitudinal studies are going to become more complicated. The analysis of change data is complex and is fraught with difficulties.

In sum, much remains to be done. The prospects and challenges, however, are exciting. Further, as our population ages, the need for valid and reliable information regarding our elderly population becomes increasingly important.

REFERENCES

Alexopoulos G, Young R, Holt J (1988). Geriatric depressive disorders. In J Mann (ed), Phenomenology of Depressive Illness. New York, Human Science Press.

American Psychiatric Association (APA) (1987). Diagnostic and Statistical Manual of Mental Disorders, 3rd ed. Washington, DC.

American Psychiatric Association (APA) (1980). Diagnostic and Statistical Manual of Mental Disorders, 3rd ed. Washington, DC.

Andreason N, Grove W, Shapiro R, Keller M, Hirshfeld R, McDonald-Scott P (1981). Reliability of lifetime diagnosis: A multicenter collaborative perspective. Arch Gen Psychiatr 38:400–405.

Aneshensel C, Estrada A, Hansell M, Clark V (1987). Social psychological aspects of reporting behavior: Lifetime depressive episode reports. J Health Soc Behav 28:232–246.

Anthony J, Folstein M, Romanoski A, Von Korff M, Nestadt G, Chahal R, Merchant A, Brown C, Shapiro S, Kramer M, Gruenberg E (1985). Comparison of lay Diagnostic Interview Schedule and a standardized psychiatric diagnosis: Experience in eastern Baltimore. Arch Gen Psychiatr 42:667–775.

Bandura A (1989). Regulation of cognitive processes through perceived self-efficacy. Dev Psychol 25:729–735.

Blazer D, Houpt J (1979). Perception of poor health in the healthy older adult. J Am Geriatr Soc 27:330–334.

Blazer D, Bachar J, Hughes D (1987a). Major depression with melancholia: A comparison of middle-aged and elderly adults. J Am Geriatr Soc 35:927–932.

Blazer D, Bachar J, Manton K (1987b). Suicide in late life: Review and Commentary. J Am Geriatr Soc 34:519–525.

Blazer D, Hughes D, George L (1987c). The epidemiology of depression in an elderly community population. Gerontologist 27:281–287.

Blazer D, Swartz M, Woodbury M, Manton K, Hughes L, George L (1988). Depressive symptoms and depressive diagnoses in a community population: Use of a new procedure for analysis of psychiatric classification. Arch Gen Psychiatr 45:1078–1084.

Blazer D, Woodbury M, Hughes D, George L, Manton K, Bachar J, Fowler N (1989). A statistical analysis of the classification of depression in a mixed community and clinical sample. J Affective Disord 16:11–20.

Bradurn N, Rips L, Shevell S (1987). Answering autobiographical questions: The impact of memory and inference on surveys. Science 236:157–161.

Bromet E, Dunn L, Connell M, Dew M, Schulberg H (1986). Long-term reliability of diagnosing lifetime major depression in a community sample. Arch Gen Psychiatr 43:435–440.

Burke J, Sartorius N (1988). Development of the Composite International Diagnostic Interview. DIS Newsletter 5:1–2.

Ciarlo J, Shern D, Tweed D, Sachs-Ericsson N (1986). Estimating need for mental health and substance abuse services: Social indicators versus directly surveyed need. DIS Newsletter.

Dohrenwend B, Dohrenwend B (1969). Social Status and Psychological Disorder: A Causal Inquiry. New York, Wiley.

Dupuy H (1973). Developmental rationale, substantive, derivative, and conceptual relevance of general well-being. Washington, DC, National Center for Health Statistics (Working Paper).

Edgerton J, Bentz W, Hollister W (1970). Demographic factors and responses to stress among rural people. Am J Public Health, 60:1065–1071.

Endicott J, Spitzer R (1978). A diagnostic interview. Arch Gen Psychiatr 35:837–844.

Feighner J, Robins E, Guze S, Woodruff R, Winokur G, Munoz R (1972). Diagnostic criteria for use in psychiatric research. Arch Gen Psychiatr 26:57–63.

Feinstein A (1970). The pre-therapeutic classification of co-morbidity in chronic disease. J Chronic Disability 23:455–468.

Goodwin D, Guze S (1989). Psychiatric Diagnosis. New York, Oxford University Press.

Haug M, Belgrave L, Gratton B (1984). Mental health and the elderly: Factors in stability and change over time. J Health Soc Behav 25:100–115.

Helzer J, Robins L, McEvoy L, Spitznagel E, Stoltzman R, Farmer A, Brockington I (1985). A comparison of clinical and diagnostic interview schedule diagnoses. Arch Gen Psychiatr 42:657–666.

Herzog A, Dielman L (1985). Age differences in response accuracy for factual survey questions. J Gerontol 40:350–357.

Hing E (1987). Use of nursing homes by the elderly: Preliminary data from the 1985 National Nursing Home Survey. Advance data from Vital and Health Statistics, No. 135, National Center for Health Statistics, DHHS Pub. No. (PHS) 87–1250.

Kendell R (1988). What is a case?: Food for thought for epidemiologists. Arch Gen Psychiatr 45:374–376.

Kendell R (1989). Clinical validity. Psychol Med 19:45–55.

Klerman G (1985). Diagnosis of psychiatric disorders in epidemiologic field studies. Arch Gen Psychiatr 42:723–724.

Klerman G (1986). Historical perspectives on contemporary schools of psychopathology. In T Millon, G Klerman (eds.), Contemporary Directions in Psychopathology: Toward the DSM-IV. New York, Guilford Press.

Klerman G (1988). The current age of youthful melancholia: Evidence for increase in depression among adolescents and young adults. Br J Psychiatr 152:4–14.

Klerman G (1989). Psychiatric diagnostic categories: Issues of validity and measurement. J Health Soc Behav 30:26–32.

Klerman G, Lavori P, Rice J, Reich T, Endicott J, Andreason N, Keller M, Hirschfield R (1985). Birth-cohort trends in rates of major depressive disorder among relatives of patients with affective disorder. Arch Gen Psychiatr 42:689–693.

Koenig H, Meador K, Cohen H, Blazer D (1988). Depression in elderly hospitalized patients with medical illness. Arch Gen Med 148:1929–1936.

Langner T (1986). What do instruments like the 22-item screening score measure?: A look at correlates and a review of construct validity. In M Weissman, J Mycrs, C Ross (eds), Community Surveys of Psychiatric Disorders. New Brunswick, NJ, Rutgers University Press.

Leenaars A (1989). Are young adult suicides psychologically different from those of other adults? (the Shneidman Lecture). Suicide and Life Threatening Behavior 19:249–263.

Manton M, Blazer D, Woodbury M (1987). Suicide in middle age and later life: Sex and race specific life table and cohort analyses. J Gerontol 42:219–227.

Meehl P (1986). Diagnostic taxa as open concepts: Metatheoretical and statistical questions about reliability and construct validity in the grand strategy of nosological revision. In T Millon, G Klerman (eds), Contemporary Directions in Psychopathology: Toward the DSM-IV. New York, Guilford Press.

Millon T (1986). On the past and future of DSM-III: Personal recollections and projections. In T Millon, G Klerman (eds), Contemporary Directions in Psychopathology: Toward the DSM-IV. New York, Guilford Press.

Mortimer J, Schuman L, French L (1983). Epidemiology of dementing illness. In J Mortimer, L Schuman (eds), The Epidemiology of Dementia. New York, Oxford University Press.

Murphy J, Monson R, Oliver D, Sobol A, Leighton A (1987). Affective disorders and mortality: A general population study. Arch Gen Psychiatr 44:473–480.

Newman F, Griffin B, Black R, Page S (1989). Linking level of care to level of need: Assessing the need for mental health care in nursing home residents. Am Psychologist 44:1315–1324.

Nunnally J (1967). Psychometric Theory. New York, McGraw-Hill.

Paffenbarger R, King S, Wing A (1966). Chronic disease in former college students: IX. Characteristics in youth that predispose to suicide and accidental death in later life. Am J Public Health 59:900–908.

Parmalee P, Katz I, Lawton M (1989). Depression among institutionalized aged: Assessment and prevalence estimation. J Gerontol 44:1722–1729.

Regier D, Boyd J, Burke J, Rae D, Myers J, Kramer M, Robins L, George L, Karno M, Locke B (1988). One-month prevalence of mental disorders in the United States: Based on five epidemiologic catchment area sites. Arch Gen Psychiatr 45:977–986.

Regier D, Myers J, Kramer M, Robins L, Blazer D, Hough R, Eaton W, Locke B (1985). The NIMH epidemiologic catchment area program: Historical context, major objectives, and study population characteristics. Arch Gen Psychiatr 41:934–941.

Robins L (1985). Epidemiology: Reflections on testing the validity of psychiatric interviews. Arch Gen Psychiatr 42:918–924.

Robins L (1989). Diagnostic grammar and assessment: Translating criteria into questions. Psychol Med 19:57–68.

Robins L, Helzer J, Croughan J, Ratcliff K (1981). National Institute of Mental Health Diagnostic Interview Schedule: Its history, characteristics and validity. Arch Gen Psychiatr 38:381–386.

Robins L, Helzer J, Ratcliff K, Seyfried W (1982). Validity of the Diagnostic Interview Schedule, Version II: DSM-III diagnoses. Psychol Med 12:855–870.

Robins R, Helzer J, Weissman M, Orvaschel H, Gruenberg E, Burke J, Regier D (1984). Lifetime prevalence of specific disorders in three sites. Arch Gen Psychiatr 41:949–958.

Ross C, Mirowsky J (1984). Socially desirable response and acquiescence in a cross-cultural survey of mental health. J Health Soc Behav 25:189–197.

Sawyer-Radloff L, Locke B (1986). The community mental health assessment survey and the CES-D scale. In M Weissman, J Myers, C Ross (eds). Community Surveys of Psychiatric Disorders. New Brunswick, NJ, Rutgers University Press.

Schwab J, Fennel E, Warheit G (1974). The epidemiology of psychosomatic illnesses. Psychosomatics 15:88–93.

Shekelle R, Raynor W, Ostfeld A, Garron D, Bieliauskas L, Liu S, Maliza C, Paul O (1981). Psychological depression and 17-year risk of death due to cancer. Psychosom Med 43:117–125.

Smyer M (1989). Nursing homes as a setting for psychology practice: Public policy prospectives. Am Psychologist 44:1307–1314.

Spitzer R, Endicott J, Robins L (1978). Clinical criteria for psychiatric diagnosis and the DSM-III. Am J Psychiatr 132:1187–1192.

Srole L, Fischer A (1986). The Midtown Manhattan Longitudinal Study: Aging, generations and genders. In M Weissman, J Meyers, C Ross (eds), Community Surveys of Psychiatric Disorders. New Brunswick, NJ, Rutgers University Press.

Sussman N (1988). Diagnosis and drug treatment of anxiety in the elderly. Geriatr Med Today 7:37–52.

Swartz M, Blazer D, Woodbury M, George L, Landerman D (1986). Somatization disorder in a US southern community: Use of a new procedure for analysis of medical classification. Psychol Med 16:595–609.

Tsuang M, Simpson J (1985). Mortality studies in psychiatry: Should they stop or proceed? Arch Gen Psychiatr 49:28–103.

Tweed D, Ciarlo J, Blazer D (in progress). Age and the prevalence of depression: A potential artifact.

Von Korff M, Anthony J (1982). The NIMH Diagnostic Interview Schedule modified to record current mental status. J Affective Disord 4:365–371.

Warheit G (1976). The mental health of a rural county: An epidemiologic overview. In R Reynolds, S Banks (eds). The Health of a Rural County: Perspectives and Problems. Gainsville, University of Florida Press.

Weinert F, Knoph M, Barann G (1983). Metakognition und Motivation als Determinanten von Gedachtnisleistungen im hoheren Erwachsenenalter. Sprache & Kognition 2:71–87.

Weissman M, Myers J (1978). Rates and risks of depressive symptoms in a United States urban community. Acta Psychiatr Scand 57:219–231.

Williams J, Endicott J, Spitzer R (1989). Some biometrics contributions to assessment: PSS, CAPPS, SADS-L/RDC, and DSM-III. In M Weissman, J Meyers, C Ross (eds), Community Surveys of Psychiatric Disorders. New Brunswick, NJ, Rutgers University Press.

Woodbury M, Manton K (1982). A new procedure for analysis of medical classification. Meth Inform Med 21:210–220.

Zung W (1967). Depression in the normal aged. Psychosomatics 8:287–292.

14

Epidemiologic Research on Nursing Home Populations

DANIEL J. FOLEY

Epidemiologic investigations conducted in older populations need to address the representativeness of the study population as early in the design of the study as possible. Some of the oldest members of a community may be residents in local nursing homes, domiciliary-care homes, or other facilities for long-term care. Data are presented here on the size and scope of the nursing home population nationwide, the reasons for admission, and the health status of the residents. Epidemiologic research on risk factors for institutionalization and on the geriatric conditions predominant in the nursing home population is discussed in the context of a growing number of residents.

SOURCES OF DATA

The National Master Facility Inventory Surveys (NMFI), conducted periodically by the National Center for Health Statistics, establish lists and summary statistics on the number of nursing and related-care facilities and beds in the United States (Roper, 1986; Sirrocco, 1989; Strahan, 1984). The most recent NMFI, conducted in 1986, was called the Inventory of Long-Term Care Places because the scope of coverage was expanded to include facilities for mental retardation.

To be classified as a nursing or related-care home in the NMFI, a facility needed to have at least three beds and provide nursing care, or provide personal care and/or custodial care to the residents. Eligible facilities were classified further as either a nursing home or a residential-care facility based on certification by an accrediting agency for Medicare and/or Medicaid program reimbursements. Facilities certified as skilled nursing facilities (SNFs), intermediate-care facilities (ICFs), or both, were called nursing homes. Facilities licensed by the state as nursing homes, but not certified under the Medicare and Medicaid programs, were also categorized as nursing homes. The remainder were called residential-care facilities.

The next NMFI is scheduled for completion in 1991 and will further expand the scope of coverage to include hospice facilities and home health care agencies. Furthermore, a change in federal regulations has established new standards that replaced the ICF–SNF distinction for nursing homes. This policy will result primarily in an upgrading of many ICF facilities for continued certification under the Medicare and Medicaid programs (US House of Representatives, 1987).

In addition to its function as an inventory, the NMFI provides a sampling frame for the ad hoc National Nursing Home Surveys (NNHS) conducted by the National Center for Health Statistics in 1973, 1977, and most recently in 1985 (Hing et al, 1989; Sutton, 1977; Van Nostrand et al, 1979). The next survey will not be conducted until 1993. The NNHS provide nationally representative data on characteristics of the facilities, the current residents, the discharged residents, and the staff. The NNHS does not include board-and-care homes or facilities providing only residential care. An updated listing of facilities enumerated in the 1982 National Master Facility Inventory served as the sampling frame for the 1985 NNHS. Data about the facility are based on an interview with the administrator or some other designated person. Information about the sampled current resident is based on data from the medical record in conjunction with an interview with the staff member most familiar with the resident's care (usually a nurse). Data on a sample of discharges that occurred in the year prior to the survey are based on an interview with a staff member most familiar with the medical record for the discharged resident. Data about the nursing staff are based on questionnaires filled out and returned by a sample of registered nurses and on the administrator's interview questionnaire.

PREVALENCE AND INCIDENCE OF INSTITUTIONALIZATION

The 1986 NMFI included data on 16,388 free-standing nursing homes, 734 hospital-based nursing homes, and 9258 residential-care facilities that supported a total of 1,767,497 beds. The free-standing and hospital-based nursing homes accounted for 85 percent and 4 percent of the nation's nursing home beds, respectively. The residential-care facilities represented the remaining 11 percent of beds (Sirrocco, 1989).

The 1985 NNHS data estimated that about 1.3 million people age 65 and over (about 5 percent of the older population) were residents of the free-standing and hospital-based nursing homes. This number represented an 18 percent increase over the 1.1 million residents in 1977 and a 37 percent increase over the 960,000 elderly residents in 1973 (Hing, 1989a). The 5 percent prevalence rate for nursing home residency has remained fairly constant over the years as the increase in the number of elderly nursing home residents has kept pace with a concurrent increase in the population age 65 and over.

The 1986 NMFI data showed that the certification, supply of beds, and number of residents per 1000 population varied considerably by state. For example, in the three states of Iowa, Minnesota, and South Carolina, more than 7 percent of persons over the age of 65 were residing in nursing homes compared to less than 3 percent in Hawaii, Arizona, Florida, Nevada, New Mexico, and West Virginia. The remaining states had a prevalence rate between 3 and 7 percent (Sirrocco, 1989).

State policies on administration of the Medicaid program, including waivers for local options to nursing home admission, influence the number of nursing home beds licensed and certified statewide (Foley, 1980; Harrington and Swan, 1987; Madans, 1981). Aside from direct out-of-pocket pay, Medicaid reimbursement is the principal source of funding for nursing-home care nationwide and covers about 40 percent of annual expenditures (Schneider and Guralnik, 1990).

The probability of using nursing-home care at some time before death (i.e., the lifetime risk) is much higher than the probability for being a nursing-home resident on any given day (i.e., the prevalence rate). Assuming no change in the current prevalence rates, over half the women and nearly one third of the men who turn age 65 in 1990 can expect to enter a nursing home at some time prior to their death (Murtaugh et al, 1990). The lifetime risk will vary from community to community relative to the supply of beds and the different cultural and ethnic views about institutionalization predominant in the community.

Incidence data on nursing-home admissions are not well established at the national level and exist only for a few communities at the subnational level. A one-year followup of medical records on a sample of noninstitutionalized Medicare enrollees in 1977 showed that about 3 percent subsequently received physician services in a nursing home. This annual incidence rate was considered an underestimate for nursing home admission since some residents may not have been visited by a physician in the nursing home during the period of the study. The authors conclude that the actual annual incidence rate may be as high as 5 percent (Cohen et al, 1986a). Community-based studies have reported three-year incidence rates for nursing-home admissions ranging from 4 percent to a high of 12 percent in a rural area of Iowa (Kelman and Thomas, 1990; Foley et al, 1992).

REASONS FOR ADMISSION

In 1985, an estimated 1.3 million persons were admitted to nursing homes, and for many of them it would not be the first time. The 1985 NNHS reported that about 38 percent of the residents in nursing homes had a prior stay at either the same facility or another nursing home. Over one third of the admissions entered from a private or semiprivate residence, another third were admitted from a general or short-stay hospital, and about 12 percent were admitted from another nursing home. Nearly three fourths of the persons discharged from nursing homes were alive at the time (72 percent), with about half of them going to a hospital (49 percent) and another 30 percent to a private or semiprivate residence. The remainder went to other types of health facilities including mental hospitals and other nursing homes. Among those discharged to hospitals and other health facilities, about 13 percent were known to have died at that facility (Hing et al, 1989).

The reasons for admission to nursing homes are based primarily on the loss of physical and cognitive function and a lack of caregiver support at home (Weissert and Cready, 1989; Morris et al, 1988; Wingard et al, 1987). As part of the 1985 NNHS, interviews were conducted with an available next-of-kin to provide information on the reasons for admission and the resident's state of health before admission. Alzheimer's disease and other mental disorders, stroke, musculoskeletal disease, and hip fracture contributed heavily to the case mix of residents in nursing homes. At least two out of three of the residents were admitted because the person "required more care than household members could give"; because the person had "problems in doing everyday activities"; and also because there was "no one at home to provide care." Although nearly one in five residents was suddenly ill or injured before admission, the majority of residents (52 percent) were reported to have had gradually worsening health before admission (Hing et al, 1989).

Research on the dynamics of the nursing home population has shown that there are basically two types of users, short-stay residents and long-stay residents (Keeler et al, 1981; Kelman and Thomas, 1990). Short-stay users, in general, are younger, more likely to be married, and less likely to have cognitive deficits in comparison to long-stay residents. Reasons for admission of short-stay residents are more likely to be associated with extended care for rehabilitation and recovery from acute care, or specifically for terminal care. Reasons for admission of long-stay residents are more likely to be associated with impaired cognitive and physical function and a poor prognosis for improvement. These general types of users have been observed in clinical practice (Kane et al, 1989; Ouslander, 1989).

Most nursing home residents need assistance in performing the activities of daily living (ADL): the ability of the resident to bathe, dress, use the toilet (including incontinence care), transfer from bed to chair, and eat. The ADL were validated in assessing rehabilitation among patients recovering primarily from strokes and hip fractures (Katz et al, 1963).

About one third of the nation's nursing home residents over the age of 65 needed assistance in all the activities of daily living. On the other hand, 10 percent of the residents were well enough not to need assistance in any of these activities (Hing et al, 1989). Furthermore, about two thirds of the residents were neither visually nor hearing impaired. These findings reaffirm the fact that the nursing home population is not a homogeneous population of frail, demented persons. Rather, there is considerable diversity in the needs and the medical-care plans for each resident (Ouslander, 1989).

The nursing home population has been aging in similar fashion to the noninstitutionalized population. Between 1977 and 1985, both the median age of the nursing home population and the prevalence of limitations in the activities of daily living among the residents age 65 and over increased significantly (Hing, 1987). Several factors have contributed to these trends and include the implementation of the Medicare prospective payment plan for hospital care, which resulted in more functionally dependent patients being discharged to nursing homes (Hing, 1989b; Meiners and Coffey, 1985; Sager et al, 1987); the dramatic growth in medical home-health care (Council Report, 1990); and state initiatives to screen Medicaid applicants for cost-effective alternatives to institutionalization (Nocks et al, 1986).

EPIDEMIOLOGIC RESEARCH

Epidemiologic studies that focus on the transition from community to nursing home address models for targeting long-term care services (Morris et al, 1988; Weissert et al, 1989), for defining predisposing risk factors (Branch and Jette, 1982; Cohen et al, 1986b; Shapiro and Tate, 1985), and for characterizing the types of users and expected length of stay (Keeler et al, 1981; Kelman and Thomas, 1990). These studies are useful in establishing more effective policies to meet the medical- and supportive-care needs of an aging population.

Epidemiologic investigations among the residents in nursing homes generally focus on the factors associated with or contributing to medical conditions and syndromes prevalent in this population such as urinary incontinence (Resnik et al, 1989), decubitus ulcers (Spector et al, 1988), disruptive behavior (Jackson et al, 1989), falls (Tinetti, 1987), infections (Garibaldi et al, 1981), and misuse of drugs (Ray et al, 1980). Epidemiologic methods also cover evaluation research to address issues in effectiveness of specialized units (Ohta and Ohta, 1988), annual clinical examination (Irvine et al, 1984) and laboratory testing (Levenstein et al, 1987), or treatment policy (Glasser et al, 1988).

These types of studies increased considerably as part of an NIA initiative for establishment of teaching nursing homes to improve our knowledge of medical care for geriatric patients (Butler, 1981; Schneider, 1983). Earlier work in specialty hospitals established the foundation for this initiative (Libow, 1976; Williams, 1976). Currently, there are about 15 research institutes affiliated with nursing homes in this country. A recent survey of these institutes summarizes the goals and the wide variety of research topics being addressed by these programs (Cohen-Mansfield et al, 1990).

Traditional epidemiologic methods may not hold up well in investigations of nursing home residents. Many unexpected problems may confront the protocol that an investigator outlines for the study, including difficulties in obtaining informed consent, lack of staff cooperation, incomplete or inadequate medical record information, an unexpectedly high dropout rate since many residents are in their last months of life, or ethical dilemmas that were not fully considered in the development of the study. Fortunately, an increasing body of literature is emerging to assist investigators in successfully developing criteria and protocols for research among nursing home residents (Annas and Glantz, 1986; Cassel, 1985; Cohen-Mansfield et al, 1988).

SUMMARY

Long-term care for older persons in the United States is primarily thought of as nursing home care. In more general terms, however, long-term care can be viewed as a program of comprehensive supportive and medical care designed to sustain a high quality of life for an aging individual. In nursing homes, an organized staff of professionals and others provide basic medical care for the geriatric needs of frail residents. In the family setting, the geriatric needs of the frail person are met by one (often the spouse) or more family members with or without the support of medical and nonmedical home-care services. Epidemiologic research is needed to reduce the need for geriatric care and improve the care given to patients with complex conditions and syndromes in either facilities or their own homes.

Already, epidemiologic studies are producing a wealth of data that will improve our knowledge about effectively meeting the needs of an aging population, including new strategies for disease prevention and health promotion; however, the challenge is formidable. In 1985, there were about 2.5 million persons age 85 and over and about half of them were either in nursing homes or at home and dependent on another person for daily care (Schneider and Guralnik, 1990). The population of persons age 85 and over will about double by the year 2000 (Spencer, 1989). This means an additional 1 million persons may need geriatric care before the turn of the century.

Public health policymakers will have to consider the following: In the year 2020 will half of those age 85 and over (about 4 million persons) require nursing care? Will we have the resources, especially in trained personnel, to meet this demand? What can we do now to reduce the geriatric nursing care needs of tomorrow's older population, especially among those age 85 and over? Increased epidemiologic research on nursing home residents today may provide many solutions and innovations to reduce the burden of morbidities at advanced ages in the years to come.

REFERENCES

Annas G, Glantz L (1986). Rules for research in nursing homes. New Engl J Med 315:1157–1158.

Branch L, Jette A (1982). A prospective study of long-term care institutionalization among the aged. Am J Public Health 72:1373–1379.

Butler R (1981). The teaching nursing home. JAMA 245:1435–1437.

Cassel C (1985). Research in nursing homes: Ethical issues. J Am Geriatr Soc 33:795–799.

Cohen MA, Tell EJ, Wallack SS (1986a). The lifetime risks and costs of nursing home use among the elderly. Med Care 24:1161–1172.

Cohen MA, Tell EJ, Wallack SS (1986b). Client-related risk factors of nursing home entry among elderly adults. J Gerontol 41:785–792.

Cohen-Mansfield J, Kerin P, Pawlson G, Lipson S, Holdridge K (1988). Informed consent for research in a nursing home: Processes and issues. Gerontologist 28:355–359.

Cohen-Mansfield J, Lawton MP, Riskin C (1990). Research institutes affiliated with nursing homes: Strengths and developmental issues. Gerontologist 30:411–416.

Council Report (1990). Home care in the 1990s. JAMA 263:1241–1245.

Foley DJ (1980). Nursing home utilization in California, Illinois, Massachusetts, New York and Texas. Vital and Health Statistics, Series 13, No. 48, National Center for Health Statistics, DHHS Pub. No. (PHS) 81-1799.

Foley DJ, Ostfeld AM, Branch LG, Wallace RB, McGloin J, Cornoni-Huntly JC (1992) (in press). The risk of nursing home admission in three communities. Aging & Health.

Garibaldi RA, Brodine S, Matsuyama S (1981). Infections among patients in nursing homes. N Engl J Med 305:731–735.

Glasser G, Zweibel NR, Cassel CK (1988). The ethics committee in the nursing home: Results of a national survey. J Am Geriatr Soc 36:150–156.

Harrington C, Swan JH (1987). The impact of state Medicaid nursing home policies on utilization and expenditures. Inquiry 24:157–172.

Hing E (1987). Use of nursing homes by the elderly: Preliminary data from the 1985 National Nursing Home Survey. Advance data from Vital and Health Statistics, No. 135, National Center for Health Statistics, DHHS Pub. No. (PHS) 87-1250.

Hing E (1989a). Nursing home utilization by current residents: United States, 1985. Vital and Health Statistics, Series 13, No. 102, National Center for Health Statistics, DHHS Pub. No. (PHS) 89-1763.

Hing E (1989b). Effects of the prospective payment system on nursing homes. Vital and Health Statistics, Series 13, No. 98, National Center for Health Statistics, DHHS Pub. No. (PHS) 89-1759.

Hing E, Sekscenski E, Strahan G (1989) The National Nursing Home Survey: 1985 summary for the United States. Vital and Health Statistics, Series 13, No. 43, National Center for Health Statistics, DHHS Pub. No. (PHS) 89-1758.

Irvine PW, Carlson K, Adcock M, Slag M (1984). The value of annual medical examinations in the nursing home. J Am Geriatr Soc 32:540–545.

Jackson ME, Drugovich ML, Fretwell MD, Spector WD, Sternberg J, Rosenstein RB (1989). Prevalence and correlates of disruptive behavior in the nursing home. J Aging Health 1:349–369.

Kane RA, Ouslander JG, Abrass IB (1989). Nursing home care. Essentials of Clinical Geriatrics, 2nd ed. McGraw-Hill, New York.

Katz SC, Ford AB, Moskowitz RW, Jackson BA, Jaffe MW (1963). Studies of illness in the aged: The index of ADL, a standardized measure of biological and psychosocial function. JAMA 185:914–919.

Keeler EB, Kane RL, Solomon DH (1981). Short- and long-term residents of nursing homes. Med Care 19:363–369.

Kelman HR, Thomas C (1990). Transitions between community and nursing home residence in an urban elderly population. J Community Health 15:105–122.

Levenstein MR, Ouslander JG, Rubenstein LZ, Forsythe SB (1987). Yield of routine annual laboratory tests in a skilled nursing home population. JAMA 258:1909–1915.

Libow L (1976). A geriatric medical residency program: A four year experience. Ann Intern Med 85:641–647.

Madans JH (1981). Long-term care for the elderly in five states. In Health, United States, 1981, DHHS Pub. No. (PHS) 82-1232, pp. 47–53.

Meiners MR, Coffey RM (1985). Hospital DRGs and the need for long-term care services: An empirical analysis. Health Serv Res 20:359–384.

Morris JN, Sherwood S, Gutkin CE (1988). Inst-Risk II: An approach to forecasting relative risk of future institutional placement. Health Serv Res 23:511–536.

Murtaugh CM, Kemper P, Spillman BC (1990). The risk of nursing home use in later life. Med Care 28:952–962.

Nocks BC, Learner RM, Blackman D, Brown TE (1986). The effects of a community-based long term care project on nursing home utilization. Gerontologist 26:150–157.

Ohta RJ, Ohta BM (1988). Special units for Alzheimer's disease patients: A critical look. Gerontologist 28:803–808.

Ouslander JG (1989) Medical care in the nursing home. JAMA, 262:2582–2590.

Ray WA, Federspeil CF, and Schaffner W (1980). A study of antipsychotic drug use in nursing homes: Epidemiologic evidence suggesting misuse. Am Public Health 70:485–491.

Resnick NM, Yalla SV, Laurino E (1989). The pathophysiology of urinary incontinence among institutionalized elderly persons. N Engl J Med 320:1–7.

Roper DA (1986). Nursing and related care homes as reported from the 1982 National Master Facility Inventory Survey. Vital and Health Statistics, Series 14, No. 32, National Center for Health Statistics, DHHS Pub. No. (PHS) 86-1827.

Sager MA, Leventhal EA, Easterling DV (1987). The impact of Medicare's prospective payment system on Wisconsin nursing homes. JAMA 257:1762–1766.

Schneider EL (1983). The teaching nursing home. N Engl J Med 308:336–337.

Schneider EL, Guralnik JM (1990). The aging of America: Impact on health care costs. JAMA 263:2335–2340.

Shapiro E, Tate RB (1985). Predictors of long term care facility use among the elderly. Can J Aging 4:11–19.

Sirrocco A (1989). Nursing home characteristics: 1986 Inventory of Long-Term Care Places. Vital and Health Statistics, Series 14, No. 33, National Center for Health Statistics, DHHS Pub. No. (PHS) 89-1828.

Spector WD, Kapp MC, Tucker RJ, Sternberg J (1988). Factors associated with presence of decubitus ulcers at admission to nursing homes. Gerontologist 28:830–834.

Spencer G (1989). Projections of the population of the United States, by age, sex, and race: 1988 to 2080. Current Population Reports, Series P-25, No. 1018. U.S. Bureau of the Census, Washington, D.C.

Strahan GW (1984). Trends in nursing and related care homes and hospitals: United States, selected years 1969–80. Vital and Health Statistics, Series 14, No. 30, National Center for Health Statistics, DHHS Pub. No. (PHS) 84-1825.

Sutton JF (1977) Utilization of nursing homes. Vital and Health Statistics, Series 13, No. 28, National Center for Health Statistics, DHEW Pub. No. (HRA) 77-1779.

Tinneti M (1987). Factors associated with serious injury during falls by ambulatory nursing home residents. J Am Geriatr Soc 35:644–648.

US House of Representatives (1987). Omnibus Budget Reconciliation Act of 1987. Report 100-495, pp. 190–91.

Van Nostrand JF, Zappolo A, Hing E, Bloom B, Hirsch B, Foley D. (1979). The National Nursing Home Survey: 1977 summary for the United States. Vital and Health Statistics, Series 13, No. 43, National Center for Health Statistics, DHEW Pub No. (PHS) 79-1794.

Weissert WG, Cready CM (1989). Toward a model for improved targeting of aged at risk of institutionalization. Health Serv Res 24:485–510.

Williams TF, Izzo AJ, Steel RK (1976). Innovations in teaching about chronic illness in a chronic disease hospital. In Clark DW, Williams TF (eds). Teaching of Chronic Illness and Aging. Bethesda, MD, Fogerty International Center, NIH, pp. 21–30.

Wingard DL, Jones DW, Kaplan RM (1987). Institutional care utilization by the elderly: A critical review. Gerontologist 27:156–163.

15

Types and Quality of Data Available on the Elderly in the 1990 Census

CYNTHIA M. TAEUBER

A decennial census provides rich information and geographic detail on local areas and the nation as a whole that is not attainable in a sample survey. Census counts by age, sex, and race are used as the denominator of epidemiologic measures. Thus, the quality of census data is critical. First, we shall discuss the quality of data available on the elderly population, particularly as it affects denominators in epidemiologic measures. Second, we shall discuss some of the types of data available from the 1990 census and evaluation studies.

DATA QUALITY

In 1712, the Chinese emperor Tsing Shen Tsu complained, "I have examined the census reports of the viceroys of the provinces and have found them inaccurate." Data were not perfect then and are not now, although there have been vast improvements. Data users should carefully consider the quality of the information they are taking from censuses, surveys, and vital statistics. All data, whether from a complete enumeration of the population or from a sample, are subject to coverage and content errors. Data based on a sample are also subject to sampling error. Data on the older population have some particular problems with respect to these sources of error.

Errors in the data are of two types: sampling errors and nonsampling errors. Sampling error affects those items collected from a sample of the population (see part II of Table 15.1). Sampling error occurs when a portion of the population is surveyed to represent the entire population. Data based on a sample are estimates that would differ somewhat from data based on a complete enumeration of all households or persons in group quarters. Sampling error can be measured based on the actual sample observed. In the census, about one in six households and one in six persons in group quarters received the sample form.

The deviation of the sample estimate from the average of all possible samples (which approximates a complete enumeration) is called sampling error. The sampling

Table 15-1 Items in the 1990 Census

Population	Housing
I. Information collected from all households*	
Population	*Housing*
Household relationship	Number of units in structure
Sex	Number of rooms in unit
Race	Own or rent housing
Age	Business at residence
Marital status	Value of owned unit or rent paid
Spanish/Hispanic origin	Congregate housing (meals included in rent)
	Vacancy characteristics
II. Information collected from a sample of households*	
Population	*Housing*
Social Characteristics	Year moved into residence
Place of birth, citizenship, year of entry	Number of bedrooms
Education—enrollment and attainment	Plumbing and kitchen facilities
Ancestry	Telephone
Migration, residence 5 years ago	Autos, light trucks and vans
Language spoken at home, ability to speak English	Fuel use
Military status	Source of water and method of sewage disposal
Disability limiting work, ability to go outside, or care for personal needs	Age of building
Fertility	Condominium or mobile home status
Economic Characteristics	Farm residence
Employment and unemployment, year last worked	Shelter costs, including utilities
Place of work and commuting to work	Real estate taxes and insurance
Occupation, employer, and type of work	Mortgages and loans
Work experience, income in 1989, and sources of income	

*Persons in group quarters, including institutions, are asked population items only.

error is a function of the observed sampling size; as the sample size becomes smaller, sampling error increases. Thus, for local areas with a small population, or when the group of interest is small, such as the population 85 years and over, sampling error may be quite large and should be accounted for in analysis. Each census report with sample data contains an appendix explaining the calculation of sampling error and its interpretation.

Nonsampling errors occur in the collection and processing of data. They are often difficult to measure and identify. Nonsampling errors may be random or may have a consistent direction that biases the data. Nonsampling errors are of two basic types: coverage and content errors. Coverage errors result in persons being missed or counted erroneously (e.g., counted more than once). Content errors include errors by respondents and interviewers, processing errors, and those occurring when the data item is not completed (i.e., nonresponse). Errors in age data include misstatement of age, a preference for giving an age or year of birth that ends in 0 or 5, and ages that are not known or not given.

Coverage errors occur when whole households are missed and when persons within households are missed or counted more than once. For example, an older couple may be traveling in their trailer and not receive their census form in the mail. In another type of coverage error, the same household may be counted twice. This might occur, for example, when a retired couple from the Northeast goes to Florida to spend the winter in their second home ("snowbirds"). There are census procedures to catch persons who may be traveling and to avoid counting in both places, but such errors do occur.

Evaluation studies performed after the 1980 census showed that there was actually a net overcount of persons in the age groups 65 to 69 and 70 to 74, for both blacks and whites. Some of this was probably due to errors in reporting age as well as coverage error. At ages 75 and over, the studies concluded there was a net undercount of 0.6 percent for black males, 6.4 percent for black females, 0.9 percent for white males, and 2.6 percent for white females (Bureau of the Census, 1988).

Some nonsampling errors occur during data collection and processing. The Census Bureau mails forms to most households. In most households, one household member fills out the questionnaire even though they may not know accurate information (such as age) for every household member. Sometimes, census takers visit respondents door to door. If a census taker does not understand a question, he or she may give seemingly authoritative but incorrect advice to respondents on how to answer. This can affect the data. In institutions such as nursing homes, the questionnaires are often filled out by staff using administrative records and their own knowledge and guesses. In larger institutions, the extra work can be a tedious, burdensome process and nonresponse to particular questions is often quite high. Clerical processing of forms in census offices can also lead to errors if workers make clerical errors or do not follow procedures. For the 1990 census, much of the processing has been automated to reduce clerical error.

Questionnaires may be returned with incomplete or inconsistent information. Nonresponse may be total (the respondent does not complete any items on the questionnaire) or partial (only some questions that should have been answered actually are answered). In institutions, such as nursing homes, the information may not be available in the administrative records, and nonresponse rates, especially for social and economic characteristics, may be unusually high. For example, neither a patient nor the institution staff may be aware of an income source that goes directly to the patient's family.

If efforts to obtain missing information fail, the computer "imputes," or fills in, the missing or inconsistent information. This imputation for missing data is based on the observed responses of a household with similar characteristics such as household size and race. In group quarters, it is based on the responses of others in the group quarters. In the 1980 census, if there had been no imputation for missing data, 11.1 percent of the population for which age was observed would have been shown as aged 65 or older; after imputation, however, the proportion of the population aged 65 or older increased to 11.3.

Nonresponse can introduce bias into the data, as the characteristics of the nonrespondents have not been observed directly and may be different from those imputed. Each census report contains an appendix with a table showing the percentage of responses to particular items that were imputed. Data users should consult these appendixes, especially when using information subject to nonresponse or misreporting, such as income. A high percentage of allocation indicates that particular caution is warranted in using the information.

Additional errors occur that affect the quality of census data. A respondent may misreport information, either intentionally or by misunderstanding the intent of the question. For example, respondents may misreport income intentionally. Or they may simply not have understood that they should have included income amounts from a particular source such as self-employment.

Errors in the statement of age may affect total error in data for the elderly more than coverage errors. This is especially true in data before the 1980 census around age 65 and among the oldest old (especially centenarians) because of the misreporting of age. In modern censuses, "year of birth" is asked in addition to "age," which has reduced this error considerably. Sometimes people misreport their age because they do not know or remember their age. Some give a "rounded-off" age and numbers ending in 0 or 5 occur more frequently than they should, a phenomenon known as "age heaping."[1] These errors are especially important when data are for single years of age and less important when grouped in five- or 10-year age groups. Historical data may need to be adjusted as the errors are often sufficient to affect death rates.[2]

Age seems to be exaggerated the most at the oldest ages and among those with lower levels of education. This affects both census and mortality data on the extreme aged. Traditionally, death rates have been unreliable for persons 85 years and older. There have, however, been improvements in these data and we can expect vast improvements as more people reach these ages with higher education and with birth certificates that document year of birth. Plenty of room for additional improvement remains. Census processing errors have produced unreliable data for counts of persons 90 years and over since at least 1960 (Rosenwaike, 1985; Spencer et al, 1987). For 1990, improvements in the edits have greatly reduced processing errors.[3]

Census error is measured by reinterviews, record matching studies, and demographic analysis. In addition, reinterviews and matching studies are one way to partially measure the effect of imputations for missing data. Another way is to compare the reported census age with death certificate information for those who die close to the time of the census. Neither method is a perfect check, as age may be misstated both in a reinterview and on death certificates. Demographic analysis develops estimates of population largely from administrative records such as vital statistics, Medicare data, and immigration statistics (Robinson et al, 1990; Shryock et al, 1971, pp. 212–228). For example, census age distributions can be compared with those from demographic analysis to determine whether systematic errors have skewed the distribution.

In summary, data users should be aware of the errors to which the data are subject. Users should review the data to make sure they make sense historically. Census estimates can often be compared with survey estimates to see whether the results differ

[1]In some cultures, certain numbers are particularly avoided (such as 13 in the West and 4 in the Orient). For a discussion of the various indexes of age preference and methods of adjusting reported single-year-of-age data, see Shryock et al (1971, pp. 205–211).

[2]Greville developed an adjustment technique described in Speigelman (1968). Speigelman discusses an adjustment technique developed by Greville for historical age data (p. 67) and a blending method for age heaping (pp. 71–75). For death rates, Spiegelman recommends choosing an age grouping for which the death rates would be essentially correct if both population and deaths were biased in the same direction and in about the same proportion.

[3]For example, the reported year of birth and age are tested for consistency, which corrects for reporting the wrong century. Additionally, no "child" of a householder can be over age 90 and no "grandchild" over age 75. Relationship and marital status are also compared with age for consistency.

significantly. Although census operations include procedures to minimize errors, it is impossible to avoid some data problems, such as adamant refusal to respond to the census form. Some census procedures themselves, such as clerical checking and computer editing and imputation, introduce error into the data. Knowledge of the types and extent of errors that may be present contributes to understanding the census results.

TYPES OF DATA AVAILABLE

The census asks everyone basic demographic questions on household relationship, sex, race, age, marital status, and Hispanic origin and social and economic questions of a sample of households and persons in group quarters. For the 1990 census, counts of persons by sex, race, and Hispanic origin will appear for single years to the end category "105 years and over" for the United States, and for statistical and political divisions within each state.

There will be nine main report series from the census as well as summary tape files and public-use microdata files. Public-use microdata samples (PUMS) are computer data files that contain the edited responses from a sample of individual households. The records contain no identifying information and large geographic areas to protect the confidentiality of respondents. In addition to PUMS for the entire population, a file that focuses specifically on the population 60 years and over will be produced (referred to as PUMS-O).

Finally, there will be reports issued that evaluate the quality of the 1990 census data. Initial reports will focus on coverage. Some content evaluation reports will provide tabulations by age and will provide additional insight into the uses and limitations of data on America's older population. These reports include a Content Reinterview Study (response bias and variance); the Integrated Evaluation of Error Study (evaluates the magnitude of all sources of error, including item nonresponse); Coverage Sampling Research (alternative coverage questions to improve coverage within households); the Master Trace Sample (impact of processing on data); the Outreach Survey (respondent attitudes toward the census); and ethnographic studies on response and coverage problems.

REFERENCES

Bureau of the Census, The coverage of population in the 1980 Census, Evaluation and Research Reports, PHC80-E4. (Washington, DC., US Government Printing Office, 1988), table 3.3.

Robinson JG (1990). Das Gupta P, Ahmed B (1990). Evaluating the quality of estimates of coverage based on demographic analysis, paper presented at the 1990 annual meeting of the Population Association of America, May 3–5, 1990.

Rosenwaike I. (1985). The Extreme Aged in America. Westport, CT, Greenwood Press, Ch. 2.

Shryock HS, Siegel JS, et al (1971). The Methods and Materials of Demography. Washington, DC, US Government Printing Office.

Speigelman (1968). Introduction to Demography, rev. ed. Cambridge, MA, Harvard University Press.

Spencer G, Taeuber CM, Goldstein A (1987). America's centenarians, Current Population Reports, Series P-23, No. 153, Washington, DC, US Government Printing Office, September.

16

Data Sets for Research in Aging: The National Center for Health Statistics

TAMARA B. HARRIS AND MARY GRACE KOVAR

Although there is a compelling need for information on the associations among risk factors, disease, and disability in older persons, there has been a dearth of epidemiologic data. The past decade has seen a partial remedy of this lack through the development of population studies such as the Established Populations for Epidemiologic Studies of the Elderly (Cornoni-Huntley et al, 1986), the Cardiovascular Health Study (Fried, 1991), and the Study of Osteoporotic Fractures (Cummings et al, 1990). The first large-scale clinical trials designed specifically for older persons have taken place as well (European Working Party, 1985; Systolic Hypertension, 1988). In addition, new funds have been directed to coordinated clinical studies of particular syndromes of importance in old age such as urinary incontinence (Ouslander and Resnick, 1990) and frailty (Zylke, 1990).

There has also been a concomitant growth in the collection of health data on older persons by the National Center for Health Statistics (NCHS), a component of the Centers for Disease Control. This growth in data has been facilitated in part by the mandate of the National Center, which by law includes collection of statistics on the extent and nature of illness and disability in the United States, including life expectancy, determinants of health, utilization of health care resources, and costs of services used (Kovar, 1989; NCHS, 1990a); in part by the force of demographic trends with the rapid growth of the older population, especially the old-old (Schneider, 1990); and in part by a growing focus on research at NCHS in areas related to aging (Havlik, 1987; Cornoni-Huntley et al, 1990; Harris et al, 1989a,b). This chapter provides an overview of data systems from the National Center for Health Statistics focused on the more important data sets for aging research.

USE OF DATA FROM THE NATIONAL CENTER FOR HEALTH STATISTICS: BENEFITS AND LIMITATIONS

The data on older populations collected by NCHS directly benefits the academic research community because all data are in the public domain. This is true of not only published data (NCHS, 1990a), but also data sets on tape, which investigators may use for their own analyses (NCHS, 1990b). These national data sets, some of which are longitudinal studies, include relatively large samples of older persons and have undergone intensive methodologic scrutiny, including evaluation of nonresponse bias. In addition, because these studies are designed to address issues of public health importance, they generally contain information on multiple chronic diseases, which facilitates examination of the impact of co-morbidity as well as of specific risk factor–disease associations. Many investigators involved in more geographically restricted studies have used NCHS data to estimate the generalizability of their own populations in terms of selected characteristics comparable between the NCHS data and their studies.

Although these data are a tremendous resource, there are limitations. Even though most of the data sets are large and allow for the use of computer modeling techniques, investigators may encounter analytic problems for several reasons. The type of sampling may make the data sets inappropriate for some studies of particular areas or groups of people. This may be particularly true for studies of small-area variation or of geographic localities that are sparsely populated and consequently seldom selected for an NCHS survey. It may also be a problem for studies of minority populations because, in general, the proportion of minorities in the sample is the same as the proportion in the U.S. population.

The data sets are relatively complex and require methodological sophistication to develop appropriate analytic models, to create linkages, and to assess the quality of the data. Investigators often use the data to evaluate hypotheses that the data were not specifically designed to test, and issues related to multiple testing must be considered. In addition, all participants in NCHS surveys are guaranteed confidentiality and there are no personal or institutional identifiers on the data sets. The care taken to preserve confidentiality may mean that items needed for linkage or for identification of specific geographic areas are not available.

Lastly, there may be a significant lag in the time between data collection and data release to investigators in academic centers. In general, most data sets are available to analysts within two years of the end of data collection. This may vary, however, depending on the complexity of the survey and the resources available for editing and documentation of computer files.

One key concept is that data collection systems of the National Center for Health Statistics are designed to produce national estimates. With the exception of the Vital Statistics Registration System and the Master Facility Inventory (Kovar, 1989), *all other data sets are based on complex, stratified samples,* and they include the weights needed to produce national estimates. The weights generally reflect three factors: (1) the likelihood of being chosen for participation, (2) an adjustment for the actual participation, and (3) an adjustment to increase the sample estimate to the national one, although other factors that relate to differential sampling and differential response may be incorporated as well. The weights, which act as multipliers, are used to obtain national prevalence estimates, to estimate the standard errors, and sometimes to model associations among variables. There is no consensus on the need for using weights in analytic epidemiology, but there is agreement that they should be used in descriptive epidemiology.

Researchers will also need to decide whether the complex multistage probability sample design utilized in the surveys needs to be incorporated into the computation of variance estimates in their analyses. There is no simple answer, and the decision should be dependent on the type of analysis (descriptive or analytic) and the particular survey, in consultation with a statistician.

DATA COLLECTION SYSTEMS AT THE NATIONAL CENTER FOR HEALTH STATISTICS

Although the population of interest to the National Center for Health Statistics includes the entire population of the United States, this section focuses only on those data sets most relevant to older persons. The descriptions are organized into four sections corresponding to four critical focuses of health status measurement in older persons: (1) as people age in noninstitutionalized settings in the community [the National Health Interview Survey, with the 1984 Supplement on Aging and the Longitudinal Study on Aging; the National Health and Nutrition Examination Surveys (NHANES) with the NHANES Epidemiologic Followup Study]; (2) as people enter the hospital and health care system (the National Ambulatory Care Survey and the National Hospital Discharge Survey); (3) as people enter, live in, and leave nursing homes (the National Nursing Home Survey and Followup); and (4) as people die (the Mortality from the Vital Statistics Registration System and National Mortality Followback Survey). For each data collection system, brief descriptions of purpose of the system, the sample (if pertinent), and the content are included.

Older Persons Living in the Community: The National Health Interview Survey

The National Health Interview Survey (NHIS) is a continuing nationwide sample survey in which data are collected on the incidence of acute illness and injuries, the prevalence of chronic conditions and impairments, the extent of disability, the utilization of health care services, and other health-related topics (NCHS, 1989). The survey consists of two parts: (1) a set of basic health and demographic items that are included every year, and (2) one or more sets of questions on selected health topics (Table 16.1) that are included for a short time, usually one year.

The sampling plan of the National Health Interview Survey follows a multistage probability design that permits continuous sampling of the civilian noninstitutionalized population residing in the United States, and includes approximately 10,000 persons over the age of 65 (Table 16.2). Since 1985, the black population has been oversampled to increase the precision of estimates for that population. The survey is designed in such a way that the sample scheduled for each week is representative of the civilian noninstitutional population living in the United States and the weekly samples are additive over time (Kovar, 1989). The response rate is generally upward of 90 percent.

For researchers in gerontology, a particular value of the NHIS lies in the use of the data to examine time trends in disability, including restricted activity and bed disability days, and long-term limitations of activity resulting from chronic disease or impairments and associated conditions. In addition, the supplement and the longitudinal study based on it is the Longitudinal Study of Aging.

Table 16-1 Supplements to the National Health Interview Survey, 1982–1992

1982	Preventive Care
	Health Insurance
1983	Alcohol/Health Practices
	Bed Days and Dental Care
	Doctor Service Supplement
	Health Insurance (Quarters 3 and 4)
1984	Health Insurance
	Supplement on Aging
1985	Health Promotion and Disease Prevention
	Smoking History During Pregnancy
	Child Safety/Infant Feeding
1986	Vitamin and Mineral Supplement Intake
	Dental Services
	Longest-Held Job
	Functional Limitations
	Health Insurance
1987	Adoption
	AIDS Knowledge and Attitudes
	Cancer
1988	Child Health
	AIDS Knowledge and Attitudes
1989	Diabetes
	Dental Health
	Digestive Disorders
	Health Insurance
	Immunizations
	Orofacial Pain
	Mental Health
	AIDS Knowledge and Attitudes
1990 Goals	Health Promotion and Disease Prevention—1990
	Assistive Devices
	Podiatric Services
	AIDS Knowledge and Attitudes
1991	Health Promotion and Disease Prevention—Year 2000 Goals
	AIDS Knowledge and Attitudes
	Illicit Drug Use

The Longitudinal Study of Aging, a collaborative project of the National Center for Health Statistics and the National Institute on Aging, is a study based on the Supplement on Aging (SOA) to the 1984 National Health Interview Survey (Kovar, 1989). The SOA was designed to obtain extensive information on family structure and frequency of contacts with children; housing—including barriers to movement, length of time in residence, ownership and rental information; use of community and social supports; occupation and retirement—including sources of retirement income; ability to perform work-related functions; conditions and impairments; functional limitations—Activities of Daily Living and Instrumental Activities of Daily Living—including conditions causing disability as well as information on providers of help. Information was obtained for 16,148 persons aged 55 and older (96 percent of the eligible

Table 16-2 Numbers of Persons Age 65 or Older in Selected Data Sets from the National Center for Health Statistics

	Age			
Data set	Total 65+	65–74	75–84	85+
1984 National Health Interview Survey	11,984	7,344	3,698	852
1985 National Health Interview Survey	10,703	6,625	3,308	770
Supplements to the National Health Interview Survey				
1984 Supplement on Aging	11,497	7,093	3,578	826
1985 Health Promotion, Disease Prevention	6,403	3,790	2,148	465
1987 Cancer Risk Factor Supplement	8,513	5,009	2,842	662
Longitudinal Study of Aging (based on 1984 Supplement on Aging)	(age 70+) 7,527	(age 70–74) 3,131	3,572	824
National Health and Nutrition Examination Survey I (1971–75)	3,853	—	—	—
NHANES I Epidemiologic Followup Study (1982–84)	5,172	1,411	2,009	1,752
National Health and Nutrition Examination Survey III (projected examinees by age)	5,179	(age 60–69) 2,219	(age 70–79) 1,672	(age 80+) 1,288
1985 National Ambulatory Medical Care Survey (patient visits)	16,750	9,600	5,932	1,218
1986 National Hospital Discharge Survey (discharges)	54,090	25,877	20,363	7,850
1985 National Nursing Home Survey				
Current residents	4,650	729	1,774	2,147
Discharged residents	5,393	901	2,168	2,324
1986 Vital Statistics Number of Deaths	1,488,161	475,539	575,149	427,473
1986 Mortality Followback Survey	10,148	3,498	3,892	2,758

people in the interviewed households in the NHIS) (Table 16.2). Ninety-two percent answered all questions for themselves (Fitti and Kovar, 1988).

Longitudinal follow-up consisted of two phases. The first involved linkage with administrative records, including Medicare files and the National Death Index for all survey participants who gave permission. After the death was established through the linkage, cause-of-death information was obtained from the multiple cause-of-death tapes. This made possible the study of survival and death in relation to social, economic, and demographic factors, family support, and health conditions.

The second phase involved reinterviews every two years. The first follow-up reinterview included all persons aged 80 and older, all black persons aged 70 and older, one half of all other persons aged 70–79 years, and all persons aged 70–79 living with someone already selected. This sample, which consisted of 5151 persons aged 70 and over, was interviewed in 1986 using computer-assisted telephone interviews with mailed questionnaires for those who could not be contacted by telephone. The 1986 interview was designed to measure change in functioning (work function items, Activities of Daily Living, Instrumental Activities of Daily Living) and providers of help; change in living arrangements; and use of medical and nursing home care. Overall, less than 4 percent of this initial follow-up group was lost to follow-up, and 92 percent (4734) participated in the reinterview.

The 1988 and 1990 interviews were also conducted using computer-assisted telephone interviewing and mail questionnaires. The major change between 1986 and 1988 was that the sample was enlarged to include *all* persons who were aged 70 or older in the original survey in 1984; this increased the effective sample size to 7527. In 1986, questions regarding children were added, and in 1990, a supplement on economics was added to assess the impact of alternative proposals for provision of health services to the oldest-old.

Older Persons Living in the Community: the National Health and Nutrition Examination Surveys

The National Health and Nutrition Examination Survey (NHANES) is unique among national surveys in that the methods of data collection include medical and dental examinations, physiologic measurements, and analysis of biochemical and hematologic parameters, in addition to an in-person interview. The goals of the survey include derivation of national population reference distributions (i.e., for weight and height), estimation of the national prevalence of diseases and risk factors, including nutritional factors, and identification of important interrelationships among health and nutritional variables (Kovar, 1989).

Since 1960, there have been five surveys; a sixth, the National Health and Nutrition Examination Survey III (NHANES III) is being conducted from 1988 through 1994 and is described later. The earliest survey, the National Health Examination Survey I, 1960–1962, concentrated on specific areas of health and included adults age 18–79 years of age. The next two surveys included only children. In 1971, a nutrition surveillance component was added and the name of the survey was changed to the National Health and Nutrition Examination Survey (NHANES).

The first NHANES survey was conducted from 1971 to 1975 (NCHS, 1977). The NHANES I target population was the civilian noninstitutionalized population 1–74 years of age, excepting persons living on reservations, sampled in a multistage stratified probability design. Older Americans, those in poverty, and women of child-bearing age were oversampled. Household interviews were conducted for more than 96 percent of the 28,043 persons selected for the NHANES I sample, and about 75 percent (20,749) were examined (see Table 16.2). The major purpose was to measure and monitor indicators of the nutritional status of the American people through dietary intake data, biochemical tests, physical measurements, and clinical assessments for evidence of nutritional deficiency, including examination by dentists, ophthalmologists, and dermatologists (Kovar, 1989). In addition, data were obtained for a subsample of adults on overall health care needs and behavior, and more detailed examination data were collected on cardiovascular, respiratory, and arthritic conditions. The value of the data were greatly enhanced when a longitudinal follow-up was initiated in the early 1980s.

The NHANES I Epidemiologic Folowup Study (NHEFS) was jointly initiated by the National Center for Health Statistics and the National Institute on Aging in collaboration with other National Institutes of Health and other Public Health Service agencies (Madans et al, 1986). The primary purpose of the study was to investigate the longitudinal relationship between physiologic, nutritional, behavioral, and demographic characteristics collected through the NHANES I and subsequent disability, morbidity, or mortality from specific diseases and conditions (Kovar, 1989).

The first phase of the follow-up study was conducted in 1982–1984 and included the 14,407 persons aged 25–74 years at the time of the NHANES I survey, of whom 93 percent were successfully traced (Cohen, 1987). Personal interviews, focused on identification of incident morbidity outcomes and disability, were conducted with traced, surviving subjects, including those living in institutions (see Table 16.2). All respondents who could cooperate had measurement made of weight, pulse, and blood pressure. Interviews with proxy respondents were conducted if the subject was deceased or incapacitated. Death certificates were obtained for decedents and both underlying and multiple-cause-of-death information were coded.

A major feature of the longitudinal follow-up has been an effort to identify all hospitalizations or nursing home stays and to obtain medical abstracts for each stay. All diagnoses from the discharge summary as well as all major surgical procedures have been coded according to ICD-9 criteria. This has been invaluable in case ascertainment for incident diagnoses such as heart disease (Harris et al, 1991) or cancer (Schatzkin et al, 1987). Linkages have been made to Medicare files, and methodological work is ongoing to compare the two record systems.

Two additional waves of follow-up have been conducted and a fourth is planned for the early 1990s. The 1986 interview was focused on persons 55–74 years of age at the time of NHANES I (Finucane et al, 1990), whereas the interview in 1987 was for the entire cohort. These additional interviews have been conducted by computer-assisted telephone. Both surveys included questions on disability and morbidity status, and enumeration of interim hospitalizations or nursing home stays. Again, health facility abstracts and death certificates were obtained.

As with the Longitudinal Study on Aging, the data from the NHEFS are useful for examination of change in disability patterns over time and factors related to these changes. The NHEFS can also be related to physiologic measures of health from the baseline 10 years earlier, which offers a variety of analytic opportunities related to specific diseases or mortality.

For the National Health and Nutrition Examination Survey II (NHANES II), conducted from 1976 through 1980, the nutrition component remained nearly identical to that of NHANES I (McDowell et al, 1981). Primary emphasis in the interview and examination was placed on diabetes, cardiovascular disease, kidney and liver function, allergy, and speech pathology. The NHANES II target population was the U.S. civilian noninstitutionalized population 6 months through 74 years of age, with oversampling of persons six months through five years of age, those 60–74 years of age, and those living in poverty areas. A sample of 27,801 persons was selected for NHANES II, with a 73.1 percent (20,322) examination rate (Kovar, 1989). A match of these participants to the National Death Index is planned and death certificate data will be obtained for decedents.

In 1982–1984, a special survey was conducted among three Hispanic groups within the United States: Mexican Americans, Cuban Americans, and Puerto Ricans (Maurer, 1985). The general structure of the Hispanic Health and Nutrition Examination Survey (HHANES) was similar to the previous NHANES, as was the general survey content. Although this is a landmark study, the age structure of the HHANES sample reflects that of the Hispanic population in the United States, leading to a comparatively small number of persons 65–74 years of age in the survey.

The National Health and Nutrition Examination Survey III (NHANES III) represents major changes in the coverage, content, and design of the NHANES (Woteki et al, 1988; Harris et al, 1989b). These changes will create a unique and unusually comprehensive group of health assessment data on a random sample of the U.S. population of older persons. The NHANES III will be in the field from 1988 to 1994; it will visit 81 counties in 26 states. The sample will be drawn from two three-year national probability samples, with over 30,000 persons expected to participate in examinations. NHANES III does not have an upper age limit and will encompass individuals aged six months upward. Older persons have been targeted for oversampling and it is planned that about 5200 persons aged 60 or older will be examined, including about 1300 persons aged 80 or older (see Table 16.2). Unlike the other NHANES surveys, where follow-up was initiated at a later date, a longitudinal component has been an important planned extension of NHANES III; efforts are under way to initiate death index matches, obtain death certificates, and, for those 65 or older, obtain Medicare administrative records for matching. A special dietary follow-up of those aged 50 or older with two additional 24-hour recalls, funded by the National Institute on Aging, is ongoing, and reexamination or reinterview of the entire cohort is possible.

The real value of the survey lies in the content. The survey represents efforts to ascertain the prevalence of most important chronic diseases that cause mortality or disability in the U.S. population. This focus will make the survey a valuable resource for the study of comorbidity. The content areas for NHANES III include cardiovascular disease; musculoskeletal disease (osteoporosis and osteoarthritis); pulmonary function; diabetes and thyroid assessments; sensory impairments; dental disease (caries and periodontal disease); nutritional assessment, including anthropometry, body composition, food frequency, dietary adequacy, nutritional biochemistries, and hematologies; and 24-hour recall. To these disease or risk factor measures have been added measures of functional health status, including measures of cognitive status (an abbreviated Minimental Status test and a memory task), social function, and physical function, both self-reported and performance-based. Figure 16.1 gives some idea of how information from each part of the survey could contribute to a comprehensive overview of glucose intolerance and aging; and Figure 16.2 suggests the further benefit of an evaluation within the context of multiple disease processes.

The NHANES surveys have always consisted of an initial interview in the home and a physical evaluation in a mobile examination center. A number of strategies have been implemented in NHANES III to gain the cooperation of older respondents for participation in the mobile examination center examination, including a home examination for persons unable to unwilling to come in for an examination. The home examination consists of a small set of measures that can be transposed with good quality control into the home setting, including physical performance, memory testing,

Risk factors:	Disease:	Disability:	Service Utilization:
Interview:	Interview:	Interview:	Interview:
Family history	Told by MD	Self-report	Physician
Weight history	Medication		Hospital
Patterns of nutrition	Special diet		Nursing Home
Examination:	Examination:	Examination:	FOLLOWUP:
Anthropometry	Fasting glucose	Performance	Hospital
Body composition	Fasting insulin	Physician estimates	Death
	C-peptide		Incident diabetes
	Hemoglobin A1C		
	Photograph of retina		
	Age 60-74		
	Glucose load-2 Hr.		

Figure 16-1 Older persons in NHANES III—Diabetes Component.

some anthropometric measures, spirometry, and drawing of blood for biochemical and hematologic evaluations. These data from the home examination will allow expansion of the data base as well as a better assessment of nonresponse bias.

Preliminary data for the first three years of NHANES III should be available by 1995.

Older Persons in the Medical Care System: The National Ambulatory Medical Care Survey

The National Ambulatory Medical Care Survey (NAMCS) is a national probability sample of patient encounters with office-based physicians. It is designed to provide data on physicians' practices, the length of time they spend with patients, the drugs they prescribe, diagnoses, and referrals (Kovar, 1989). Information is also requested for the patient's source of payment, the presenting complaint, and any diagnostic procedures performed (McLemore and DeLozier, 1987) (see Table 16.2). Beginning in 1989 NAMCS became a continuing survey, with a sample of 2500 physicians that year. In 1991, the survey will expand coverage of physician–patient encounters to include visits to hospital outpatient departments.

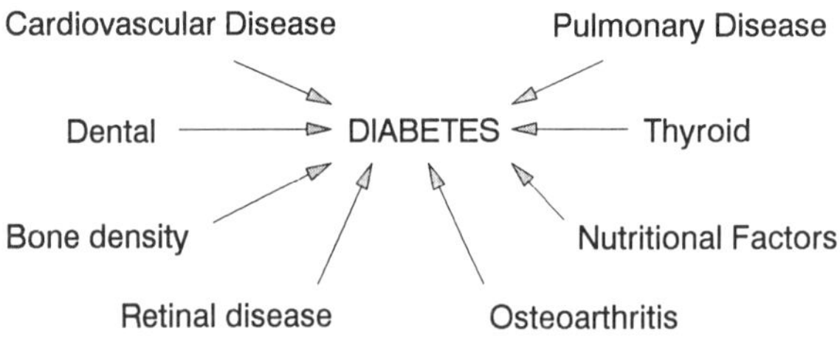

Figure 16-2 Uses of NHANES III to examine co-morbidity in relation to diabetes.

Older Persons in the Medical Care System: The National Hospital Discharge Survey

The National Hospital Discharge Survey is a continuing nationwide sample survey of discharges from short-stay nonfederal hospitals in the United States, designed to measure the volume of hospitalization, diagnoses and procedures, and changes in inpatient care. The scope of the survey encompasses patients discharged from noninstitutional hospitals, exclusive of military and Veterans Administration hospitals, located in the 50 states and the District of Columbia (NCHS, 1990a). Each year approximately 400 or more hospitals participate in the survey, with data abstracted from over 181,000 records, of which approximately one third are for persons aged 65 or older (see Table 16.2). Survey information also includes fact of death during hospitalization and whether the patient was discharged home or to another institution (Graves, 1988). The data in this survey are particularly useful in examination of age trends in particular diagnoses or in examination of time trends for a particular diagnosis over time. For example, it was this survey that documented the dramatic downward trends in inpatient hospital use following the implementation of diagnosis-related groups for adults of all ages, complementing Medicare data showing the downturn for people aged 65 and over. For the study of rarer diagnoses or emerging trends, several years of data can be aggregated.

Older Persons in Institutions: The National Nursing Home Survey

Although older persons living in nursing homes incur major medical expenses (Kovar, 1986), there are few studies that describe the nursing home population as a whole. Three sample surveys, in 1974, 1977, and 1985, have been conducted by the National Center for Health Statistics to obtain information on nursing homes, including the number and characteristics of residents and staff and expenditures for care of residents. The recent surveys have collected information on expenditures and characteristics of a sample of discharged patients as well.

The nursing home survey design is a stratified two-stage probability sample, with a first-stage selection of a sample of facilities and a second-stage selection of samples of residents, discharges, and RNs (Kovar, 1989; NCHS, 1990a). Data sources vary by type of questionnaire. Data on each facility are collected by interviews with administrators. Data about the nursing staff are collected by interviews or mail-in questionnaires. Data about current and discharged residents are collected by interviews with a nurse most familiar with the care provided to the resident, with the use of medical records during the interview. To supplement the information gathered on current and discharged residents from the nurse in the nursing home, a next-of-kin component obtains data not readily available from the nursing facilities, such as information on the subject's health during the period immediately preceding the nursing home admission and information on previous nursing home utilization.

Data for prior nursing home surveys are published (Kovar, 1989; Van Nostrand et al, 1979) and this section focuses on the 1985 National Nursing Home Survey. It included all types of nursing homes, including personal care and domiciliary-care homes (Hing et al, 1989; Kovar, 1989). Data were obtained from over 1000 facilities; over 2500 registered nurses; and over 10,000 current residents and discharged residents (see Table 16.2), including information from the next of kin.

The data in this survey are unique in their importance in describing a population of frail elders. The survey includes information on number of nursing home residents by age, sex, and race, source of resident payments, current and admission diagnoses, cognitive and physical functional status, and, for discharged residents, duration of stay as well as bed type and size of facilities, number and types of employees, per diem expenses. The value of these data for health services research has been further enhanced by a longitudinal follow-up of all those with a next-of-kin interview at baseline.

The National Nursing Home Followup collects additional information on the flow of the sampled residents in and out of long-term care facilities and hospitals (Kovar, 1989). It extends the period of observation for utilization patterns by 18–24 months. Respondents for all subjects not known to be deceased at the time of the National Nursing Home Survey were interviewed in 1987 (approximately 6000 cases) and again in 1988 using computer-assisted telephone interviewing. The questionnaire includes items on vital status, disability, nursing home and hospital utilization since the last contact, current living arrangements, and source of payment. In addition, linkages have been made to death data. The follow-up and the data linkages will allow examination of impairments among a group of older persons at very high risk of poor outcomes, as well as a more complete summary of health care utilization, particularly of institutional resources.

OLDER PERSONS AND DEATH STATISTICS: THE NATIONAL VITAL STATISTICS SYSTEM

Although investigators may be primarily interested in manipulation of survey microdata, published data is an equally important resource. Published data may be particularly useful for examination of time trends or ecologic studies. For instance, mortality data on underlying cause of death has been published yearly since 1933, through the National Vital Statistics System (Kovar, 1989), to complement the data tapes that are also available for investigators. Data in the Vital Statistics System are collected and published on births, deaths, marriages, and divorces in the United States, with almost complete registration of deaths (see Table 16.2). This important set of data is discussed elsewhere in this volume, so this description is brief. Cause of death is coded according to the International Classification of Disease promulgated by the World Health Organization at the most detailed (four-digit) level. Since 1968, information has been available for both underlying and multiple cause of death. Beginning with data year 1984, information is available on the usual occupation and industry of the decedent for 16 states as well (Kovar, 1989). One utility for these published data is examination of time trends for particular causes of death (Sempos et al, 1988). Data of this type also finds a major utility in cost–benefit modeling of the effect of intervention programs on all-cause or cause-specific mortality (Weinstein et al, 1987).

Older Persons and Death Statistics: The National Mortality Followback Survey

It is well known that medical expenses increase in the last year of life (Kovar, 1986). Because of this, the antecedents of death are of great interest to health care economists and epidemiologists. The National Mortality Followback Survey (NMFS) is designed to address this issue, as well as to examine the reliability of items such as age, race, occupation, and industry reported on the death certificate through comparison of death certificate information and information from the survey respondent. The 1986 survey included information on the utilization of hospitals and institutions during the last year of the decedent's life, household composition, education, income and residence of the decedent, hospital and surgical insurance coverage, charges for hospital care and source of payment, surgeons' bills and source of payment, and smoking habits (Kovar, 1989).

The 1986 NMFS was based on a sample of about 18,500 death certificates of persons aged 25 years and older, with the next of kin identified on the death certificate or some other knowledgeable informant as the respondent (see Table 16.2) (Kapantais and Powell-Griner, 1989). Additional data on admission dates, diagnoses, and procedures were collected from those health facilities the decendent used in the last year of life.

SUMMARY

This chapter has provided an overview of data systems at the National Center for Health Statistics relevant to research on aging. Every other year, to encourage the utilization of these resources and to interact with the research community in terms of priorities for data collection, NCHS holds a data users conference in which the latest data available from the NCHS are reviewed, including discussion of statistical techniques for analysis of these data. In addition, the National Center for Health Statistics publishes several series of reports based on the data sets (Havlik et al, 1987), which can be used to examine time trends, perform ecologic analysis, or provide models for forecasting or cost–benefit analysis. From the continued use of the health statistics data that are available and from data collected in the future, strategies aimed at prevention of frailty and disability in older persons will continue to be developed.

REFERENCES

Adams PF, Hardy AM (1989). Current estimates from the National Health Interview Survey, 1988. Vital and Health Statistics, Series 10, No. 173. NCHS, Washington, DC.

Cohen BB, Barbano HE, Cox CS, Feldman JJ, Finucane FF, Kleinman JC, et al (1987). Plan and operation of the NHANES I epidemiologic followup study, 1982–84. Vital and Health Statistics, Series 1, No. 22. NCHS, Washington, DC.

Cornoni-Huntley J, Brock DB, Ostfeld AM, Taylor JO, Wallace RB (eds) (1986). Established

populations for epidemiologic studies of the elderly, resource data book. National Institutes of Health, Washington, DC.
Cornoni-Huntley J, Huntley RR, Feldman JJ (eds) (1990). Health status and well-being of the elderly. National Health and Nutrition Examination Survey I-Epidemiologic Follow-up Study. Oxford University Press, New York.
Cummings SR, Black DM, Browner WS, Cauley JA, Genant HK, Mascioli SR, et al. (1990). Appendicular bone density and age predict hip fracture in women. JAMA 263:665–668.
European Working Party on High Blood Pressure in the Elderly (1985). An international trial of antihypertensive therapy in elderly patients. Objectives, protocol and organization. Arch Int Pharmacodyn Ther 275:300–334.
Finucane FF, Freid VM, Madans JH, Cox CS, Kleinman JC, Rothwell ST, et al. (1990). Plan and operation of the NHANES I Epidemiologic Followup Study, 1986. Vital and Health Statistics, Series 1, No. 25. NCHS, Washington, DC.
Fitti J, Kovar MG (1988). The 1984 supplement on aging. Vital and Health Statistics, Series 1, No. 21. NCHS, Washington, DC.
Fried LP, Borhani NO, Enright P, Furberg CD, Gardin JM, Kronmal RA, et al (1991). The Cardiovascular Health Study: design and rationale. Ann Epidemiol 1:263–276.
Graves EJ (1988). Utilization of short-stay hospitals: Annual summary, United States, 1986. Vital and Health Statistics, Series 13, No. 96. NCHS, Washington, DC.
Harris T, Kovar MG, Suzman R, Kleinman JC, and Feldman JJ (1989a). Longitudinal study of physical ability in the oldest-old. Am J Public Health 79:698–702.
Harris T, Makuc DM, Kleinman JC, Gillum RF, Curb JD, Schatzkin A, et al (1991). Is the cholesterol–ischemic heart disease relationship modified by activity level in older persons? J Am Geriatric Society 39:747–754.
Harris T, Woteki C, Briefel R, Kleinman JC (1989b). NHANES III for older persons: Nutrition content and methodological considerations. Am J Clin Nutr 50:1145–1149.
Havlik RJ, Liu BM, Kovar MG, Suzman R, Feldman JJ, Harris T, Van Nostrand J (eds) (1987). Health statistics on older persons, United States, 1986. Vital and Health Statistics, Series 3, No. 25. NCHS, Washington, DC.
Hing E, Sekscenski E, Strahan G (1989). The National Nursing Home Survey: 1985 summary for the United States. Vital and Health Statistics, Series 13, No. 97. NCHS, Washington, DC.
Kapantais G, Powell-Griner E (1989). Characteristics of persons dying of diseases of heart: Preliminary data from the 1986 National Mortality Followback Survey. Advance Data from Vital and Health Statistics, No. 172. NCHS, Washington, DC.
Kovar MG (1986). Expenditures for the medical care of elderly people living in the community in 1980. Milbank Quart 64:100–132.
Kovar MG (1989). Data systems of the National Center for Health Statistics. Vital and Health Statistics, Series 1, No. 23. NCHS, Washington, DC.
Madans JH, Kleinman JC, Cox CC, Barbano HE, Feldman JJ, Cohen B, et al (1986). 10 Years after NHANES I: Report of initial followup, 1982–84. Pub Health Rep 101:465–473.
Maurer K (1985). Plan and operation of the Hispanic Health and Nutrition Examination Survey, 1982–84. Vital and Health Statistics, Series 1, No. 19. NCHS, Washington, DC.
McDowell A, Engel A, Massey JT, Maurer K (1981). Plan and operation of the Second National Health and Nutrition Examination Survey, 1976–80. Vital and Health Statistics, Series 1, No. 15. NCHS, Washington, DC.
McLemore T, DeLozier J (1987). 1985 summary: National Ambulatory Medical Care Survey. Advance Data from Vital and Health Statistics, No. 128. NCHS, Washington, DC.
National Center for Health Statistics (1977). Plan and operation of the Health and Nutrition Examination Survey. 1971–73. Vital and Health Statistics, Series 1, No. 10b. NCHS, Washington, DC.

National Center for Health Statistics (1990a). Health, United States, 1989. NCHS, Washington, DC.

National Center for Health Statistics (1990b). Catalog of Electronic Data Products. NCHS, Washington, DC.

Ouslander JG, Resnick NM (eds) (1990). National Institutes of Health Consensus Development Conference on Urinary Incontinence. J Am Geriatr Soc 38:263–386.

Schatzkin A, Taylor PR, Carter CL, et al (1987). Serum cholesterol and cancer in the NHANES I epidemiologic followup study. Lancet ii:298–301.

Schneider EL, Guralnik JM (1990). The aging of Ameria. JAMA 263:2335–2340.

Sempos CT, Cooper RS, Kovar MG, McMillen MM (1988). Divergence of recent U.S. trends in coronary mortality for the four major sex–race groups. Am J Public Health 78:1422–1427.

Systolic Hypertension in the Elderly Program (SHEP) Cooperative Research Group. (1988). Rationale and design of a randomized clinical trial on prevention of stroke in isolated systolic hypertension. J Clin Epidemiol 41:1197–1208.

Van Nostrand JF, Zappolo A, Hing E, et al (1979). The National Nursing Home Survey, 1977 Summary for the United States. Vital and Health Statistics Series 13, No. 43. NCHS, Washington, DC.

Weinstein MC, Coxson PG, Williams LW, Pass TM, Stason WB, Goldman L (1987). Forecasting coronary heart disease incidence, mortality, and cost: The Coronary Heart Disease Policy Model. Am J Public Health 77:1417–1426.

Woteki C, Briefel R, Kuczmarski R (1988). Contributions of the National Center for Health Statistics. Am J Clin Nutr 47:320–328.

Zylke JW (1990). As nation grows older, falls become greater source of fear, injury, death. JAMA 263:2021–2023.

17

The Quality and Application of Death Records of Older Persons

RICHARD J. HAVLIK AND HARRY M. ROSENBERG

The death certificate is the basic source of information for mortality statistics. Various types of death statistics, as generated from governmental jurisdictions or epidemiologic research studies, provide fundamental information on the ultimate effects of the aging process and its relationship with various diseases prominent in older persons. However, the usefulness of this information depends on the quality of the original death records.

A great deal of attention has been paid to the validity of cause-of-death statistics, relationships of certificate entries to autopsy findings, multiple cause-of-death analyses, and programs to improve the quality of death records; but much more effort is necessary (Israel et al, 1986; Kircher et al, 1985; Moriyama, 1989; Rosenberg, 1989; Sirken et al, 1987). This chapter will review these issues for investigators using cause-of-death data in studies of the epidemiology of aging and present examples of data and analyses relevant to these issues.

As background, in 1987, a total of 2,123,323 deaths were registered in the United States, the largest number ever recorded (National Center for Health Statistics, 1989). The reasons for this large number of deaths were population growth and the increasing proportion of older persons in the population, where the majority of these deaths occur. However, if the effects of aging of the population are eliminated through age adjustment, the death rate for this same year was the lowest recorded. About two thirds, or 1,509,686, of the 1987 deaths occurred among those 65 years of age and older. Almost 70 percent of these deaths of older persons result from the top three causes—heart diseases, malignant neoplasms, and cerebrovascular diseases (Table 17.1). For these older persons, the relative order of causes does not change for age subgroups until ages 85 years and over, when cerebrovascular disease replaces malignant neoplasms as the second leading cause.

Such cause-of-death information from death certificates is a simple example of their potential usefulness in characterizing the health status of older persons. Researchers and public health officials have used mortality statistics for trend analysis, geographic comparisons, testing of etiologic hypotheses, clinical trial end points, and so on. However, it is the obligation of the epidemiologist to be aware of the strengths and weaknesses of death records in order to use them properly.

Table 17-1 Deaths and Death Rates for the 10 Leading Causes of Death, Age 65 Years and Over: United States, 1987 (rates per 100,000 population in specified group)

Rank order	Cause of death (Ninth Revision International Classification of Diseases, 1975)		Number	Rate
	All causes		1,509,686	5059.9
1	Diseases of heart	390–398, 402, 404–429	618,989	2074.6
2	Malignant neoplasms, including neoplasms of lymphatic and hematopoletic tissues	140–208	316,199	1059.8
3	Cerebrovascular diseases	430–438	129,784	435.0
4	Chronic obstructive pulmonary diseases and allied conditions	490–496	64,451	216.0
5	Pneumonia and influenza	480–487	60,542	202.9
6	Diabetes mellitus	250	28,377	95.1
7	Accidents and adverse effects	E800–E949	25,838	86.6
–	Motor vehicle accidents	E810–E825	6,781	22.7
–	All other accidents and adverse effects	E800–E807, E826–E949	19,057	63.9
8	Atherosclerosis	440	21,372	71.6
9	Nephritis, nephrotic syndrome, and nephrosis	580–589	18,249	61.2
10	Septicemia	038	15,868	53.2
	All other causes	Residual	210,017	703.9

Source: Extracted from National Center for Health Statistics, 1989.

QUALITY OF DEMOGRAPHIC DATA ON DEATH RECORDS

Studies have been conducted on the reliability of information other than cause of death on the death certificate. A major study was carried out for 1960 by comparing the information from a large sample of death records (340,000) with information from manually matched census records for the same individuals (National Center for Health Statistics, 1968). Regarding accuracy of age, a total of 69 percent of the decedents had the same age on the two records, and 87 percent agreed within one year of each other. When the records were combined into five- and 10-year age groups, as normally tabulated, the levels of agreement were, respectively, 86 and 90 percent. Agreement levels were somewhat higher for the white than for the nonwhite population, and they were higher for males than for females. A similar study carried out in Great Britain using their 1951 census showed 80 percent agreement on exact age, a much higher rate than for the United States in 1960 (Great Britain General Register Office, 1958). Stratification by age shows only slightly better agreement for the younger than for the older population.

The U.S. study also provided information on the reliability of other variables, such as marital status, race, and nativity (National Center for Health Statistics, 1969). With respect to agreement on marital status, approximately 94 percent of the matched records for decedents aged 15–74 years showed the same marital status on both records, as compared with 98 percent for a similar study carried out in Great Britain for the census of 1961 (Great Britain General Register Office, 1968). With respect to race, the agreement between the two records by specified race was as follows: white, 99.8 percent; black, 97.7 percent; American Indian, 79.2 percent; Japanese, 97.0 percent; Chinese, 90.3 percent; Filipino, 72.6 percent; and all other races, 60.4 percent. It was found that a relatively large percent of the records for the smaller race groups on the census was assigned to the white race category on the death certificate. With respect to nativity, the agreement rates for native-born and foreign-born were both in excess of 98 percent.

A number of studies have been done on the accuracy of reports of occupation and industry on the death certificate by comparing this information with other sources. Such studies indicate a level of agreement in the range of 50–80 percent (National Office of Vital Statistics, 1961; California Department of Health Services, 1979–1981; and Schade and Swanson, 1988). Among the problems noted in the study are reporting the last occupation rather than the "usual" occupation, which is requested on the death certificate; the "upgrading" of the occupation; and the use of vague and imprecise descriptions. It has been pointed out that for many people who have different jobs throughout their work life, it may be difficult to designate any single occupation as the usual one. This can be particularly true of women, who may have been housewives and held a variety of other jobs both before and after being a homemaker.

It can be assumed that the degree of reliability of the demographic items reported on the death certificate is improving over time as a result of concerted efforts on the part of federal and state officials. These efforts take the form of (1) improved edit procedures at the data-processing level to ensure consistency among certain items, such as date of birth and reported age of the decedent, and cause of death and sex of decedent; (2) educational efforts exemplified by handbooks, video and audio aids, and so on, aimed at the funeral directors who report this information on decedents; and (3) querying respondents from whom responses on these items are ambiguous, unclear, or inconsistent with other reported information. Also contributing to improvements over this time is simply the increasing educational attainment and sophistication of the public. Thus, a generation ago, for some segments of the population there may have been a real question of age at death, because no birth certificate may have been filed. Over time, that segment of the population has diminished as the practice of birth registration has become universal.

QUALITY OF CAUSE-OF-DEATH DATA

The validity of cause-of-death data has been a concern because of the importance and wide use of these data at national, state, and local levels. Also, it is the means for comparison of mortality statistics with other countries. Because of its importance, the medical certification section of the death certificate is standardized through an agreement with the World Health Organization. The International Classification of Diseases (ICD) stipulates the general format of the certificate, the attending physician as responsible for completion of the certificate, and a coding structure to process this information (World Health Organization, 1977). The United States has developed a standard certificate of death, which with minor variations is used by most States (Figure 17.1).

TYPE/PRINT IN PERMANENT BLACK INK FOR INSTRUCTIONS
SEE OTHER SIDE AND HANDBOOK

LOCAL FILE NUMBER

U.S. STANDARD
CERTIFICATE OF DEATH

STATE FILE NUMBER

DECEDENT

1. DECEDENT'S NAME *(First, Middle, Last)*
2. SEX
3. DATE OF DEATH *(Month, Day, Year)*
4. SOCIAL SECURITY NUMBER
5a. AGE—Last Birthday *(Years)*
5b. UNDER 1 YEAR: Months | Days
5c. UNDER 1 DAY: Hours | Minutes
6. DATE OF BIRTH *(Month, Day, Year)*
7. BIRTHPLACE *(City and State or Foreign Country)*
8. WAS DECEDENT EVER IN U.S. ARMED FORCES? *(Yes or no)*
9a. PLACE OF DEATH *(Check only one; see instructions on other side)*
HOSPITAL: ☐ Inpatient ☐ ER/Outpatient ☐ DOA
OTHER: ☐ Nursing Home ☐ Residence ☐ Other *(Specify)*
9b. FACILITY NAME *(If not institution, give street and number)*
9c. CITY, TOWN, OR LOCATION OF DEATH
9d. COUNTY OF DEATH
10. MARITAL STATUS - Married, Never Married, Widowed, Divorced *(Specify)*
11. SURVIVING SPOUSE *(If wife, give maiden name)*
12a. DECEDENT'S USUAL OCCUPATION *(Give kind of work done during most of working life. Do not use retired.)*
12b. KIND OF BUSINESS/INDUSTRY

SEE INSTRUCTIONS ON OTHER SIDE

13a. RESIDENCE - STATE
13b. COUNTY
13c. CITY, TOWN, OR LOCATION
13d. STREET AND NUMBER
13e. INSIDE CITY LIMITS? *(Yes or no)*
13f. ZIP CODE
14. WAS DECEDENT OF HISPANIC ORIGIN? (Specify No or Yes - If yes, specify Cuban, Mexican, Puerto Rican, etc.) ☐ No ☐ Yes Specify
15. RACE—American Indian, Black, White, etc. *(Specify)*
16. DECEDENT'S EDUCATION *(Specify only highest grade completed)* Elementary/Secondary (0-12) | College (1-4 or 5+)

PARENTS

17. FATHER'S NAME *(First, Middle, Last)*
18. MOTHER'S NAME *(First, Middle, Maiden Surname)*

INFORMANT

19a. INFORMANT'S NAME *(Type/Print)*
19b. MAILING ADDRESS *(Street and Number or Rural Route Number, City or Town, State, Zip Code)*

DISPOSITION

20a. METHOD OF DISPOSITION
☐ Burial ☐ Cremation ☐ Removal from State
☐ Donation ☐ Other *(Specify)* ______
20b. PLACE OF DISPOSITION *(Name of cemetery, crematory, or other place)*
20c. LOCATION—City or Town, State
21a. SIGNATURE OF FUNERAL SERVICE LICENSEE OR PERSON ACTING AS SUCH ▶
21b. LICENSE NUMBER *(of Licensee)*
22. NAME AND ADDRESS OF FACILITY

SEE DEFINITION ON OTHER SIDE

PRONOUNCING PHYSICIAN ONLY

Complete items 23a-c only when certifying physician is not available at time of death to certify cause of death.
23a. To the best of my knowledge, death occurred at the time, date, and place stated. *Signature and Title* ▶
23b. LICENSE NUMBER
23c. DATE SIGNED *(Month, Day, Year)*

ITEMS 24-26 MUST BE COMPLETED BY PERSON WHO PRONOUNCES DEATH

24. TIME OF DEATH M
25. DATE PRONOUNCED DEAD *(Month, Day, Year)*
26. WAS CASE REFERRED TO MEDICAL EXAMINER/CORONER? *(Yes or no)*

SEE INSTRUCTIONS ON OTHER SIDE

CAUSE OF DEATH

27. PART I. Enter the diseases, injuries, or complications that caused the death. Do not enter the mode of dying, such as cardiac or respiratory arrest, shock, or heart failure. List only one cause on each line.
Approximate Interval Between Onset and Death
IMMEDIATE CAUSE (Final disease or condition resulting in death) ⟶ a. ______
DUE TO (OR AS A CONSEQUENCE OF):
Sequentially list conditions, if any, leading to immediate cause. Enter UNDERLYING CAUSE (Disease or injury that initiated events resulting in death) LAST
b. ______
DUE TO (OR AS A CONSEQUENCE OF):
c. ______
DUE TO (OR AS A CONSEQUENCE OF):
d. ______
PART II. Other significant conditions contributing to death but not resulting in the underlying cause given in Part I.
28a. WAS AN AUTOPSY PERFORMED? *(Yes or no)*
28b. WERE AUTOPSY FINDINGS AVAILABLE PRIOR TO COMPLETION OF CAUSE OF DEATH? *(Yes or no)*
29. MANNER OF DEATH
☐ Natural ☐ Pending Investigation
☐ Accident
☐ Suicide ☐ Could not be Determined
☐ Homicide
30a. DATE OF INJURY *(Month, Day, Year)*
30b. TIME OF INJURY M
30c. INJURY AT WORK? *(Yes or no)*
30d. DESCRIBE HOW INJURY OCCURRED
30e. PLACE OF INJURY—At home, farm, street, factory, office building, etc. *(Specify)*
30f. LOCATION (Street and Number or Rural Route Number, City or Town, State)

SEE DEFINITION ON OTHER SIDE

CERTIFIER

31a. CERTIFIER *(Check only one)*
☐ CERTIFYING PHYSICIAN *(Physician certifying cause of death when another physician has pronounced death and completed Item 23)*
To the best of my knowledge, death occurred due to the cause(s) and manner as stated.
☐ PRONOUNCING AND CERTIFYING PHYSICIAN *(Physician both pronouncing death and certifying to cause of death)*
To the best of my knowledge, death occurred at the time, date, and place, and due to the cause(s) and manner as stated.
☐ MEDICAL EXAMINER/CORONER
On the basis of examination and/or investigation, in my opinion, death occurred at the time, date, and place, and due to the cause(s) and manner as stated.
31b. SIGNATURE AND TITLE OF CERTIFIER ▶
31c. LICENSE NUMBER
31d. DATE SIGNED *(Month, Day, Year)*
32. NAME AND ADDRESS OF PERSON WHO COMPLETED CAUSE OF DEATH (ITEM 27) *(Type/Print)*

REGISTRAR

33. REGISTRAR'S SIGNATURE ▶
34. DATE FILED *(Month, Day, Year)*

NAME OF DECEDENT: For use by physician or institution

DEPARTMENT OF HEALTH AND HUMAN SERVICES · PUBLIC HEALTH SERVICE · NATIONAL CENTER FOR HEALTH STATISTICS · 1989 REVISION

Figure 17-1 US standard certificate of death, 1989 revision.

Death Certificate Completion

The design of the death certificate is organized to obtain from the physicians the "underlying cause of death" or the disease or injury that initiated the train of events that leads directly to death or the circumstances of the accident or violence that produced the fatal injury. For public health purposes and in the prevention of death it is the underlying cause that is believed to have the most potential for breaking the chain of events leading to death. Of course, in issues related to the elderly, other information on the death certificate, such as the contributing causes of death, may be quite important. These "multiple-cause" aspects of death certification and analysis will be discussed later in the chapter.

The death certificate provides a format for entering the causes of death in a sequential manner with the underlying cause in the final position (see Figure 17.1). To reach this "bottom line" the physician is requested to enter on the top line of Item No. 27 the immediate cause. This should not be a nonspecific entry such as asystole or cardiac arrest but a disease entity associated with death. This entry is followed by one or more intermediate conditions that develop from the underlying cause, which may differ from the primary or principal diagnosis, which is often required in medical records as the reason for contact with the health care system.

Because of the physician's potential uncertainty in certifying a single underlying cause at any age, especially in the elderly, the certificate includes the words "to the best of my knowledge death occurred due to the causes listed." Ultimately, the data are based on the physician's opinion; however, the attending physician should be in the best position to make such a decision. In medical–legal cases, it is the responsibility of the coroner or medical examiner to use the best available information to complete the death certificate. Should some information be unavailable at the time of certification, such as the results from an autopsy or special tests, an amended certificate can be prepared by the physician in most states. However, in many instances this important step is not taken, or if it is, the certificate entries might be amended too late to be incorporated into official statistics.

Currently, a number of states have begun using a certificate with examples of proper completion on the reverse side (Figure 17.2). One example deals with a heart attack death and the other deals with a motor vehicle accident. Although it is too early to evaluate whether this change will have a positive effect on certification validity, this addition was made in response to recommendations by certifying physicians (Freedman et al, 1988).

Death Certificate Processing

To be aware of potential sources of bias that might occur after entries are made on the death certificate, the epidemiologist should be familiar with the process that converts the raw data entered by the physician on the death certificate into state and national mortality statistics. Also, if one needs to compare study-specific data with vital statistics, it might be advantageous to incorporate certain standard methodologies, such as the use of nosologist coding or available computer programs. In terms of collecting, processing, and maintaining the quality of cause-of-death data, the individual states have the prime responsibility. The NCHS supplies technical and other support. For example, instruction manuals, which incorporate ICD directives and changes, are circulated to the states on a regular basis. This mutually beneficial interaction, which includes uniform standards for quality control, data processing and editing, and data presentation, is called the Vital Statistics Cooperative Program. Also NCHS sponsors a National Death Certificate Registry, the National Death Index, which allows scien-

INSTRUCTIONS FOR SELECTED ITEMS

Item 9 – Place of Death
If the death was pronounced in a hospital, check the box indicating the decedent's status at the institution (inpatient, emergency room outpatient, or dead on arrival (DOA)). If death was pronounced elsewhere, check the box indicating whether pronouncement occurred at a nursing home, residence, or other location. If other is checked, specify where death was legally pronounced, such as a physician's office, the place where the accident occurred, or at work.

Items 13 a-f – Residence of Decedent
Residence of the decedent is the place where he or she actually resided. This is not necessarily the same as "home State," or "legal residence." Never enter a temporary residence such as one used during a visit, business trip, or a vacation. Place of residence during a tour of military duty or during attendance at college is not considered as temporary and should be considered as the place of residence.

If a decedent had been living in a facility where an individual usually resides for a long period of time, such as a group home, mental institution, nursing home, penitentiary, or hospital for the chronically ill, report the location of that facility in items 13a through 13f.

If the decedent was an infant who never resided at home, the place of residence is that of the parent(s) or legal guardian. Do not use an acute care hospital's location as the place of residence for any infant.

Items 23 and 31 – Medical Certification
The PRONOUNCING PHYSICIAN is the person who determines that the decedent is legally dead but who was not in charge of the patient's care for the illness or condition which resulted in death. Items 23a through 23c are to be completed only when the physician responsible for completing the medical certification of cause of death (Item 27) is not available at time of death to certify cause of death. The pronouncing physician is responsible for completing only items 23 through 26.

The CERTIFYING PHYSICIAN is the person who determines the cause of death (Item 27). This box should be checked only in those cases when the person who is completing the medical certification of cause of death is not the person who pronounced death (Item 23). The certifying physician is responsible for completing items 27 through 32.

The PRONOUNCING AND CERTIFYING PHYSICIAN box should be checked when the same person is responsible for completing Items 24 through 32, that is, when the same physician has both pronounced death and certified the cause of death. If this box is checked, items 23a through 23c should be left blank.

The MEDICAL EXAMINER/CORONER box should be checked when investigation is required by the Post Mortem Examination Act and the cause of death is completed by a medical examiner or coroner. The Medical Examiner/Coroner is responsible for completing items 24 through 32.

Item 27 – Cause of Death
The cause of death means the disease, abnormality, injury, or poisoning that caused the death, not the mode of dying, such as cardiac or respiratory arrest, shock, or heart failure.

In Part I, the immediate cause of death is reported on line (a). Antecedent conditions, if any, which gave rise to the cause are reported on lines (b), (c), and (d). The underlying cause, should be reported on the last line used in Part I. No entry is necessary on lines (b), (c), and (d) if the immediate cause of death on line (a) describes completely the train of events. ONLY ONE CAUSE SHOULD BE ENTERED ON A LINE. Additional lines may be added if necessary. Provide the best estimate of the interval between the onset of each condition and death. Do not leave the interval blank, if unknown, so specify.

In Part II, enter other important diseases or conditions that may have contributed to death but did not result in the underlying cause of death given in Part I.

See examples below.

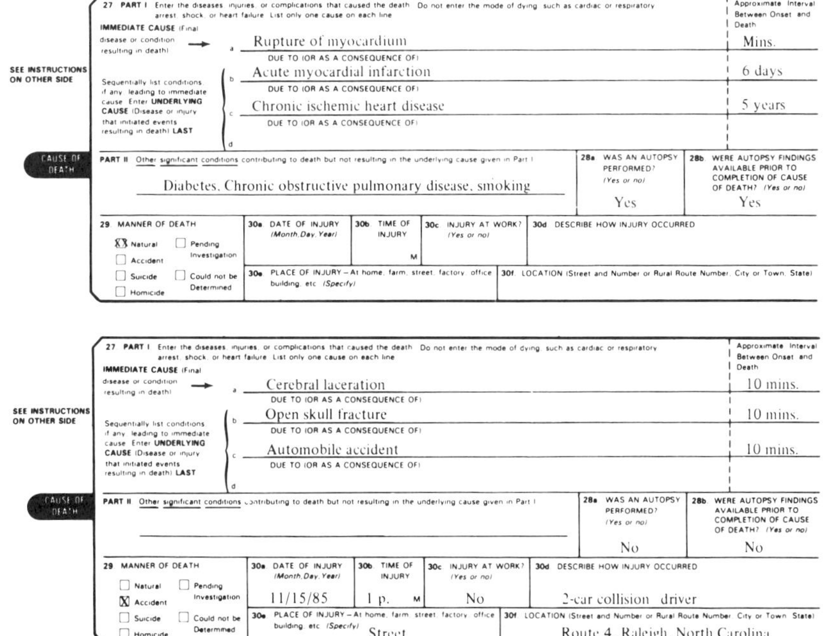

SEE INSTRUCTIONS ON OTHER SIDE

CAUSE OF DEATH

27. PART I. Enter the diseases, injuries, or complications that caused the death. Do not enter the mode of dying, such as cardiac or respiratory arrest, shock, or heart failure. List only one cause on each line.

IMMEDIATE CAUSE (Final disease or condition resulting in death) → a. Rupture of myocardium — Approximate Interval Between Onset and Death: Mins.

DUE TO (OR AS A CONSEQUENCE OF):

Sequentially list conditions, if any, leading to immediate cause. Enter UNDERLYING CAUSE (Disease or injury that initiated events resulting in death) LAST

b. Acute myocardial infarction — 6 days

DUE TO (OR AS A CONSEQUENCE OF):

c. Chronic ischemic heart disease — 5 years

DUE TO (OR AS A CONSEQUENCE OF):

d.

PART II. Other significant conditions contributing to death but not resulting in the underlying cause given in Part I: Diabetes, Chronic obstructive pulmonary disease, smoking

28a. WAS AN AUTOPSY PERFORMED? (Yes or no): Yes

28b. WERE AUTOPSY FINDINGS AVAILABLE PRIOR TO COMPLETION OF CAUSE OF DEATH? (Yes or no): Yes

29. MANNER OF DEATH: [X] Natural [ ] Accident [ ] Suicide [ ] Homicide [ ] Pending Investigation [ ] Could not be Determined

30a. DATE OF INJURY (Month, Day, Year) | 30b. TIME OF INJURY M | 30c. INJURY AT WORK? (Yes or no) | 30d. DESCRIBE HOW INJURY OCCURRED

30e. PLACE OF INJURY – At home, farm, street, factory, office building, etc. (Specify) | 30f. LOCATION (Street and Number or Rural Route Number, City or Town, State)

SEE INSTRUCTIONS ON OTHER SIDE

CAUSE OF DEATH

27. PART I. Enter the diseases, injuries, or complications that caused the death. Do not enter the mode of dying, such as cardiac or respiratory arrest, shock, or heart failure. List only one cause on each line.

IMMEDIATE CAUSE (Final disease or condition resulting in death) → a. Cerebral laceration — Approximate Interval Between Onset and Death: 10 mins.

DUE TO (OR AS A CONSEQUENCE OF):

Sequentially list conditions, if any, leading to immediate cause. Enter UNDERLYING CAUSE (Disease or injury that initiated events resulting in death) LAST

b. Open skull fracture — 10 mins.

DUE TO (OR AS A CONSEQUENCE OF):

c. Automobile accident — 10 mins.

DUE TO (OR AS A CONSEQUENCE OF):

d.

PART II. Other significant conditions contributing to death but not resulting in the underlying cause given in Part I:

28a. WAS AN AUTOPSY PERFORMED? (Yes or no): No

28b. WERE AUTOPSY FINDINGS AVAILABLE PRIOR TO COMPLETION OF CAUSE OF DEATH? (Yes or no): No

29. MANNER OF DEATH: [ ] Natural [X] Accident [ ] Suicide [ ] Homicide [ ] Pending Investigation [ ] Could not be Determined

30a. DATE OF INJURY (Month, Day, Year): 11/15/85 | 30b. TIME OF INJURY: 1 p. M | 30c. INJURY AT WORK? (Yes or no): No | 30d. DESCRIBE HOW INJURY OCCURRED: 2-car collision driver

30e. PLACE OF INJURY – At home, farm, street, factory, office building, etc. (Specify): Street | 30f. LOCATION (Street and Number or Rural Route Number, City or Town, State): Route 4, Raleigh, North Carolina

Figure 17-2 Reverse side, US standard certificate of death, 1989 revision.

tific investigation in prospective studies by identifying where copies of the actual death certificate are filed for use by researchers (Curb et at, 1985).

Although the physician designates the underlying cause of death, certain rules based on the classification structure and other considerations in the ICD are applied systematically by the responsible vital statisticians to all the information on the certificate. These rules contribute to comparability and uniformity of cause-of-death statistics among different parts of the country and compensate somewhat for the known variation in certification practices by individual physicians. There is a reasonable amount of consistency between the underlying cause of death as reported by the physician on the death certificate and the underlying cause selected by the nosologist. Studies by NCHS have shown that even with the most specific classification categories there was agreement for three of every four deaths. It needs to be pointed out that the ICD nomenclature underemphasizes certain gerontologically oriented areas, such as physical and other functions, and this lessens the usefulness of such less specific categories in death certification.

Although for many years the selection of the underlying cause of death was done manually by highly trained medical coders in a successful manner, currently the selection is done using a computer algorithm called ACME (Automated Classification of Medical Entities), using all the medical conditions on the death certificate keyed into the computer by medical coders. The benefits of the new procedure are more uniform and rapid processing of the data, more consistency in selecting the underlying cause of death, and the routine production of multiple cause-of-death data for the United States. The production of multiple-cause data (contributing or non–underlying-cause-of-death data) requires the application of additional software called TRANSAX (Translation of Axes). A system termed MICAR (Mortality Medical Information, Coding, and Retrieval System) was tested during 1990 in a few states. This system ultimately should allow the direct entry of the written physician statements on the death certificate and their automated conversion into cause-of-death codes that can be used subsequently with both ACME, for selection of underlying cause of death, and TRANSAX, for the production of multiple-cause data. MICAR promises to reduce considerably the requirements for trained medical coders, who would only be required to adjudicate situations the computer software cannot handle and to make possible retrieval of the exact wording used by the physician to characterize the medical conditions contributing to or causing death, conditions whose specificity is now often lost in the broad categories of the International Classification of Disease.

Measuring Validity

A recent review of the nature and accuracy of cause-of-death data has been completed (Rosenberg, 1990). The development of protocols that permit the ascertainment of accuracy of death certificates is challenging. Some clinical studies have side-stepped this problem by using physician panel review of mortality end-point results and the substantiating historical documents in order, at least, to apply consistent criteria for establishing the cause of death. Part of the difficulty is determining what is a "true" cause of death. This, then, would be used as a gold standard to compare with the certifying physician's best judgment as to the cause of death. Various studies have proposed the use of available clinical information and/or postmortem findings. However, there is the all too frequent situation of having a panel of clinicians second-guess the attending physician. Many times this is on the basis of the same set of medical records. In fact, because of these difficulties, some have concluded that there are probably no completely representative studies that provide valid estimates of the "true error" in national mortality statistics. An annotated bibliography of cause-of-death validation studies on selected populations and covering 128 references for approximately 25 years ending in 1980 has been prepared (National Center for Health Statistics, 1982). In general, those diseases that were more readily detected, especially neoplasms, were more accurately reported than others, such as cardiovascular diseases. However, there was variability of diagnoses both with cancer sites and cardiovascular diseases. Also, results cited in this report varied by whether clinical validation or autopsy findings were used.

Recent Clinical Validation Studies

Since the publication of the NCHS bibliography, there have been attempts to address different aspects of the validity issue. For example, investigators studied potential systematic biases in death certification in Maryland (Sorlie and Gold, 1987). The study was prompted by an apparent major shift in cardiovascular deaths in the state with the initiation of the revised mortality classification, ICD-9, in 1979. The observed change in cardiovascular mortality for Maryland was much greater than would have been indicated by the national comparability studies, which contrast mortality statistics based on the previous and the new ICD versions (ICDA-8 and ICD-9, respectively). Their innovative study suggested that the use of generalized cardiovascular terms, rather than specific diagnoses related to the heart, by medical examiners and other physicians in Maryland resulted in an apparent distortion of cardiovascular trends. The discontinuity resulted from general terms being coded in one manner in ICDA-8 and differently in ICD-9. Thus, in examining long-term trends in morbidity and mortality the epidemiologist cannot be concerned only about the death certificate entries themselves. He or she must also consider the potential interaction with changing disease classification structures. This suggests that in studies of small areas epidemiologists may need to do their own validation studies to be sure that gross distortions are not occurring unexpectedly.

Another strategy that can be used to obtain an estimate of the validity of death certificate entries is comparing them to a separate data source. A recent example is instructive in giving the principles of such clinical validation studies (Rosenberg et al, 1991). In this case the independent source was a survey of informants who were asked to respond to questions about the health history of the decedent in a mortality followback survey. By comparing the responses from the survey with the cause of death on the certificate, the investigators could get an indication of the extent to which the certificate reflected the medical history of the decedent and whether any correlation was stronger for younger than for older individuals.

For this study two sources of NCHS data were used: the underlying cause-of-death data for U.S. deaths in a sample drawn from 1986 and the medical data from the 1986 National Mortality Followback Survey (Kapantais and Powell-Griner, 1989). This survey obtained a history from the informant on important characteristics of the decedent that may have affected mortality. These characteristics included, for example, various health services experienced prior to death. This additional history supplemented the information obtained from death records. The sample consisted of data for 18,753 decedents. The survey data were obtained from a mailed questionnaire or interview with the person identified as the informant on the death certificate. The analysis was limited to six conditions (hypertension, heart attack, stroke, cancer, diabetes, and asthma) for sample size considerations, although other information was collected. The presence of each of these conditions in the health history of the decedent from the survey was compared with selected underlying causes of death from the certificate. The categories of cause of death were determined on the basis of their similarity to the condition identified in the survey or because of already-known etiologic relationships. For example, hypertension on the survey was compared separately with either diseases of heart or major cardiovascular diseases on the death certificate.

Since it was hypothesized that the associations would diminish with age, each relationship was examined by age subgroup. Such an age interaction might be expected, since older persons would generally have more morbid conditions present, which could lead to more possible causes of death. The actual analysis was done using an odds ratio statistic. For example, contingency tables were constructed for cardiovascular diseases as an underlying cause and a reported history of hypertension from the followback by age (Table 17.2). The ratio of those with and without the condition was compared by whether or not they had cardiovascular disease. The survey showed an association between medical history on the survey and underlying cause of death from the certificate for each of the conditions. However, the degree to which the history raised the likelihood varied. At the very oldest ages, the underlying cause was not strongly related to the antecedent history, except for stroke, where there was much more of a relationship.

Several factors may have accounted for this finding. It is possible that for younger persons the antecedent medical condtions may have been more acute and more directly associated with death. So for the young cardiovascular death a history of

Table 17-2 Percent of Deaths Due to Cardiovascular Diseases as Underlying Cause on the Death Certificate, with or without Reported History of Selected Conditions, with Odds and Odds Ratios, by Age: United States, 1986

History of specified condition reported on survey	Percent dying of cardiovascular diseases on death certificate					Odds and odds ratios			
	25–64 years	65–74 years	75–84 years	85 years and over		25–64 years	65–74 years	75–84 years	85 years and over
Cardiovascular diseases (total)	32.9	46.2	53.0	62.7	Odds ratio	2.83	1.98	1.57	1.39
Cardiovascular diseases									
with hypertension	46.8	54.0	58.6	67.0	Odds	0.88	1.17	1.41	2.03
without hypertension	23.7	37.2	47.3	59.3		0.31	0.59	0.90	1.46

Source: Extracted from Rosenberg (in press, a).

hypertension may be indicative of a much more malignant course than in an older person, who may have had treated hypertension for many years. Another possible reason for the weakening association with increasing age is poorer diagnosis of causes of death for the elderly population as compared with decedents of a younger age. For the very old person in long-term care facilities medical diagnosis and certification of cause of death may be handled with much less completeness than in a hospital setting (Gross et al, 1988). Also, staff may not be cognizant of previous illnesses and less diagnostic information would be available. The interpretation of death certificate validation studies in the elderly is very demanding; however, observers have suggested that the situation could be improved by more autopsy-based investigative studies being done.

Recent Autopsy Validation Studies

A number of commentators, principally pathologists, have emphasized the importance of the autopsy as the "gold standard" for studies and a way to improve the quality of cause-of-death statistics. An editorial by Carter is a good example of this viewpoint (Carter, 1985). An important factor in evaluating the potential usefulness of autopsies is the reality that the number of autopsies in the country has been dropping and in 1987 was about 12 percent (National Center for Health Statistics, 1989). Also, there is variation in rates, depending on premorbid diagnoses. They are particularly low for the three major causes of death but quite high for medical–legal cases. In addition, the frequency of autopsies decreases with age. Thus, there are selective factors that lessen the representativeness of validation results that rely on autopsy data.

As an example of a typical autopsy study, Kircher et al examined the extent of agreement between underlying cause of death on the certificate and the autopsy results using 272 randomly selected autopsy reports in Connecticut (Kircher et al, 1985). They found disagreements for about one third of the cases for the major ICD categories. In about a fourth of the cases the disagreement was in the specific diseases; for example, an acute myocardial infarction should have been reported as a ruptured aortic aneurysm. As expected, neoplasms showed a high rate of agreement, but so did circulatory diseases as a general category; however, consistency for respiratory diseases was lower. Because of the relatively select and small sample size of the study population, dichotomization by age was apparently not possible.

In another study by Shottenfeld et al (1982), autopsy findings for 575 deaths were compared with clinical information and with the death certificate cause. Discrepancies were reduced considerably when autopsy information was available and used for completing the cause of death on the certificate. Confirmation rates without autopsy were 95 percent for neoplasms, 86 percent for vascular disease, but only 60 percent for respiratory and digestive diseases. When the autopsy report was available at the time of certification, the results were better. Thus, the use of autopsy during the certification process was beneficial to the certificate validity. Unfortunately, again no separate age data were available.

A recent autopsy study in a university hospital compared the results of 87 subjects of age over 64 years with 75 younger adults (Middleton et al, 1989). The cases were studied retrospectively by six internists to determine if diagnostic errors were quantitatively or qualitatively different between two age subgroups, and if the cause of any errors was age-related. The frequency of major clinical autopsy discrepancies was found to be similar to those in previous studies, about 35 percent. There were significantly more unexpected minor discrepancies in the older patients, believed to be due to the multiplicity and complexity of their problems. Generally, however, there was no difference in terms of frequency or errors in the diagnostic accuracy regarding cause of death between the geriatric and other adult groups. It should be emphasized that this study was in a university hospital, and the results should not be generalized to other settings. Although autopsy validation might have some limitations, there is no doubt that use of all available information at the time of certification can only improve the quality of the data.

Diagnostic Completeness on the Death Certificate

It might be postulated that the precision of diagnostic information on the death certificate would decline with increased age of the decedent. With an older age of the decedent the medical certifier may be more likely to characterize the cause of death on the death certificate with terms that are vague and imprecise, such as natural causes or old age. In fact, Kohn has taken the extreme position, recommending that causes of death for the very old person without clear etiology should be reported as "senescence" (Kohn, 1982). For example, this term would be used when deaths in debilitated members of the aged population cannot be clearly attributed to specific causes. Certainly, Kohn's recommendation goes against the need for more specificity in diagnoses at all ages; still, it serves as a caution when considering the quality of cause-of-death data in the elderly.

However, in fact, if one measures diagnostic completeness in national data by using the number of deaths assigned the ICD-9 category of "symptoms, signs and ill-defined conditions," where entries such as "natural causes," "stopped breathing", and "old age" would be assigned, this was not the case (Rosenberg et al, 1991). In Table 17.3 the number and percentage of deaths with vague diagnoses in persons 25 years and older by age subgroups are shown. The percentage declines with age except at the oldest ages. There is some discrepancy between percentages in whites and blacks at all ages with more use of these terms for black decedents (not shown). This situation is

Table 17-3 Number and Percent Distribution by Age (25 Years and Over) for All Deaths and Deaths Due to Symptoms, Signs, and Ill-defined Conditions, by Race and Sex: United States, 1985

			Male		Female	
Age (years)	Total deaths (numbers)	Total Ill-defined deaths (percent)	Total deaths (numbers)	Ill-defined deaths (percent)	Total deaths (numbers)	Ill-defined deaths (percent)
25–34	51,852	3.19%	37,354	3.03%	14,498	3.60%
35–44	65,815	2.26%	43,494	2.39%	22,321	2.01%
45–54	116,634	1.48%	73,320	1.57%	43,314	1.33%
55–64	286,480	1.16%	177,711	1.26%	108,769	1.00%
65–74	482,646	1.00%	283,017	1.04%	199,629	0.94%
75–84	568,848	0.98%	279,872	1.01%	288,976	0.96%
85 and over	419,051	1.23%	141,653	1.21%	277,398	1.24%
Not stated	877		491		386	

most likely the result of less access to care and, therefore, of less knowledge of specifics of preexisting conditions.

MULTIPLE CAUSE-OF-DEATH DATA: CURRENT PRACTICE AND RESEARCH OPPORTUNITIES

Since the findings of clinical and autopsy validation studies have raised questions about the validity of the underlying cause as a true indicator of health status in the older persons, multiple cause-of-death analysis has been proposed as a means for overcoming the known limitations of using a single underlying condition for characterizing each death, especially for older persons (Israel et al, 1986). Multiple causes of death represent all conditions reported on the death certificate as contributing to death, including "other significant conditions" (see Figure 17.1). These designations are without regard to whether they were selected to be the underlying cause. Such an approach is more consistent with the disease realities in older persons, where the effects of a number of conditions often combine to result in death. Kohn has described death in the older persons as an "increasing collection of diseases" (Kohn, 1982).

Among older persons, death might be considered to be somewhat "opportunistic," with the presence of many chronic conditions providing competition to be the actual cause of death. Compared to younger persons in which there may be a clearly defined etiologic pathway, in the elderly the particular cause may be an almost random event occurring on top of an older person's more generalized disease processes. These have reduced the reserve to respond to acute problems. Such environmental challenges and variations may be as important as the underlying conditions in terms of the actual terminal event. For example, the older person with chronic congestive failure, chronic lung disease, and diabetes would be quite vulnerable to death from viral pneumonia accompanying an influenza outbreak. Other stresses may include temperature, medications, or small changes in disease status.

Data on the number of chronic conditions contributing to death by age are available from the NCHS tapes for multiple causes of death. As indicated in the chapter section on validity, these data are generated using various computer programs, especially TRANSAX (National Center for Health Statistics, 1986). Each condition on the death certificate is listed on these tapes in two formats: (1) in the order in which it appeared on the death certificate (called the "disease entity axis") and (2) a "record axis," in which each condition has been subjected to a systematic editing and recombination of certain codes to resolve inconsistencies.

For this illustrative example of the potential usefulness of multiple cause-of-death data (Rosenberg et al, 1991), the analysis is based on final mortality data for all U.S. residents occurring in 1985. In this study each medical condition reported on the death certificate is counted one time. For example, if a physician reported three nonredundant conditions in Part I and two other conditions in Part II of the certificate, a total of five reported conditions would be used for this analysis. Because deaths caused by trauma are characterized by both the "manner of death" (e.g., accident, homicide, or suicide) and the nature of the injury, these cases were excluded from the analysis. The average number of reported conditions remained relatively constant at about 2.5 for those 25–54 years of age and then steadily increased to about 2.9 for persons aged 85 years old and over (Table 17.4). This rise was similar for both sexes and the major races. If the increasing number of conditions with age are considered as a frequency distribution, the percentage with one condition decreases from about 24 percent for decedents less than 65 years of age to about 14 percent in the oldest old. The percent with four or more conditions is 28 percent in the oldest subgroup compared to 22 percent at younger ages. Although these are not dramatic changes with increasing age and may not represent the full extent of diseases present at older ages, the analysis is consistent with the notion that, on the average, two additional causes beyond the underlying cause are present for older persons.

With more conditions being included on the death certificate there is a question of the effect on the relative ranking of causes as in Table 17.1. Using multiple-cause instead of underlying-cause data for 1978, generally, the rankings of leading cause of death remain similar (National Center for Health Statistics, 1984). In that year arteriosclerosis replaced influenza and pneumonia as the fourth most frequent cause, and septicemia and avitaminosis replaced cirrhosis and nephritis, respectively in positions 9 and 10.

As another analytic strategy, the frequency that a certain cause of death is mentioned anywhere on the death certificate can be compared to the number of times it is the underlying cause. This can be expressed as a ratio (Israel et al, 1986). A ratio of 1 would indicate that such a diagnosis would infrequently be reported as anything other than an underlying cause. Trauma, such as motor vehicle accidents or homicide, has a low ratio. Even with a relatively low ratio such as the 1.2 for ischemic heart disease, this can be important in an absolute sense of the number of diagnoses, since it is so frequent in older persons. An example of a diagnosis with a relatively high ratio is diabetes. Because of its association with a number of chronic diseases, to which the certifying physician gives precedence as an underlying cause, diabetes is relatively underrepresented when only underlying cause of death is presented as the basis for cause-of-death statistics. The ratio for diabetes increases substantially in older persons. For example, the ratio was 2.2 for those aged 35–44 and 4.1 for those aged 75–84. These results emphasize the importance of using both multiple- and underlying-cause data for investigating diabetes-related deaths.

Table 17-4 Average Number of Medical Conditions Reported on Death Certificates[a], by Age (25 Years and Over), Race, and Sex: United States, 1985

	All races			White			Black		
Age (years)	Total	Male	Female	Total	Male	Female	Total	Male	Female
25–34	2.52	2.52	2.53	2.51	2.51	2.52	2.54	2.53	2.54
35–44	2.51	2.50	2.52	2.48	2.48	2.50	2.57	2.56	2.58
45–54	2.52	2.50	2.56	2.50	2.49	2.52	2.58	2.52	2.67
55–64	2.63	2.62	2.66	2.63	2.62	2.65	2.66	2.61	2.73
65–74	2.78	2.77	2.80	2.79	2.78	2.80	2.75	2.70	2.81
75–84	2.89	2.88	2.89	2.89	2.89	2.89	2.82	2.78	2.85
85 and over	2.89	2.91	2.88	2.89	2.92	2.88	2.81	2.79	2.82

Source: NCHS, National Vital Statistics System, 1985. Extracted from Rosenberg (in press).
[a]Excludes death that list external "E" codes as underlying cause.

Examples of Other Analyses

Aubert et al (1987) used multiple cause-of-death data to explore trends in the frequency of Alzheimer's disease (AD) at death. Because a chronic condition, such as AD, might not be listed as the underlying cause of death, the investigators considered not only all reported AD but also trends in senile dementia, a surrogate diagnosis in the Mental Diseases Chapter of ICD. Their primary source of data was the NCHS multiple cause-of-death tape for 1968–1983. Using the data from the record axis as described previously, age- and sex-adjusted trends and prevalence rates were reported. There was a nearly 20-fold increase in reported prevalence over the time period. An important question was whether this rise resulted from a shift from the entity "senile dementia." In the years from 1968 to about 1975 there was some tendency for senile dementia to decrease and AD to increase. With an analysis by state it was determined that most of this early shifting occurred mainly in New York State. However, during recent years, when the rise had been greater, both senile dementia and AD increased. The authors concluded that there was no national trend toward shifting diagnoses as an explanation for the increase in AD.

National multiple-cause data for AD are available for 1987. These are shown in Figure 17.3. The multiple-cause mentions added 14,639 beyond the underlying count of 11,311 for AD (ICD-9 Code 331.0) and 17,699 to the 4,683 for senile and presenile dementia (ICD-9 Code 290.0–290.3, 290.8, 290.9). Senility (ICD-9 Code 797) was reported about 1193 times, with an additional 16,719 deaths with multiple causes. However, it should be recognized that it would be inappropriate to add these numbers together for an upper-limit frequency estimate because there may be some overlap

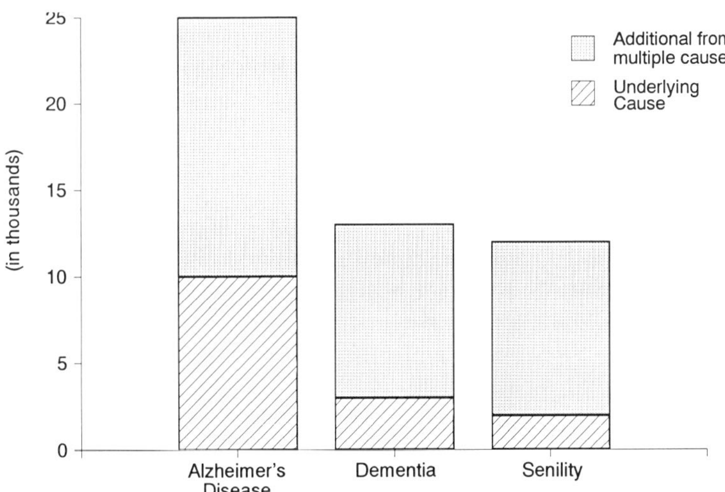

Figure 17-3 Number of deaths from Alzheimer's disease, dementia, and senility, as underlying or multiple-cause listing (for all ages, United States 1987).

among the categories. For example, some of the same decedents with senile dementia as a multiple cause could be occurring with the subgroup of Alzheimer's disease as the underlying diagnosis.

Data from the death certificate should not be viewed as a precise indicator of disease prevalence, since the physician is asked to report *only* conditions that significantly contributed to death. Thus, for a patient dying of cancer or trauma the physician might not report the AD unless its association with underlying cause was significantly intertwined with the morbid process leading to death. Some studies have suggested that mortality statistics are a gross undercount of the frequency of AD at death (Martyn and Pippard, 1988). Thus, it is probable that mortality statistics do not provide a satisfactory indicator of AD morbidity in older persons. As the recognition and diagnosis of AD increases, physicians are likely to portray more accurately the true frequency of AD at death, especially if multiple-cause tabulations are used.

Another use of multiple cause-of-death data is in the description of associations among medical conditions present at the time of death (Israel et al, 1986). Although joint occurrence will happen randomly among common conditions, some associations may be more than expected and represent possible etiologic relationships. Examples are diabetes with cardiovascular diseases and osteoporosis with fall-related fractures. It has been suggested that cardiovascular diseases occur less frequently with Alzheimer's disease than would be expected. Although the evaluation of such relationships is complex, it is possible by creating a ratio of the number of observed to expected pairs to address some of these issues. A significant ratio greater or less than 1 would indicate a possible relationship. For example, for decedents of all ages, chronic liver disease and cirrhosis were associated with nephritis, nephrotic syndrome, and nephrosis 1.7 times the expected number of pairs of causes, as determined by the product of the frequency of underlying cause on the death certificate for the two diseases. A similar excess of pneumonia with chronic obstructive pulmonary disease was identified. Interestingly, for many diseases the interrelationship varies with age. Thus, for the combination of diabetes with chronic ischemic heart disease the ratio of actual to expected deaths was 1.2 for all ages, but there was a decrease from 3.4 at ages 25–34 to about unity for those 75 years and older. There are various possible explanations for such age relationships. They might represent an age-related difference in physician reporting patterns or a true relationship with age.

There are other potential applications of multiple-cause data. For example, Manton has used such data to study race and sex differentials in mortality (Manton, 1980). Others have used such data to differentiate various disease outcomes in smokers and nonsmokers. Because the question often arises in older persons about relationships between two diseases, the issues of competing risk must be addressed. New statistical models have been developed that supplement the usual competing risk models [e.g., the pattern-of-failure model by Manton (1976)].

Limitations of Multiple Cause-of-Death Data

Since underlying-cause data are sensitive to physician preferences in disease etiology or nomenclature, this potential problem becomes magnified when multiple listed conditions must be interpreted (Israel et al, 1986). For example, geographic differences in disease terminology or expected combinations would be compounded with multiple-cause tabulations. Also, if a physician perceives certain diseases or conditions, such as Lyme disease, as becoming more likely as fatal causes, these diseases will begin appearing on the death certificate, even if there is insufficient proof of a relationship. Time trends over long periods of time will be sensitive to changes in physician reporting practices, which would be magnified by multiple causes needing to be tracked. Finally, some have raised the question of whether the design of the current certificate, which emphasizes a sequence leading to the underlying cause, may inhibit or prevent adequate characterization of the multiple associated causes (Freedman et al, 1988).

There is a great unmet potential for use of multiple-cause data in characterizing the health status of older persons. Besides the availability of national data tapes for ongoing analyses, small area and local epidemiologic studies need to utilize the concepts of multiple causes for comparison with national data and other investigations. Especially because of questions raised about underlying-cause data and some special limitations on their use in older persons, investigations of epidemiology in the elderly should incorporate the principles of multiple cause into end-point studies.

STRATEGIES FOR IMPROVING CAUSE-OF-DEATH STATISTICS

Although the death records themselves and the resulting data from the national vital statistics system have been durable and versatile in providing important public health and etiologic information, there have been recurrent attempts to improve the system. Various commentators have made suggestions in the literature of possible improvements (Rosenberg, 1989).

Periodically, the NCHS has organized reviews of the format of the vital records with physicians and vital statisticians. Recently, a certificate with more lines in the sequencing section and instructions with examples on the back has been promulgated (see Figures 17.1 and 17.2) (Freedman et al, 1988). In addition, for a number of years NCHS has participated in the development of special followback and validity studies. Finally, guidelines for querying physicians for inadequate entries on the death certificate have been provided to the states, and many states, notably Oregon, have well-developed programs (Hopkins et al, 1989).

Recently, a workshop on "Improving Cause-of-Death Statistics" was convened to involve representatives from federal, state, and professional organizations in an evaluation of the situation (Rosenberg, 1990). The workshop participants, after reviewing various relevant issues, many of which have been mentioned in this chapter, developed recommendations for future actions. Examples of these will be helpful both in understanding future directions and in supporting efforts for the improvement of local or study death records.

The major recommendation was that a widespread educational effort for physicians should be undertaken. This program would involve physicians at all levels of training from medical school through postgraduate training, and then as practicing physicians through continuing medical education participation. Although a training booklet is available nationally and locally in many states, modified or customized materials would be an appropriate next step. States might consider pinpointing certain institutions or certifiers for special training. Hospitals that, depending on the size, have already knowledgeable personnel for medical records review could provide more consultation to physicians to ensure completeness and plausible sequences of conditions on death records. Since almost half of deaths occur in hospitals, this association between the records administrator and the certifying physicians is likely to occur. With modest efforts such a relationship could be developed to improve death certification.

State and local jurisdictions with coordination from NCHS could enhance quality assessment programs. For example, this process might involve a review of death certificates as part of mortality reviews at hospitals. Frequency of querying programs and alternative strategies should be expanded as well. However, the positive educational aspects rather than the punitive ones would need to be maintained. Also, it should be made as easy as possible for physicians to make necessary and appropriate changes to the entries on the death certificate.

A number of clinicians and vital statisticians have commented on the need to evaluate the format of the death certificate with respect to the sequence of listing causes of death. Although the present sequence is the one required by the ICD, which the United States has agreed to follow, a study to understand what effect reversing the sequence and other format changes would have on quality may have merit. However, the design of such a study is recognized to be difficult because of problems in simulating the true circumstances of the completion situation. It should be possible to obtain more in-depth information on how physicians perceive the certificate and what thought processes they use to complete it. Of course, if the relevant data about a patient are not available, it would be unlikely that the improved accuracy could ever be achieved, no matter what the sequence.

The only area that was controversial at the workshop was the potential effect of different state policies on the release of data on the records. Some states have completely open records and others are restricted to various degrees. Usually, for bonafide research purposes it is possible to gain access after an approval process in almost all states. Although some participants in the workshop believed that restricting access would improve the accuracy of the information, others felt that secrecy did not serve the public interest in the long run. In any case, physicians need to be encouraged to complete the certificate in as accurate and complete a manner as possible. This can become an issue when perceived indirect or direct pressure is brought to bear on the physician not to indicate socially less acceptable diagnoses, such as suicide or acquired immunodeficiency syndrome. The latter case is becoming more of an issue not just for the young, but for older persons. The investigator who uses data from different states is likely to be aware of differences in ease of access but might not be aware of potential, although not proven, differences in quality, depending on the various state laws. Subsequent meetings are planned to consider this complex topic.

SUMMARY

Death records are a valuable and ultimate source of epidemiologic information on the health status of older persons. This process occurs through both the availability of aggregated vital statistics and examination of individual records, as they may be part of a specific epidemiologic study. However, there needs to be a persistent inquisitiveness on the part of users of death data about the validity of the source records, especially for older persons and for certain diseases. Although there may be limitations, undoubtedly, there will be continuing programs to improve the quality of vital records and statistics. These changes should enhance even more the usefulness of these mortality data in epidemiologic research.

REFERENCES

Aubert R, Parker R, Rothenberg R, May D (1987). Methodologic issues in the reported prevalence of Alzheimer's disease on death certificates. Proceedings of the Biennial Conference on Records and Statistics. National Center for Health Statistics, Hyattsville, MD. pp 183–187.

California Department of Health Services (1987). California Occupational Mortality, 1979–81, Riedmiller, K. Doebbert G, Lashuay N, Rudolph L, Glazer E.

Carter JR (1985). The problematic death certificate. N Engl J Med 313:1285–1286.

Curb JD, Ford CE, Presser S, Palmer M, Babcock C, Hawkins CM (1985). Acertainment of the vital status through the National Death Index and the Social Security Administration, Am J Epidemiol 121:754–766.

Freedman MA, Gay GA, Potrzebowski PW, Rothwell CJ (1988). The 1989 revision of the U.S. standard certificates of live birth and death and the U.S. standard report of fatal death, Am J Public Health 78:168–172.

Great Britain General Register Office (1958). 1951 Census of England and Wales, General Report. H.M. Stationery Office, London.

Great Britain General Register Office (1968). 1961 Census of England and Wales, General Report. H.M. Stationery Office, London.

Gross JS, Nemfeld RR, Libon LS, Gerber I, Rodstein M (1988). Autopsy study of the elderly institutionalized patient: Review of 234 autopsies. Arch Intern Med 148:173–176.

Hopkins DD, Grant-Worley JA, Bollinger TL (1989). Survey of cause-of-death criteria used by state vital statistics programs in the US and efficacy of the criteria used by the Oregon Vital Statistics Program. Am J Public Health 79:570–574.

Israel RA, Rosenberg HM, Curtin LR (1986). Analytical potential for multiple cause-of-death data. Am J Epidemiol 124:161–179.

Kapantais G, Powell-Griner E (1989). Characteristics of persons dying of diseases of heart: Preliminary data from the 1986 National Mortality Followback Survey. Advance Data from Vital and Health Statistics, No. 172, Hyattsville, MD.

Kircher T, Nelson J, Burdo H (1985). The autopsy as a measure of accuracy of the death certificate, N Engl J Med 313:1263–1269.

Kohn RR (1982). Cause of death in very old people. JAMA 247:2793–2797.

Manton KG, Tolley HD, Poss SS (1976). Life table techniques for multiple cause mortality. Demography 13:541–564.

Manton KG (1980). Sex and race specific mortality differentials in multiple cause of death data. Gerontologist 20:480–493.

Martyn CN, Pippard EC (1988). Usefulness of mortality data in determining the geography and time trends for dementia. J Epidemiol Community Health 42:138–143.

Middleton K, Clarke E, Homann S, Naughton B, Neely D, Repasy A, Yarnold PR, Yungbluth M, Webster JR (1989). An autopsy-based study of diagnostic errors in geriatric and nongeriatric adult patients. Arch Intern Med 149:1809–1812.

Moriyama IM (1989). Problems in measurement of accuracy of cause-of-death statistics. Am J Public Health 79:1349–1350.

National Center for Health Statistics (1968). Comparability of age on the death certificate and matching census records, Hambright Z, Vital and Health Statistics, Series 2, No. 29. US Department of Health, Education, and Welfare, Washington, DC.

National Center for Health Statistics (1969). Comparability of marital status, race, nativity, and country of orgin on the death certificate and matching census records, Hambright Z, Vital and Health Statistics, Series 2, No. 24. US Department of Health, Education, and Welfare, Washington, DC.

National Center for Health Statistics (1982). Gittelsohn A, Royston P, Annotated bibliography of cause-of-death validation studies, 1958–80. Vital and Health Statistics Series 2, No. 89, DHHS Pub. No. (PHS) 82-1363. Public Health Service, Washington, DC.

National Center for Health Statistics (1984). Multiple causes of death in the United States. Monthly Vital Statistics Report Vol 32, No. 10, Supp. (2), DHHS Pub. No. (PHS) 84-1120. Public Health Service, Hyattsville, MD.

National Center for Health Statistics (1986). Chamblee RF, Evans MC, TRANSAX, the NCHS system for producing mutliple cause-of-death statistics, 1968–78. Vital and Health Statistics, Series 1, No. 20, DHHS Pub. No. (PHS) 86-1322. Public Health Service, Washington, DC.

National Center for Health Statistics (1989). Advance report of final mortality statistics, 1987. Monthly Vital Statistics Report, Vol. 38, No. 5, Supp. Public Health Service, Hyattsville, MD.

National Office of Vital Statistics (1961). Comparability of reports on occupation, Kaplan DL, Parkhurst E, Whelpton PK, Vital Statistics—Special Reports, Vol. 3, No. 1. US Department of Health, Education, and Welfare, Washington, DC.

Rosenberg HM (1989). Improving cause-of-death statistics. Am. J Public Health 79:563–564.

Rosenberg HM (1990). Nature and accuracy of cause of death data. Report of Workshop on Improving Cause-of-Death Statistics. National Center for Health Statistics.

Rosenberg HM, Chevarley F, Powell-Griner E, Kochanek K, and Feinleib M et al. (1991). Causes of death among the elderly: Information from the death certificate. Proceedings of 1988 International Symposium on Data on Aging. Feinleib, M. (ed). National Center for Health Statistics Series 5, Vital and Health Statistics.

Schade WJ, Swanson G (1988). Comparison of death certificate occupation and industry with lifetime occupational histories obtained by interview: Variations in the accuracy of death certificate entries. Am J Ind Med 14:121–136.

Schottenfeld D, Eaton M, Sommers SC, Alonso DR, Wilkenson C (1982). The autopsy as a measure of accuracy of the death certificate. Bull NY Acad Med 58:778–794.

Sirken MG, Rosenberg HM, Chevarley FM, Curtin LR (1987). The quality of cause-of-death statistics. Am J Public Health 77:137–139.

Sorlie PD, Gold EB (1987). The effect of physician teminology preference on coronary heart disease mortality: An artifact uncovered by the 9th Revision, ICD. Am J Public Health 77:148–152.

World Health Organization (1977). Manual of the International Statistical Classification of Diseases, Injuries, and Causes of Death, based on the recommendations of the Ninth Revision Conference, 1975. World Health Organization, Geneva.

18

Assessing Income and Resources of the Elderly

WILLIAM S. CARTWRIGHT

Income and wealth are often central factors in epidemiologic studies, and their assessment can be critical to investigations of health and aging. Both conceptually and pragmatically, income and wealth have at least two important general applications. First, they are used as surrogates or indicators of socioeconomic status (SES) and class. Despite occasional misapplication of these notions, it is clear that many elements of health status are related to one's social standing and SES, although the causal pathways tend to be complex and uncertain. Second, income and wealth serve as important measures of access to goods and services, including food, clothing, shelter, and medical services. Further, certain levels of income, wealth and other resources serve as triggers for receipt of helping services and thus need to be clearly defined for administrative purposes, a difficult task.

The distribution of income and wealth has many components. The most obvious one is the flow of money to the recipient on a periodic basis. In-kind benefits can be valuable additions to one's salary. The period of time may be as varied as one week for a salary check to one year for an interest payment on a savings instrument. Both salary and in-kind benefits represent income. In contrast, wealth represents a stock of assets with various degrees of liquidity (the ease with which they may be translated into payment for goods and services). Over time, wealth may be increased by reducing consumption below income so as to generate savings. A typical listing of these income and wealth components follows:

- Income
  - Earnings from full-time and part-time employment
  - Social Security
  - Employer benefit plans
  - Interest income from assets
  - Public assistance programs
    - Supplemental Security Income
    - Worker's Compensation
    - Medicare
    - Medicaid
    - Food stamps

Housing
Energy assistance
Family transfers
Cash
Medical assistance
Care-giving

Wealth
IRA and Keogh plans
Annuities
Net housing worth
Business assets
Investment assets—stocks, bonds, life insurance, savings deposits, notes
Liquid assets—cash, bank deposits
Personal property—cars and household items

Some of these components have been subject to special analysis. For example, there is particular interest in determining the monetary value of in-kind benefits when assessing the general well-being of the elderly. In many cases, receipt of an in-kind benefit makes significant difference in determining the poverty status of the individual. Often of additional interest is the eligibility status of the individual for a particular public subsidy or helping program. One could make a case that in any survey work, some operating procedure will be necessary to address whether an elderly participant is eligible for an important government benefit, is in desperate economic need, or requires assistance to apply for some benefit. Such an operating procedure is analogous to the requirement that participants be referred to their physician if a screening uncovers unattended medical problems.

In examining the income status of a family or a household, a consistent concept and definition of income must be used. Income may be defined as accretion, or the increase in net worth (assets minus liabilities) plus consumption during a given period. In empirical research, not all income is realized in the period of definition. The difficulty is apparent when considering a professional athlete who receives a current income payment from his club but has deferred annuity payments in future years after retirement. When should the income be counted—in the current year, or when it is realized? Consumption also can be ambiguous. It includes outlays for current consumer goods as well as durable goods that can be consumed over a particular period of time in the form of services. A consistent concept is necessary to standardize measures of well-being. In economics, a great deal of work in income measurement is related to defining the appropriate income base to levy taxes upon so that equity may be obtained between equals and across the distribution.

The change in net worth, an important component of income, can be measured by comparing net worth at market prices at the beginning and ending of a period. This is usually done in the context of net wealth surveys, such as those conducted by the Federal Reserve Board and the 1980 President's Commission on Pension Policy. Unfortunately, the epidemiologist cannot wholly use this approach because it requires a survey time of two to two and one half hours to probe for ownership of all assets such as those detailed earlier. Individuals require a considerable amount of prompting and referral to records to enumerate all the items of wealth. Assigning a value to real estate and business assets can be very difficult because such properties have not been exchanged on the market so that no realized value is available. Pension values are particularly difficult to assess. Although corporations have actuaries to value their pension plans, individual researchers usually do not have access to such sophisticated techniques. Valuation of these assets is independent of any problems related to recall of specific assets and their value.

With such difficulty in collecting wealth data, more attention is usually focused on earnings from various sources. Wage earnings appear to be somewhat less difficult to value than wealth, but unfortunately, not all wage payments are made in cash. Fringe benefits have grown enormously since World War II. Because of favorable tax treatment, it is often preferable to receive additional wage compensation in the form of a fringe benefit rather than cash payment. The difficulty in valuing economic status may be illustrated in the example of two individuals who both earn $2000 per month.

The second of the two has a vested pension to which the employer deposits $200 per month. Who is better off? The second individual is certainly better off than the first. However, if you queried them as to what their monthly income is, they both would probably answer $2000.

Additional problems may develop when the value of health insurance varies in benefit packages offered to workers. In this case, employers may make different contributions, plans may have different coverages, and future retirement benefits may or may not include access to the health plan. In some studies, health insurance status may be an even more important valuable than income status, since health insurance provides access to medical care and cushions the loss of income from ill health.

The source of the income may also determine the actual availability. For example, two individuals over age 65 may be receiving equal pension benefits, but one individual may pay taxes on half the benefit received and another may be taxed on the complete pension income. In this case, the concept of taxable income gives a better measure of the control over consumption opportunities. Indeed, given federal, state, and local tax laws, considerable variation in after-tax income may be created by the area in which the individual lives.

An example of a national study collecting information on income is the Panel Study of Income Dynamics (Survey Research Center, 1976). Its purpose is to measure on a consistent basis changes in the well-being of the family. Income was gathered in the questionnaire for each year. Typically, one asks, "How much did you (Head of family) receive from wages and salaries in 1989—that is, before anything was deducted for taxes or other things?" Then any income from "bonuses, overtime, or commissions" is queried. Then one probes for all other sources of income that may involve government welfare payments, Social Security, pensions, asset income, alimony and gifts, and so on. One may then ask for money income for the spouse and other members of the family or household.

Since occupation and work earnings are so important in many social studies, the occupation, weeks worked, and hours worked per week are also gathered for individuals in the family unit. The survey then generates a total Family Money Income based on the taxable income and total transfers of all members of the family. In generating an income, variable imputations and editing are done to achieve the final result.

A less burdensome approach is used by the investigators of the Established Populations for Epidemiologic Studies of the Elderly (NIA, 1986). Motivated by fear that at the point in the survey in which the elderly are asked about their income refusals to participate in further survey questions would threaten the study, the investigators placed the income question at the end of their survey. In New Haven and East Boston, the interviewer was asked to show a card to the individual and ask the following:

> Please look at this card. Which of these income groups represents your (and your spouse's) income for the past month/year? Include income from all sources such as wages, salaries, Social Security or retirement benefits, help from relatives, rent from property, and so forth.

	Monthly income
A.	$ 0–$ 166
B.	167– 249
C.	250– 333
D.	334– 416
E.	417– 583
F.	584– 833
G.	834– 1249
H.	1250– 1666
I.	1667– 2499
J.	2500– 3333
K.	3334 and over

In Iowa, before asking a minor variant of this question, the interviewer reassured the interviewee of the confidentiality of the responses and prompted for the receipt of 13 sources of income. In the Duke Piedmont Survey investigators probed for four sources of income before asking the general question. This approach has the advantage of jogging the memory of the responder for all the various sources, without collecting actual information leading to the generation of total money income from the various sources.

In designing the actual form of the income question, a number of decisions must be made by the investigator. For example, the selection of the actual income categories must be done to facilitate the research goals. If the researcher is interested in comparing the income statistics to national surveys, the appropriate survey should be obtained and the income cutpoints utilized. However, if there is a considerable time between the comparison survey and the new survey, consideration must be given to dealing with the problem of inflation. New cutpoints may be generated by using the Consumer's Price Index to deflate the index. Unfortunately, precise use of the CPI necessitates abandoning the nice rounding characteristics, which have great aesthetic appeal for both the interviewer and interviewee. Some compromise may be achieved by judicious rounding of income values to the nearest thousand dollars.

If the investigator is interested in determining poverty levels, the income categories should be created with a cutpoint to permit accurate determination of the numbers in poverty. Most likely, the investigator would choose the cutpoints to keep in mind that the poverty level varies according to size and composition of the household. For most elderly households, the poverty line for two-couple households will be different than that for single-person households. In family studies with children or other dependents present, other cutpoints are relevant. If income data are collected without reference to predetermined categories, the investigator is then free to construct a poverty variable against the continuous measure of income, as is done in many survcys.

Consumption and saving patterns of the elderly differ from those of the nonelderly. In a recent study of consumption, Anderson (1984) found significant differences in saving and consumption patterns according to demographic categories, with the age of the head of household an important determinant. McConnel and Deljavon (1983) compared the consumption patterns of families with retired to the nonretired heads of households. Upon retirement, different consumption patterns are noted as work-related expenses and are eliminated, and other expenses become more important. In both studies medical care expenditures were a particularly important item of increase in elderly budgets. Besides the consumption patterns of disposable income, consumption is affected by a number of governmental and social environmental aspects. For example, the elderly are eligible for subsidized medical care through both the Medicare and Medicaid programs. Housing expenses will vary according to the living arrangement, whether in their own home, with relatives, in sheltered housing, or in a long-term care institution. Older persons may be receiving a subsidized rent while living in certain housing units. In health consumption, considerable variation may be generated by the ownership of supplementary health insurance, for which the elderly may have to pay full cost or receive a subsidy from a previous employer. Different rates of reimbursement may exist for individuals in their consumption of hospital services, physician services, and drugs. Recognition of this factor may be particularly important to epidemiologists as they assess health outcomes and attempt to control for access to the medical care system and differential rates of utilization.

The investigator must also give consideration to the mode of income data acquisition: personal interview, telephone interview, or mailed questionnaire. The problem here is that in the home, one may show a prompt card; over the telephone one is restricted to verbal prompts, which may be extensive and difficult to follow. Also, given that individuals may be reluctant to compare themselves unfavorably with others, in a telephone survey one should start with the lowest category and proceed upward.

Most investigators advise placing the income items at the end of an instrument rather than at the beginning. In some science surveys, however, income questions are often asked after household structure information is obtained, usually toward the beginning of the survey. Many epidemiologists prefer to ask the question toward the end to avoid a premature refusal to participate in the whole survey. When income is not deemed of dominant importance in certain disease processes, a systematic refusal would not be important to the integrity of the study.

Because of the strength of epidemiologic methods, more health services research may be conducted in a combination with epidemiologic studies. In some cases, the medical records or other administrative records may be the key component to measuring particular disease end point and associated treatment or lack of treatment. The apparent research cost savings may generate more collaborative studies between epidemiologist and public health analysts, requiring a recognition that income may be a key independent variable in the collaborative studies. For example, lack of income may restrain use of medical services and bias the probability of a whole population group appearing in the administrative records. Hence, adjustment must be made on the basis of income to control for this potential bias. Public health policy is also greatly concerned with the distribution aspects of health services and needs to correlate income with disease processes for policy purposes. Epidemiologists and other survey researchers should judge carefully the goals of their research and the possibility that income information would expand the usefulness of their results. However, nothing should compromise the scientific accuracy of the main health hypothesis under investigation.

REFERENCES

Anderson J (1984). National Institute on Aging Macroeconomic Demographic Model. Bethesda, MD, National Institutes of Health.

Avery R et al (1984). Survey of consumer finances, 1983. Fed Reserve Bull September 679–692.

Cartwright WS, Friedland RB (1985). The President's Commission on Pension Policy Household Survey 1979: Net wealth distributions by type and age for the United States. Rev Income Wealth, 31(3):285–308.

Clark R et al (1984). Inflation and the Economic Well-being of the Elderly. Baltimore, MD Johns Hopkins Press.

Mausner JS, Kramer S (1985). I Mausner JS and Bahn A (eds), Epidemiology: An Introductory Text. Philadelphia, Saunders, pp. 127–128.

McConnel CE, Deljavon F (1983). Consumption patterns of the retired household. J Gerontol 38(4):480–490.

National Center for Health Statistics (1988). Health of an aging america: Issues on data for policy analysis, Vital and Health Statistics, Series 4, No. 25, DHHS Pub. No. (PHS)89-1488. Public Health Service, Washington, DC.

National Institute on Aging (NIA) (1986). Established populations for epidemiologic studies of the elderly, Resource Data Book, Cornoni-Huntley J, et al (ed), US Department of Health and Human Services, Public Health Service, National Institutes of Health, NIH Publication No. 86-2443.

Radner DB (1989). Net worth and financial assets of age groups in 1984. Social Security Bull 52(3):2–15.

Reno VP, Maxfield LD (1985). Distribution of income sources of recent retirees, findings from the new beneficiary survey. Social Security Bull 48(1).

Survey Research Center (1976). A panel study of income dynamics: Procedures and tape codes, 1976 interviewing year, wave IX. Ann Arbor, The University of Michigan.

Waldo DR, Lazenby HC (1984). Demographic characteristics and health care use and expenditures by the aged in the United States, 1977–1984. Health Care Financing Rev 6(1).

Waldo DR, Sonnefeld ST, McKusick DR, Arnett RH (1989). Health expenditures by age groups, 1977 and 1987. Health Care Financing Rev 10(4):111–120.

19

Epidemiologic Studies of Aging in Historically Understudied Populations

PATRICIA L. COLSHER

Gerontologists have long emphasized the heterogeneity of the elderly with regard to physical health and function, cognitive function, psychosocial behavior, and other measurable attributes; yet research on populations whose aging experience might be expected to differ from that of the "majority" is relatively new and remains sparse. Markides (1989), for example, noted the absence of adequate national data on such basic topics as the mortality of Native Americans and Hispanics. In its report "Health Status of Aged Blacks" (National Caucus and Center on Black Aged, Inc., 1989), the National Caucus and Center on Black Aged wrote of the paucity of detailed information on African-American elders. Anderson and Cohen, in a 1989 editorial on clinical research with minority elderly, reported that only 19 articles focusing on the health of minority groups had been published in the major gerontologic and geriatric journals during the previous decade. In a review of publications on minority elders, Halperin (1990) noted that, although progress had been made, many important issues remained to be addressed.

Groups defined by factors other than race or ethnicity may also merit directed research programs. For example, advances in medical care have increased the lifespan of persons with Down syndrome, the major known cause of mental retardation, resulting in a growing cohort of mentally retarded elderly (Jacobsen et al, 1985; Seltzer and Kraus, 1987). Groups defined by medical diagnoses such as end-stage renal disease or those with chronic mental illness or mental retardation may have unique aging experiences. Other populations are defined by their sociobehavioral or legal status and may also be of interest. For example, although historically they have constituted only a small percentage of the incarcerated population, the number of elderly inmates in correctional facilities is growing rapidly and constitutes an important challenge to correctional systems (Rubenstein, 1984). Similarly, although elderly persons are a small percentage of the homeless (Alstrom et al, 1975; Fischer et al, 1986), their numbers are also growing (Overbo, 1990).

There are a variety of reasons to conduct epidemiologic investigations with these historically understudied populations. One of the most basic is simply to characterize their health and functional status in order to facilitate health care and other planning and to improve utilization of existing services. Historically understudied population may have unique exposure histories as a result of socioeconomic considerations (e.g., working in certain industries), ethnic practices (e.g., dietary habits), or sociobehavioral characteristics (e.g., substance use), which permit the examination of special outcomes. As will be seen, there is evidence that some racial groups are differentially susceptible to such illnesses as hypertension, diabetes, and renal insufficiency, and this may be in part because of genetic factors. Comparisons among ethnic and racial groups may therefore be useful in assessing putative causal factors. Historically understudied groups may also have unique health outcomes, such as the Alzheimer-like changes seen in many persons with Down syndrome after age 35 (Lott, 1982).

This chapter will review some of the important considerations in studies focusing on historically understudied groups, including those defined by racial or ethnic characteristics, by medical diagnosis, and by sociobehavioral or legal status. The thesis is that, although the criteria for sound scientific research are the same, regardless of what population is studied, certain characteristics of historically understudied populations may present additional challenges to the researcher. Although an exhaustive discussion of these populations is not possible here, illustrative groups have been chosen to highlight specific ethical and methodologic issues.

RACIAL AND ETHNIC MINORITY GROUPS

As was noted earlier, studies of racial and ethnic minority groups characterizing their health and functional status are useful in health care planning, development and implementation of other supportive services, and increased utilization of existing services. Generalization from research done with whites is not a scientifically acceptable strategy (Anderson and Cohen, 1989).

The unique pressures produced by socioeconomic disadvantages and discriminatory practices may have implications for age-associated changes. For example, elderly African-American women are less likely than elderly white women to receive screening mammography (Centers for Disease Control, 1988). This clearly has implications for morbidity and mortality associated with breast cancer, and efforts have been called for to improve screening services for African-American and other minority women (Burack and Liang, 1989). The elevated cervical cancer mortality in some Native American women has been attributed in part to lower rates of screening (Horner, 1990). The high rates of alcohol abuse among Native Americans (Levy and Kunitz, 1974) also affect the elderly, although more detailed investigations are needed (Kunitz and Levy, 1989). Informal social support networks are important sources of assistance and caregiving for the elderly (Sauer and Coward, 1985), and both cultural traditions and socioeconomic pressures have been implicated in what have been described as especially strong and extensive support networks of Hispanic elders (Bastida, 1988; Sotomayer and Randolph, 1988).

In addition to societal and environmental factors, the genetic heritage of members of minority groups may influence their aging process. For example, differential susceptibility to hypertension in African Americans and type II diabetes and chronic renal insufficiency in Native Americans may be, in part, genetically determined (Garstide et al, 1984; Mohs et al, 1988; Young et al, 1989). Investigation of such conditions among minority groups is thus particularly important if adequate health care and optimization of quality of life are to be provided. Such studies may also provide important insights into the biology of these conditions.

Finally, comparisons among ethnic and racial groups may provide useful insights into aging, including survivorship patterns and their determinants. For example, Table 19.1 shows the life expectancies at birth and age 65 for African-Americans and whites (US Bureau of Commerce, 1990). The life expectancies for African-Americans at birth are markedly less than those for whites, but by age 65 the differences are much smaller. In fact, although mortality rates for minority groups exceed those for whites throughout much of the lifespan, there is a reversal or cross-over of rates among the oldest old (Jackson and Perry, 1989), and this has been attributed to the "selective survival" of the heartiest minority group members (Markides and Machalek, 1984). Presumably, factors such as poor diet, reduced access to health care, and increased exposure to accidents and interpersonal violence play a role in the excess early mortality observed in minority groups (Jackson and Perry, 1989; Kunitz and Levy, 1989; Markides, 1989).

As illustrated by this "mortality cross-over," explaining differences in outcomes, whether with regard to mortality, prevalence of specific chronic illnesses, rates of physical functional impairment, or level of cognitive function, is a scientifically complex and politically charged issue. Race or ethnicity themselves may serve as a marker for the actual causal factors and not be responsible for the differences. With regard to historically understudied minority groups in the United States such as Native Americans, African-Americans, and Hispanics, some of the most important potential confounders relate to socioeconomic status. Moreover, the discrepancies between minority groups and white Americans may be greater among the elderly than among younger persons—for example, with regard to educational attainment (US Bureau of Commerce, 1990).

Table 19.2 provides basic socioeconomic information for elderly whites, African-Americans, and Hispanics from various national surveys. As may be seen, elderly minority group members are less educated, have lower incomes, are more likely to have incomes under the poverty level, are less likely to have private insurance, and are less likely to own their own homes. Moreover, there is often a lifelong history of lower income and relative lack of health care. Any of these factors might have an impact on the types of variables generally studied by gerontologic epidemiologists, and it has been argued that it is impossible to understand racial–ethnic differences without considering these variables (Markides, 1989).

Table 19-1 Life Expectancy (in Years) at Birth and Age 65 According to Race and Gender

	Black		White	
Age	Men	Women	Men	Women
Birth	65.2	73.5	72.0	78.8
65 years	13.4	17.0	14.8	18.7

Source: US Bureau of Commerce (1990).

Table 19-2 Socioeconomic Status of White, African-American, and Hispanic Elders[a]

	White	Afro-American	Hispanic
Percent with less than high school education	43.2	76.6	77.7
Percent with zero to three years of education	4.1	20.1	29.3
Percent below 1987 poverty rate	10	34	27
Mean household income (1987 $)	21,029	12,622	15,332
Percent having *no* private insurance	19	61	[a]
Percent owning home in which they live	74	61	56

Source: Monheit and Schur (1989); US Bureau of Commerce (1990).
[a]Small sample size precluded stable estimates.

An example from a regional survey illustrates the relation between race and health care use, as modified by income. Table 19.3 shows educational attainment, income, and occupational information as well as health care service use among white and non-white (overwhelmingly African-American) participants in the Yale Health and Aging Study (conducted in New Haven, Connecticut), one of four National Institute on Aging–sponsored Established Populations for Epidemiologic Studies of the Elderly (Cornoni-Huntley et al, 1986). The pattern of racial differences seen in this study with regard to income and education (upper portion) was similar to that seen nationally. Utilization of health care by whites and nonwhites also differed (lower portion of Table 19.3). Nonwhites were less likely to have seen a dentist in the previous six months. However, the use of dental services was a function of income. Persons with higher incomes were more likely to report dental visits. When dental visits were disaggregated by income, 11 percent of white men with income less than $5000 had seen a dentist in the six months prior to interview and 48.5 percent of those with incomes exceeding $15,000 had done so. Comparable percentages for nonwhite men were 13 percent and 58 percent—somewhat higher than those for white men in the same income groups. Thus, the less frequent utilization of dental services by nonwhite men appears to be a function of income rather than of race.

Findings with regard to differences in disease prevalence may also be difficult to interpret. For example, prior to age 65, rates of coronary heart disease and coronary

Table 19-3 Comparison of White and Nonwhite Participants in the Yale Health and Aging Study

	White		Nonwhite	
	Men	Women	Men	Women
Income:				
Percent with less than $5,000	14.4	29.5	35.3	61.3
Percent with more than $15,000	21.9	10.0	4.1	2.2
Dental service use:				
Percent seen within 6 months	23.3	24.1	13.4	12.5
Percent not seen for 3 years	48.0	47.8	64.6	57.0

Source: Cornoni-Huntley et al (1986).

heart disease mortality are higher among African-Americans than whites (Roig et al, 1987). African-Americans are also more likely to smoke, have higher intakes of dietary cholesterol, and have higher body mass (Block et al, 1988; Dawson, 1988; Roland and Fulwood, 1984; Sprafka et al 1988). Social and psychological factors (e.g., discrimination, chronic unemployment) have also been implicated, and differential utilization of medical care may have an impact on the diagnosis of specific conditions (Johnson, Gobson, and Luckey, 1990; Kasl, 1984). Differences in known risk factors, however, do not appear to account entirely for differences in disease prevalence (Sprafka et al, 1988).

The validity of commonly employed scales may also be affected by the demographic confounders noted earlier. For example, performance on mental status screening examinations for gross cognitive dysfunction and disorientation is related to educational attainment (Colsher and Wallace, 1991). Although some mental status examinations include race- and education-specific norms (Pfeiffer, 1975), many do not. If persons are to be classified as "impaired" or "nonimpaired" based on a single score applied without regard to educational attainment, there may be misclassification, with the result that less-educated groups may have spuriously high rates of impairment.

Understandability of questionnaire items may also be an issue. This may again relate to educational attainment. Indexes of data quality, such as item nonresponse, have been shown to decrease with educational attainment (Colsher and Wallace, 1989). In working with groups with low educational attainment, it may be possible to reword items into simpler language, break down long questions into a series of items, or even use a "storybook" approach with simple language and illustrations (Lessler et al, 1989; Tymchuk and Ouslander, 1990). For example, in a laboratory study of the influence of cognitive factors on survey responding, response accuracy to questions about fluoridation was 43 percent when the item asked was about "public water fluoridation" but 60 percent when the phrase "fluoride added to the water" was used (Lessler et al, 1989). Providing additional information may also facilitate recall of information. Lessler and colleagues found that the inclusion of reasons for dental visits (e.g., to have teeth cleaned, to get a filling) increased reporting of dental visits (Lessler et al, 1989).

Items may need to be modified to reflect regional lay terms for illnesses, such as "low blood" for anemia or "rich," "high," or "hot" blood for hypertension. Pilot investigations, including the use of focus group discussions and debriefing interviews with individuals, are useful in developing appropriate items for specific groups (Lessler et al, 1989).

In some instances, items may need to be translated from their original language. The presence of idioms [e.g., the Center for Epidemiologic Studies Depression Scale (Radloff, 1977) item, "I could not get going"] or the use of proverb interpretation as an index of higher cognitive function clearly creates problems, but more subtle differences in language usage may also preclude verbatim translation and raise questions about the comparability of items. When repetition of a simple phrase is included as a screen for speech or language problems, simple translation may also be inappropriate. For example, in the Chinese-language version (Yu et al, 1989) of the Mini-Mental Status Examination (Folstein et al, 1975), the phrase "forty-four stone lions" in Chinese was substituted for the English phrase "no ifs, ands, or buts."

CHRONICALLY ILL PERSONS

Specific chronic conditions may provide useful models for health service delivery. For example, end stage renal disease (ESRD) is treated with transplantation, chronic hemodialysis, or chronic peritoneal dialysis. Although treatment with dialysis is successful in terms of maintaining physiologic indices within reasonable bounds, ESRD patients must follow strict care regimens and often have residual disability. This is particularly true of older ESRD patients, who may have age-associated co-morbid conditions in addition to ESRD (Berra and Nitz, 1986; Jacobs et al, 1984; Plawecki and Brewer, 1986). For example, in a study of ESRD patients 50 years of age and older, more than 50 pecent required assistance with routine self-care activities, and about 75 percent were dependent in more complex instrumental activities of daily living (Wallace et al, 1990). Over 85 percent had at least one major ESRD complication. Thus, older ESRD patients treated with dialysis are likely to require a range of services for the duration of their survival. Other chronic conditions, including liver failure and chronic obstructive pulmonary disease, may similarly provide useful models for studying the delivery of a range of services over a long period of time.

In addition, the clinical course of older persons with chronic illnesses may differ from that of middle-aged and younger persons with the same condition. The complications introduced by age-associated co-morbid conditions have already been noted with regard to ESRD and would be expected to be a factor in other chronic illnesses as well. Older persons may be at particular risk of adverse drug reactions (Ouslander, 1981; Thompson et al, 1983a, 1983b; Williamson and Chopin, 1980), including toxic dementias and other cognitive impairments (Hutchinson et al, 1986; Klein et al, 1984; Martys, 1979). Health risk appraisal may also differ for older persons. Although serum cholesterol level is an established risk factor for cardiovascular morbidity and mortality among middle-aged men (Pooling Project Research Group, 1978), the "meaning" of cholesterol levels in elderly persons is less clear (Woolf et al, 1990).

There are both ethical and methodologic issues in research with chronically ill persons. The ethical issues involve obtaining consent and limiting response burden. As is discussed in detail elsewhere in this book, it is considered possible to obtain valid consent from persons in the early stages of dementia or those with other mild cognitive impairments (American College of Physicians, 1989). When the impairment is more severe, a surrogate should be consulted, although the patient's wishes regarded participation should also be considered (American College of Physicians, 1989).

Sensitivity regarding response burden is particularly important, and there are several ways to reduce the burden of patients. It may be possible to obtain the needed information from different sources, thus reducing the length of interviews. For example, a caregiver may provide information about service utilization or medication history while the patient is asked about subjective information, such as mood, or is given physical performance or cognitive testing. Some information may be obtained in a mail questionnaire prior to interview.This may be particularly useful if detailed residential, occupational, or exposure histories are gathered. It may also be possible to conduct interviews in several brief sessions rather than in a single longer session.

Other methodological issues include obtaining an appropriate representation of the population and questions about the validity and reliability of commonly used scales. In population-based studies, it is commonly observed that nonparticipants are more likely to be ill and less functional than participants. In groups defined by the presence of a chronic illness, this tendency may be exacerbated and participation rates may be reduced.

The reliability and validity of individual item responses also may be troublesome. These issues are most clearly seen in studies of mildly or moderately demented persons. However, persons with a variety of chronic conditions—including but not limited to chronic obstructive pulmonary disease, renal failure, liver failure, diabetes, and thyroid disease—may also experience varying degrees of cognitive impairment (Tarter et al, 1988). Medications used in treating these illnesses may also produce cognitive impairment. The impairments may be of attentional processes, memory function, or information processing, and although these are not necessarily as severe as those seen in advanced dementia, they may affect survey responses.

The validity of standardized scales may also be suspect. For example, measures of depressive symptoms (Beck et al, 1961; Brink et al, 1982; Radloff, 1977; Zung, 1965) often include vegetative items, such as disturbed sleep, reduced energy level, and changed appetite. To the extent that these are also associated with chronic illness and its treatment, patients may have spuriously high depressive symptom scores. The concerns about reliability and validity of individual items also affect scales.

MENTALLY RETARDED PERSONS

Advances in medical care, including the development of antibiotics and heart surgery as well as their more aggressive use, have greatly reduced early mortality of persons with Down syndrome, the most common cause of mental retardation (Lott, 1982). Reviewing the literature, Thase (1982) concluded that there had been a 20–80 percent decrease in mortality (depending on the age group) since the 1940s. For example, mortality prior to five years of age decreased from 60 to 15 percent (Gallagher and Lowry, 1975; Record and Smith, 1954). As a result, there is a growing cohort of older persons with Down syndrome as well as other forms of mental retardation (Jacobsen et al, 1985; Seltzer and Krauss, 1987).

Although many retarded individuals are able to live independently or with only modest assistance as young adults (Jacobsen et al, 1985), age-associated changes may overload their coping resources. A nonretarded person with physical health or functional problems may be able to develop a variety of strategies to accomplish formerly routine tasks that have become physically challenging (e.g., bathing or dressing). A mentally retarded person, however, may need assistance in developing these strategies or even may become dependent in the activities. A better understanding of the health and functional status of retarded elders is also important for the planning and delivery of appropriate services.

In addition, study of mentally retarded elders may yield valuable insights into conditions affecting nonretarded elders. For example, Alzheimer-like brain changes have frequently been reported in autopsy studies of persons 30 years of age and older with Down syndrome (Lott, 1982). In neuropsychological evaluations, persons over the age of 35 with Down syndrome are more likely to have memory and other cognitive deficits similar to those seen in Alzheimer's than are younger persons with Down syndrome (Lott, 1982). There have also been reports of higher than expected rates of Down syndrome in the families of persons with Alzheimer's disease (Cook-Deegan et al, 1987).

The first challenge in doing epidemiologic research with mentally retarded elders is identification of the potential participants. Although persons with profound or severe retardation may be relatively easy to identify, since they are likely to have received state or federal assistance and/or have been institutionalized, mildly retarded individuals may be more difficult to identify. Depending on the assumed prevalence of mental retardation, only 15–40 percent of mentally retarded persons 55 years of age and older receive governmental assistance (Jacobsen, Sutton, and Janicki, 1985). Many may be undiagnosed, since the widespread use of intelligence testing is a relatively recent occurrence (Anastasi, 1976), and many of today's elders have never been evaluated with psychometric tests. They may simply have quit school very early and gone on to hold simple jobs and take care of their own needs by themselves or with the help of family members. Even moderately impaired persons may not need governmental assistance if they have sufficient informal support systems.

Obtaining consent for participation may also be an issue. Mildly retarded persons may be competent to give consent when suitably worded information summaries and consent forms are employed. With more severely impaired persons, competency is in question, and a proxy should be sought. In some cases a surviving parent may be available. However, it is possible that the parent will be frail and impaired, and the consent of a sibling or other responsible persons will need to be sought.

Various tests have been developed specifically for evaluating mentally retarded persons. Indeed, the contents of some of these tests are quite similar to geriatric functional assessment. For example, the Vineland Social Maturity Scale (Doll, 1965) and the Adaptive Behavior Scale (American Association on Mental Deficiency, 1974) both include assessment of routine self-care activities, and the Adaptive Behavior Scale includes more complex instrumental activities of daily living. However, many of the tests developed for use with mentally retarded persons did not include elders or even middle-aged persons in their normative samples. The validity and reliability of these tests with older populations thus remains to be demonstrated.

HOMELESS PERSONS

There is a general consensus that the homeless population is growing (Overbo, 1990), and although the homeless are typically relatively young, the number of homeless elders is increasing rapidly (Overbo, 1990) and may comprise over one quarter of the homeless (Cohen et al, 1988). The homeless have higher than expected mortality rates and a variety of often untreated chronic health problems (Martin, 1990). Although not universal, psychiatric illness is common. The lifetime prevalence of any psychiatric disorder is over 75 percent, with substance abuse–dependence the most common (Fischer et al, 1986). In terms of their demographic characteristics, the homeless are less educated, less likely to be employed, and more likely to be divorced or never married than persons having homes (Fischer et al, 1986).

The public health importance of studies of the homeless seems clear. The range and severity of health problems observed in this group, coupled with their lack of financial, social, and other resources, make provision of appropriate care and services to the homeless, regardless of their age, critical. Studies of the homeless are also needed to develop means for their successful reintegration into homes (Overbo, 1990) as well as programs to prevent the disintegration that leads to homelessness.

The homeless also constitute a unique group in which to study the interaction of aging with a variety of illnesses and exposures. For example, tuberculosis and other infectious illnesses are increasing among the homeless. Chronic alcoholism and the abuse of other drugs occur more commonly among the homeles than among those with homes (Fischer et al, 1986). Untreated or inadequately treated schizophrenia is observable in the homeless (Bassuk et al, 1984). The effects of inadequate diet and sanitation can also be studied.

The first two challenges to epidemiologists interested in research with the homeless elderly should be apparent: identification of potential participants and their recruitment into the study. Identification of the homeless for purposes of simply estimating the size of the population became a well-publicized issue with regard to the conduct of the 1990 U.S. Census. Even when homeless persons can be identified, they are likely to fit the classic profile of survey nonparticipants: unemployed, unmarried, and having a history of substance abuse (Bergstrand et al, 1983).

Obtaining valid consent from those who choose to participate may also be difficult: An estimated 8 percent have clinically significant cognitive impairment (Fischer et al, 1986). Thought disorders associated with schizophrenia may impair ability to give consent (Appelbaum and Roth, 1981), as may intoxication. Although remuneration might be expected to improve participation rates, it may raise questions about potential coerciveness.

There may also be questions about the reliability and validity of survey responses. The observed low levels of education and high rates of cognitive impairment would be expected to have an impact on data quality. The high rates of substance abuse suggest that participants may be intoxicated at the time of interview and unlikely to give reliable responses. Other psychiatric disorders observed more often in the homeless than in the general population may also degrade data quality. For example, persons with antisocial personality disorder may be more inclined to manipulate interviewers or portray themselves in exaggeratedly positive light. Persons who are floridly psychotic may simply be uninterviewable, but milder thought disorders may also affect the reliability and validity of responses.

INMATES IN CORRECTIONAL FACILITIES

Despite the difficulties of working with incarcerated populations, much valuable information may be gained from such research (Wallace and Colsher, 1990). The prison population may have higher levels of certain exposures (e.g., illicit drug use) than the population as a whole. Prisons may be suited for the study of psychosocial issues such as crowding. Hypertension has been observed less often in prison populations than would be expected (Ostfeld et al, 1988), and the cardiovascular reactivity of this group appears to be lessened (Raine et al, 1990). All-cause mortality rates as well as some chronic disease mortality rates are lower in prisons than in the general population (Salive et al, 1990). Investigations of these issues may provide valuable information and have implications for both the general population and inmates.

In a recent discussion of impediments to research with inmates in correctional facilities, Prout and Ross (1988) noted that corrections administration and staff, inmates, structural and organizational factors, and even the attitudes of researchers had contributed to the lack of basic investigations. For example, administration and staff may be overburdened by their work duties and not have time or may view researchers as troublesome, interfering, or intrusive. Inmates may fear disclosure of confidential information or may simply not wish to cooperate with anyone if it is not required. When medical records exist, they may be incomplete or inaccurate. If they are accessible, the records may be kept at some central location other than the facility at which the inmates are housed.

Researchers may hesitate to become involved because of ethical concerns, the added demands of such work (e.g., the logistics of interviewing in prisons), or even stereotypes of inmates and prisons. The latter issue may have contributed to the relative dearth of information on elderly inmates. The stereotype of a warm, caring grandparent is difficult to reconcile with that of a convicted criminal.

The history of occasional exploitative research with prison inmates is such that the ethical issues involved in prison research deserve special consideration. For example, the prison environment may be viewed as inherently coercive, thus complicating the consent procedure, particularly if the research is being done in collaboration with the corrections system. Financial compensation for participation may be a difficult issue. Inmate salaries are generally very low, and even small amounts of money may be considerably more than could be earned at a prison job, thus raising the possibility of coerciveness. Corrections officials may require the presence of corrections staff during interviews or may place other limitations on confidentiality. The low levels of education typically seen in inmates of all ages, but especially striking in older inmates, may also complicate the consent procedure. Simplified information summaries and consent forms may be needed.

Several methodological issues arise in working with inmates. Illiteracy and low levels of educational attainment may necessitate modified questionnaires or preclude self-administration. Standard assessment instruments may not be applicable. For example, instrumental activities of daily living, such as shopping, cooking meals, and taking medication, are commonly included in geriatric functional assessment, yet these activities may be restricted in the prison population. Other types of information, well known to those familiar with the prison population but not commonly gathered as a part of geriatric assessment (e.g., use of illicit drugs, sex with prostitutes), may be an important part of geriatric prison epidemiology.

SUMMARY AND CONCLUSIONS

This chapter has briefly reviewed some of the major considerations in epidemiologic investigations of historically understudied populations. Clearly, much is to be gained from the study of these groups, including a more complete understanding of the epidemiology of aging and a better information base from which to plan for health care and other service delivery. In addition, there are unique opportunities to address important issues such as the role of genetic factors in chronic illnesses, the interaction of substance abuse and aging, and the optimization of long-term, intensive delivery of health care services.

Both ethical and methodological issues in research with historically understudied populations were addressed. In some instances, there are concerns about obtaining consent, which, given historical incidents of inappropriate conduct involving some of these populations by researchers, must be treated with particular sensitivity. Methodological challenges arise on a number of levels, from identification of potential participants to the reliability and validity of commonly used assessment instruments and to analytic issues involving such confounders as socioeconomic status. As has been asserted, however, these issues are basic to good scientific work, not specific to the populations reviewed here. Although the initial work may be somewhat more challenging, the study of the epidemiology of aging can only be enriched by more comprehensive examination of historically understudied populations.

ACKNOWLEDGMENT

This work was supported by National Institute of Aging Grant AG-07094.

REFERENCES

Alstrom CH, Lindelius R, Salum I (1975). Mortality among homeless men. Br J Addiction 70:245–252.

American Association on Mental Deficiency (1974). Adaptive Behavior Scale. Washington, DC, American Association on Mental Deficiency.

American College of Physicians (1989). Cognitively impaired subjects. Ann Intern Med 111:843–848.

Anastasi A (1976). Psychological Testing. New York, Macmillan.

Anderson NB, Cohen HJ (1989). Editorial. Health status of aged minorities: Directions for clinical research. J Gerontol: Med Sci: 44:M1–M2.

Appelbaum PS, Roth LH (1981). Clinical issues in the assessment of competency. Am J Psychiatr 138:1462–1467.

Bassuk EL, Rubin L, Lauriat A (1984). Is homelessness a mental health problem? Am J Psychiatr 141:1546–1550.

Bastida E (1988). Reexaming assumptions about extended familism: Older Puerto Ricans in a comparative perspective. In Sotomayor M, Curiel H (eds), Hispanic Elderly: A Cultural Signature. Edinburg, TX, Pan American University Press.

Beck AT, Ward CH, Mendelson M, Mock J, Erbaugh J (1961). An inventory for measuring depression. Arch Gen Psychiatr 4:53–571.

Bergstrand R, Vedin A, Wilhelmsson C, Wilhelmsson L (1983). Bias due to non-participation and heterogeneous sub-groups in population surveys. J Chronic Dis 36:725–728.

Berra B, Nitz J (1986). The geriatric patient with ESRD. Special patients—special needs. J Nephrol Nurs Jan/Feb:5–13.

Block G, Rosenberger WF, Patterson BH (1988). Calories, fat, and cholesterol: Intake patterns in the US population by race, sex and age. Am J Public Health 78:1150–1155.

Brink TL, Yesavage JA, Lum O, Heersma PH, Adey M, Rose TL (1982). Screening tests for geriatric depression. Clin Gerontol 1:37–43.

Burack RC, Liang J (1989). The acceptance and completion of mammography by older black women. Am J Public Health 79:721–726.

Centers for Disease Control (1988). Provisional estimates from the National Health Interview Survey supplement on cancer control— United States, January–March, 1987. Morb Mortal Weekly Rev 37:417–425.

Cohen C, Teresi J, Holmes D, Roth E (1988). Survival strategies of older homeless men. Gerontologist 28:58–65.

Colsher PL, Wallace RB (1989). Data quality and age: Health and psychobehavioral correlates of item nonresponse and inconsistent responses. J Gerontol: Psych Sci: 44:P45–P52.

Colsher PL, Wallace RB (1991) Longitudinal application of cognitive function measures in a defined population of community-dwelling elders. Ann Epidemiol. 1:215–230.

Cook-Deegan RM, Mace N, Baily MA, Cahvkin D, Hawes C (1987). Confronting Alzheimer's Disease and Other Dementias. Philadelphia, Lippincott.

Cornoni-Huntley J, Brock DW, Ostfeld AM, Taylor JO, Wallace RB (1986). Established Populations for Epidemiologic Studies of the Elderly: Resource Data book. Bethesda, MD, National Institute on Aging, 1986.

Dawson DA (1988). Ethnic differences in female overweight: Data from the 1985 National Health Interview Survey. Am J Public Health 78:1326–1329.

Doll EA (1965). Vineland Social Maturity Scale: Manual of Directions. Minneapolis, American Guidance Service.

Fischer PJ, Shapiro S, Breakey WR, Anthony JC, Kramer M (1986). Mental health and social characteristics of the homeless: A survey of mission users. Am J Public Health 76:519–524.

Folstein MF, Folstein SE, McHugh PR (1975). "Mini-mental state": A practical method for grading the cognitive state of patients for the clinician. J Psychiatr Res 12:189–198.

Gallagher RR, Lowry RB (1975). Longevity in Down's syndrome in British Columbia. J Ment Defic Res 19:157–164.

Gartside PS, Khoury O, Glueck CJ (1984). Determinants of high density lipoprotein cholesterol in Blacks and Whites: The second National Health and Nutrition Examination Survey. Am Heart J 180:641–653.

Halperin RH (1990). Aging and minority cultures: A comparison of three groups. J Cross-Cultural Gerontol 5:395–404.

Horner RD (1990). Cancer mortality in Native Americans in North Carolina. Am J Public Health 80:940–944.

Hutchinson TA, Flegel KM, Kramer MS, Leduc DG, Ho Ping Kong H (1986). Frequency, severity, and risk factors for adverse drug reactions in adult out-patients: A prospective study. J Chron Dis 129:319–331.

Jackson JJ, Perry C (1986). Physical health conditions of middle-aged and aged Blacks. In Markides KS (ed), Aging and Health. Perspectives on Gender, Race, Ethnicity, and Class. Newbury Park, CA, Sage.

Jacobs C, Diallo A, Balas EA, Nectoux M, Etienne S (1984). Maintenance haemodialysis treatment in patients aged over 60 years. Demographic profile, clinical aspects, and outcome. Proc EDTA-ERA 21:477–489.

Jacobsen JW, Sutton MS, Janicki MP (1985). Demography and characteristics of aging and aged mentally retarded persons. In Janicki MP, Wisniewski HM (eds), Aging and Developmental Disabilities: Issues and Approaches. Baltimore, MD, Paul H. Brookes.

Johnson HR, Gibson RC, Luckey I (1990). Health and social characteristics. Implications for services. In Harel Z, McKinney EA, Williams M (eds), Black Aged. Understanding Diversity and Service Needs. Newbury Park, CA, Sage.

Kasl SV (1984). Social and psychological factors in the etiology of coronary heart disease in black populations: An exploration of research needs. Am Heart J 108:660–669.

Klein LE, German PS, Levine DM, Feroli R, Ardery J (1984). Medication problems among outpatients. A study with emphasis on the elderly. Arch Intern Med 144:1185–1188.
Kunitz SJ, Levy JE (1989). Aging and health among Navajo Indians. In Markides KS (ed), Aging and Health. Perspectives on Gender, Race, Ethnicity, and Class. Newbury Park, CA, Sage.
Lessler J, Tourangeau R, Salter W (1989). Questionnaire Design in the Cognitive Research Laboratory. Vital and Health Statistics, Series 6, No. 1. DHHS Pub. No. (PHS) 89-1076. Hyattsville, MD, US Department of Health and Human Services.
Levy JE, Kunitz SJ (1974). Indian Drinking: Navajo Practices and Anglo-American Theories. New York, Wiley.
Lott IT (1982). Down's syndrome, aging, and Alzheimer's disease: A clinical review. In Sinex FM, Merril CR (eds), Alzheimer's Disease, Down's Syndrome, and Aging. New York: The New York Academy of Sciences, pp. 15–28.
Markides KS (1989). Aging, gender, race/ethnicity, class, and health: A conceptual overview. In Markides KS (ed), Aging and Health: Perspectives on Gender, Race, Ethnicity, and Class. New York: Sage, pp. 9–22.
Markides KS, Machalek R (1984). Selective survival, aging, and society. Arch Gerontol Geriatr 3:207–222.
Martin MA (1990). The homeless elderly: No room at the end. In Harel Z, Erlich P, Huber R (eds), The Vulnerable Aged. New York, Springer.
Martys CR (1979). Adverse reactions to drugs in general practice. Br Med J 2:1194–1197.
Mohs ME, Leonard TK, Watson RR (1988). Interrelationships among alcohol abuse, obesity, and type II diabetes mellitus: Focus on Native Americans. World Rev Nutr Diet 56:93–172.
Monheit A, Schur C (1989). Health Insurance Coverage of Retired Persons. DHHS Pub. No. (PHS) 89-3444. National Medical Expenditure Survey research findings 2, National Center for Health Services Research and Health Care Technology Assessment. Rockville, MD, Public Health Service.
National Caucus and Center on Black Aged, Inc. (1989). Health Status of Aged Blacks. Washington, DC.
Ostfeld AM, Kasl SV, D'Atri DA, Fitzgerald EF (1988). Stress, Crowding, and Blood Pressure in Prison. Hillsdale, NJ, Lawrence Erlbaum, 1988.
Ouslander JG (1981). Drug therapy in the elderly. Ann Intern Med 95:711–722.
Overbo B (1990). Ollie Randall Symposium: Homeless elders: A growing national crisis. Gerontologist 30:142A.
Pfeiffer E (1975). A short portable mental status questionnaire for the assessment of organic brain deficit in elderly patients. J Am Psychiatr Soc 23:433–441.
Plawecki HM, Brewer S (1986). The elderly hemodialysis patient. ANNA J 13:146–149.
Prout C, Ross RN (1988). Care and Punishment. Pittsburgh, University of Pittsburgh Press, 1988.
Pooling Project Research Group (1978). Relationship of blood pressure, serum cholesterol, smoking habit, relative weight and ECG abnormalities to incidence of major coronary events. Final report of the Pooling Project. J Chronic Dis 31:210–306.
Radloff LS (1977). The CES-D scale: A self-report depression scale for research in the general population. Appl Psychol Measure 1:385–401.
Raine A, Venables PH, Williams M (1990). Relationships between central and autonomic measures of arousal at age 15 years and criminality at age 24 years. Arch Gen Psychiatr 47:1003–1007.
Record RG, Smith A (1954). The incidence, mortality, and sex distributions of mongloid defectives. Br J Prev Soc Med 9:10–15.
Roig E, Castaner A, Simmons B, Patel R, Ford E, Cooper R (1987). In-hospital mortality rates

from acute myocardial infarction by race in US hospitals: Findings from the National Hospital Discharge Survey. Circulation 76:280–288.
Roland ML, Fulwood R (1984). Coronary heart disease risk factor trends in Blacks between the first and second National Health and Nutrition Examination Surveys, United States, 1971–1980. Am Heart J 108:771–779.
Rubenstein D (1984). The elderly in prison: A review of the literature. In Newman ES, Newman DJ, Gerwitz ML (eds), Elderly Criminals. Cambridge, MA, Oelgeschlager, Gunn, & Hain, pp. 153–168.
Salive ME, Smith GS, Brewer TF (1990). Death in prison: Changing mortality patterns among male prisoners in Maryland, 1979–1987. Am J Public Health 80:1479–1480.
Sauer WJ, Coward RT (1985). Social Support Networks and the Care of the Elderly. New York, Springer.
Seltzer MM, Krauss MW (1987). Aging and Mental Retardation. Washington, DC, American Association on Mental Retardation.
Sotomayor M, Randolph S (1988). A preliminary review of caregiving issues and the Hispanic family. In Sotomayor M, Curiel H (eds), Hispanic Elderly: A Cultural Signature. Edinburg, TX, Pan American University Press.
Sprafka JM, Folsom A, Burke GL, Edlavitch SA (1988). Prevalence of cardiovascular disease risk factors in Blacks and Whites: The Minnesota Heart Survey. Am J Public Health 78:1546–1549.
Tarter RE, Van Thiel DH, Edwards KL (1988). Medical Neuropsychology: The Impact of Disease on Behavior. New York, Plenum Press, 1988.
Thase ME (1982). Longevity and mortality in Down's syndrome. J Ment Defic Res 27:177–192.
Thompson TL, Moran MG, Nies AS (1983a). Psychotropic drug use in the elderly. Part I. New Engl J Med 308:134–138.
Thompson TL, Moran MG, Nies AS (1983b). Psychotropic drug use in the elderly. Part II. New Engl J Med 308:194–199.
Tymchuk AJ, Ouslander JG (1990). Optimizing the informed consent process with elderly people. Educ Gerontol 16:245–257.
US Bureau of Commerce (1990). Statistical Abstract of the United States. Washington, DC: US Government Printing Office.
Wallace RB, Colsher PL (1990). The prison environment as a model for the study of community problems. Presented at the meeting of the American Public Health Association, New York.
Wallace, RB, Colsher PL, Schadle J (1990). End-stage renal disease in the elderly: Health and functional impact. Paper presented at the meeting of the American Public Health Association, New York.
Williamson J, Chopin JM (1980). Adverse reactions to prescribed drugs in the elderly: A multicentre investigation. Age and Ageing, 9:73–80.
Woolf SH, Kamerow DB, Lawrence RS, Medalie JH, Estes EH (1990). The periodic health examination of older adults: Recommendations of the U.S. Preventive Services Task Force. Part II. Screening tests. J Am Geriatr Soc 38:933–942.
Young TK, Kaufert JM, McKenzie JK, Hawkins A, O'Neil J (1989). Excessive burden of end-stage renal disease among Candian Indians: A national survey. Am J Public Health 79:756–758.
Yu ESH, Liu WT, Levy P, Zhang M-Y, Katzman R, Lung C-T, Wong S-C, Wang Z-Y, Qu G-Y (1989). Cognitive impairment among elderly adults in Shanghai, China. J Gerontol (Soc Sci) 44:S97–S106.
Zung WWK (1965). A self-rating depression scale. Arch Gen Psychiatr 12:63–70.

20

Cross-cultural Research on Aging and Health

JERSEY LIANG AND GINA M. JAY

This chapter provides a discussion of generic issues in comparative research. First, four types of analytical approaches in conducting cross-cultural research are presented. Second, the current state of the comparative literature on aging is characterized. Third, two major concerns related to comparative research are examined: cross-cultural comparability of measures, and organizational issues in establishing linkages with foreign investigators and institutions. These two concerns receive more detailed discussion because they illustrate particularly well the unique character of cross-cultural comparative research. Finally, an agenda for future research is offered.

ANALYTICAL APPROACHES

Because different nations tend to have distinct cultures, investigators often use the terms *cross-national research* and *cross-cultural studies* interchangeably, however, they are not identical. A nation may contain several distinct cultures, whereas several nations may share a common cultural heritage. For convenience, we shall use the term *cross-cultural research* throughout this chapter.

According to Kohn (1987) there are four ways to conduct cross-national comparative research. The first type of research treats nation or culture as the object of study. The primary interest is to attain an in-depth understanding of aging within one or more given cultures, although the findings may have implications beyond the cultures studied. Examples of such research include studies by Davis-Friedman (1983) and Palmore (1975) on the Chinese and Japanese elderly. Studies of aging and health in a single culture or subculture are comparative only implicitly. For a direct and explicit quantitative comparison, data from at least two different cultures are required. The second type of comparative research views culture as the context of observed phenomena and relations. The purpose is to establish the generalizability of findings and validity of interpretations beyond one culture. An example of such research is the international comparison of the epidemiology of dementia conducted by Mortimer (1988). The third type of comparative research views the nation or culture as the unit of analysis. The goal is to examine the relationships between the characteristics of cultures and aging. In such studies, one no longer speaks of cultures or nations by name but classifies them along one or more dimensions. An illustration of this approach is the analysis of population aging in 31 countries conducted by Torrey, Kinsella, and Taeuber (1987). Finally, a given culture can be conceptualized as part of an international system. Relationships among the characteristics of various cultures are examined by assuming that these cultures are integrated parts of a system. For example, the relationship between population health and economic development in Latin American countries can be analyzed within the capitalist world-system.

CURRENT STATE OF COMPARATIVE RESEARCH ON AGING AND HEALTH

As noted by Palmore (1983), there are relatively few truly comparative cross-cultural studies of social gerontology. Most of the existing studies are primarily descriptive and contain little theory, generalization, or quantitative comparison with other cultures. Indeed, the majority of social gerontological research published in English deals only with the dominant white Anglo-Saxon Protestant culture in the United States. In a similar vein, Cowgill (1986) observed that much of the comparative research on aging consists of disparate case studies with no uniformity of definition, method, sample, or range of subject matter. The failure to provide adequate and systematic attention to conceptual and methodological problems undoubtedly contributes to a lack of meaningful and interpretable data, which in turn poses significant risks of misinterpretation. Cowgill argues eloquently that to advance comparative aging research, one should undertake parallel studies using comparable techniques, covering the same subject matter, and employing comparable concepts in distinct cultures. He acknowledges that such research has not yet been done and would be exceedingly complex, time-consuming, and costly.

With reference to cross-cultural studies of health and illness, Angel and Thoits (1987) suggested that two traditions exist, the epidemiologic and ethnographic approaches. The epidemiologic tradition seeks to understand the etiology, progress, and consequences of diseases in different populations. The ethnographic tradition, which is largely anthropological and sociological in nature, attempts to understand the illness-labeling and help-seeking process. Investigators of the ethnographic tradition often overlook or deemphasize the significance of diseases and related medical facts (Pflanz, 1976). On the other hand, proponents of the epidemiologic approach frequently do not recognize that cross-cultural differences in health and illness reflect not only genuine variation in the incidence and prevalence of morbidity, disability, and mortality, but also the social processes by which these data were generated. These processes may be far removed from the biological reality (Kleinman, 1978). Accordingly, a sensible strategy requires the adaptation of a combination of epidemiologic and ethnographic approaches. Such practice has been rare in the comparative research on aging and health.

MEASUREMENT ISSUES

A major issue in comparative epidemiologic research on the aged is the equivalence of measures. One must establish that the variables measured in different cultures are sufficiently similar in terms of construct validity and measurement properties, to treat them as the same phenomena and to warrant a meaningful comparison. One must consider at least three types of measurement equivalence (Hui and Triandis, 1983; Kalimo et al, 1970). The first is *semantic or operational* equivalence under which research materials or behaviors have the same meaning in two or more cultural systems. The second is *metric* equivalence, which implies that a given measurement specification can be applied to different cultures. Specifically, the observable indicators have the same relationship with the theoretical construct across different cultures. The third is *structural* equivalence, which refers to the fact that the causal linkages between a given construct (e.g., dementia) and its causes and consequences are invariant across different cultures. Cross-cultural comparability is, therefore, a matter of degree rather than an either–or proposition.

A wide variety of measures and data sources are used in epidemiologic research with the elderly, including interview items, self-report questionnaires, archival records (e.g., from a hospital or clinic), and various biological and physiologic measures (e.g., electroencephalograms, blood tests). There are several concerns regarding the comparability of such measures. Some issues apply to all studies; some, only to those utilizing biological or physiologic measures; and others, to those using survey or questionnaire items.

Issues of concern in all cross-cultural epidemiologic studies include differences in modes of data collection, in how a given condition has been defined or a variable operationalized, and in the reliability of data sources. For example, comparison of self-report questionnaire data with clinical data may lead to over- or underestimation of cultural differences, simply because the information being compared is not truly comparable. One illustration of how mode of data collection can affect study results is found in Iwatt (1987). This research found a much lower prevalence of hemorrhoids in England when examining clinical data than when relying on verbal responses to interview questions. Even when the mode of data collection is the same, subtle differences in how key study variables are defined may also affect study results. Finally, one must be concerned with the reliability of the data being analyzed. In cross-cultural research it is common to use secondary data for at least one culture, since the expense of collecting multicultural primary data is prohibitive. As such, one must rely on the documentation for a given data set to indicate data quality. Since differences generally exist in data collection practices between countries, the data for one culture may be more reliable than those for another. The reliability and validity of archival data (e.g., medical records) are also of concern, since some countries, and institutions within countries, keep more accurate and comprehensive records than others. Comparing data differing greatly in reliability may also lead to over- or underestimation of cultural differences.

Issues of particular importance for studies utilizing biological or physiologic measures concern the actual measure or test employed, and accuracy of diagnoses. Cross-cultural differences identified in a given study may actually be artifacts of different laboratory or clinical tests used to assess a given condition. For example, Reed et al (1988) compared two different methods of measuring atherosclerosis in a sample of men and found that the two approaches produced very different results. They concluded that estimates of the extent of atherosclerosis and its relation to various risk factors depend on the method used to measure it and that studies utilizing only one measure may overlook important risk factor associations.

The same test conducted in different countries could also yield different results. Van Saase and colleagues (1989) reported differences in levels of radiologic osteoarthritis in 11 different populations. They concluded, however, that some of the differences found may be due in part to interobserver variation in the interpretation of the radiographs used to assess the condition. That is, investigators in one country may be more inclined to score a given radiograph higher or lower than those in another country, thereby using slightly different criteria to determine the presence of the disease. This is yet another example of how method differences may introduce artificial cultural differences into the data.

One must also be concerned with possible variation in the accuracy of diagnoses of a given condition. Many conditions are complex and difficult to diagnose, thereby increasing the likelihood of variation in diagnosis within and between countries. Parkinson's syndrome, for example, can result from a variety of factors (e.g., medication side effects, exposure to toxins, lesions on the basal ganglia), making it difficult to distinguish between idiopathic Parkinson's disease and secondary Parkinsonism (Schoenberg, 1986). Also, since Parkinson's disease is most common in the elderly, very careful evaluation is required to distinguish symptoms of the disease from others often observed in the elderly patient (e.g., slowing or hesitancy of movement due to arthritis). When diagnostic criteria are not comparable across countries, study results may be misleading.

Issues of particular importance for studies using questionnaire or survey items include wording of items and item translation. For example, one study comparing health promotion in Canada and the United States found that they were probably underestimating differences in physical activity between the two countries because of differences in item wording (Schoenborn and Stephens, 1988). The U.S. item asked if respondents exercised or played sports regularly, whereas the more rigorous Canadian item asked about engaging in physical activity for at least 15 minutes three or more times each week.

Item translation is a critical component in cross-cultural research methodology. Questions that are valid and reliable in one language often "lose something" in translation (Palmore, 1983). Moreover, even with an accurate translation, the problem of different connotations and nuances implied in different cultures by apparently similar concepts may not be resolved. On the other hand, as Brislin (1976) notes, in the development of an instrument researchers often take advantage of common experiences. However, the source of the common experiences may be culture dependent; therefore, some questions may have limited usefulness in another culture, where the same experiences, or values attached to experiences, differ. Consequently, a critical evaluation of the substantive equivalence of survey instruments is essential for any cross-cultural comparison.

Several approaches have been used to ensure the equivalence of questionnaire and survey variables and to identify culture-universal (i.e., meaningful across cultures) and culture-specific (i.e., meaningful only within a given culture) items. To address the issue of equivalence, a combination of methods is required (Jackson et al, 1982). A triangulation of quantitative and qualitative methods is useful for ensuring the meaningfulness of items within cultures, and their measurement equivalence across cultures. In particular, survey questionnaires must be extensively evaluated through such qualitative procedures as back-translation, random probe (Schuman, 1966), and in-depth interviews.

In back-translation a researcher prepares material in one language and asks a bilingual person to translate it into another language. A second bilingual person translates the material back into the original language. The quality and accuracy of translation are then evaluated by comparing the two original language forms. Random probe refers to the supplementation of quantitative survey responses with open-ended descriptive responses provided by the respondent. This qualitative information may then be used to assess the respondent's understanding of the survey questions, to validate survey data, to decipher puzzling responses, and to interpret statistical results. In-depth interviews involve probing responses to many, and sometimes all, survey questions. The qualitative data resulting from even a small number of in-depth interviews may produce a wealth of new insights to complement the quantitative data in defining research questions, designing instruments, illustrating the range of meaning attached to statistical findings, and suggesting hypotheses and plausible explanations for observed cross-cultural similarities and differences. The preceding procedures have recently been applied by James Jackson and his associates (1982) in the study of the black aged, and by Liang and his colleagues (1989) in a comparative analysis of health and well-being among the elderly in the United States and Japan.

The quantitative approach of structural equation modeling can also be employed to evaluate equivalence in measurement and causal linkages. Metric equivalence can be assessed by factor-analyzing data obtained in different cultures and comparing the factor structures that emerge (Hui and Trandis, 1983; Miller et al, 1981). In this regard, the least defensive, but very frequently used, method is the "pseudoetic" approach (Davidson et al, 1976). Emic measures (developed in a single culture), usually developed in North America, are simply assumed to be etic (appropriate for use across diverse cultures). That is, instruments composed of items reflecting Western cultures are translated and used in other cultures with little regard for the conceptual and metric equivalence across different cultures (Fry and Ghosh, 1980). Mean differences found between cultural groups are assumed to be cultural differences. However, this approach rarely yields useful results, since the validity of the measures across cultures has never been established.

Even when factorial structures of a given instrument are compared across cultures, many problems persist. When exploratory factor analysis is used, this is less than satisfactory because ad hoc comparisons often are made (Hofstede and Bond, 1984). As suggested by Blalock (1982), an explicit auxiliary measurement model is required to address the issue of comparability of measurement and to determine the precise nature of potential noncomparability of measures across settings, time periods, or different populations. Without an explicit formulation, the claim of comparability is inherently untestable. Using a structural equation modeling approach, Liang and his associates (1988) have recently outlined a procedure for analyzing factorial invariance across cultural groups. In particular, basic measurement models are developed separately within each cultural group. Once these models are developed, simultaneous factor analysis involving the explicit comparison of common elements is undertaken. This involves the examination of changes in goodness of fit by applying equivalence constraints across two or more cultural groups. If cross-cultural differences exist, a residualized convariance matrix is computed by adjusting for the influences of factors thought to be contributing to the observed nonequivalence. This matrix is then subjected to multiple group factor analysis. The logic of this strategy is straightforward: If differences in the parameter estimates can be attributed to certain factors such as age and sex, then those differences should disappear once the input covariance matrix has been purged of their influence (see Liang et al 1988).

Given that the construct validity of a given measure may vary across cultures, this may lead to the use of different indicators of the same concept in different social contexts (Kalimo et al, 1970). This is a provocative and controversial position (Pflanz, 1976). However, if this is to be pursued, the distinction of culture-general component from the culture-specific component must be maintained. The linkages between the culture-general and culture-specific components have to be explicated. The ethnographic perspective and qualitative research techniques are particularly useful in identifying culture-specific indicators.

Cross-cultural variations of structural equivalence in causal linkages can be analyzed with similar methodology used to ensure metric equivalence of instruments and concepts. These same comments are applicable to research on aging in racial and ethnic groups within societies, where most studies have been based on data collected within one ethnic or cultural group; comparisons are at best implicit. When two or more groups have been explicitly compared, descriptive and analytical techniques have been applied without addressing issues concerning conceptual, metric, and causal equivalence. Presently, relatively little is known about the cross-cultural comparability of many widely used instruments in social gerontology (for exceptions, see Liang et al, 1987a; Liang et al, 1987b). Even less is understood about the cross-cultural equivalence in causal linkages.

General concerns for study comparability not specifically linked to measurement include the representativeness of the populations under study and the timing of the data collection. Cross-cultural differences or similarities identified in studies using different types of samples (e.g., regional, national) may be misleading. If regional-level data in one country are compared with national-level figures in another country, over- or underestimation of differences is possible. Similarly, comparison of data collected at two different times (e.g., 1970s and 1980s) may also be problematic, particularly if changes occurring at a societal or national level have influenced the variables under study.

ORGANIZATIONAL ISSUES

The importance of a sound organizational foundation on which high-quality comparative research can be implemented must be emphasized. Given the relatively unique conditions within each country or culture, the input and collaboration of investigators who are familiar with the native language, social system, and cultural values are imperative in ensuring the sensitivity and meaningfulness of the research operations and the proper interpretation of the findings. At the same time, the comparability of research design and instrumentation must be maintained and comparative analyses must be conducted. This calls for the close collaboration of researchers and at least one research organization within each of the cultures involved in the comparative study. This network of investigators and research organizations will certainly improve the quality of research, produce more reliable findings, and allow the investigation of phenomena that formerly could not be explored.

Such an organization is difficult to accomplish in that it requires a great deal of personal and institutional connections as well as resources. The massive scale of the operation and the high costs involved in data collection, processing, and analysis in conjunction with the reality of limited funds available for research inevitably restrict the number of cross-cultural comparative research projects to only a few. Consequently, it is critical to view a comparative research data base as a valuable resource that can be shared and utilized by many investigators. In this way, the utility of scarce resources is increased, opportunities to undertake comparative research are extended, and scientific productivity is expanded.

In the following, strategies in establishing international ties are reviewed in terms of three major modes of activities: exchange of personnel, collaborative research, and joint conferences and workshops. The discussion will be illustrated with our experience in working with investigators in East Asian countries such as Japan, China, and Taiwan. In addition, organizational concerns in the planning and execution of comparative research will be examined.

Establishing Ties

Exchange of Personnel

Exchanges of personnel can be short-term (e.g., one month) or long-term (e.g., two months to one year). Each serves a somewhat different purpose. The exchange of short-term visits by representatives who are in leadership positions and/or who are potential collaborators is critical in establishing good contacts and winning support for future cooperation. Long-term visits are more appropriate for training and implementing joint research. The costs of exchange should be divided between the organizations involved. Given the shortage and tight control of foreign exchange in some countries (e.g., China), foreign researchers often need substantial assistance from their American counterparts in raising travel funds.

Although this type of exchange is an excellent way to establish contacts and rapport with investigators, one needs to be selective and cautious in identifying individuals who are genuinely interested and committed to gerontological research. Other countries may have very different ideas about scientific research and its role within the general organizational context. Accordingly, they may have a different agenda and priorities. For instance, many Chinese institutions are much more interested in training and curriculum development than in original empirical research. This is understandable in view of the tremendous damage suffered by the higher educational system as a result of the Cultural Revolution. Moreover, China has a Russian-style two-tier system, in that universities are primarily teaching institutions and academies of sciences and social sciences are responsible for research. Many Chinese researchers unrealistically expect that substantial funding can be obtained easily in the United States and all costs of research can be borne by Americans. The role of the U.S. government in supporting research and the competitive nature of the peer review process associated with the allocation of research funds are frequently unfamiliar to many Chinese investigators. One good way to recruit potential collaborators is to work with visiting scholars and foreign graduate students who are already in the United States. They are likely to be well trained in the latest technology, knowledgeable about research practices in the United States, and may soon be placed in leadership positions in their organizations.

Collaborating in Research

Although many foreign investigators are likely to respond enthusiastically to the prospect of collaborative research, one must be aware of potential obstacles. In addition to the different conceptions of research, the role of government in controlling research in some countries is often incomprehensible to many American researchers. For example, in China the infrastructure for conducting research leaves much to be desired. Communications and transportation are not well developed particularly in the rural areas. There is often a shortage of trained personnel and adequate facilities. Thus, American investigators are often required to train the research staff and to build the research organization. Accordingly, those who are interested in conducting research in the Chinese mainland should realize that this is a somewhat risky undertaking that requires sufficient resources and a strong commitment over a relatively long period of time. Although conditions are more hospitable in other countries, gerontological interests and expertise may not be in an advanced stage of development. Consequently, similar concerns may also apply.

What should one do to overcome these obstacles? A generally useful approach may involve a carefully prepared long-term plan that calls for a series of preliminary studies and the accomplishment of a number of intermediate goals before making any substantial investment. Thus, it is frequently desirable to compile published data and statistics and to write one or more preliminary papers before undertaking primary data collection. In addition, one may analyze data already collected or undertake pilot studies. These are very appealing options in that they involve modest investments and provide an excellent way for the investigator to assess the feasibility of planned research. By working with foreign researchers on these pilot studies, one would get a fairly realistic understanding of the capabilities of the collaborators and their organizations. Furthermore, one can learn whether there are resources that may be contributed by these investigators and their institution.

Conferences and Workshops

Conferences and workshops serve several useful functions. First, they enable investigators with gerontological interests to meet to facilitate exchanges in research and practice. Second, they help to generate some visibility for the aging cause in various nations and to reinforce the support of gerontological research. Third, they provide excellent opportunities for disseminating research findings, training new researchers, and recruiting established investigators in the field of gerontology.

There are at least two ways by which international exchanges can be accomplished through conferences and workshops. A very efficient way is to organize specific paper sessions or symposiums on topics of mutual interest within the program of annual meetings of established professional associations. For example, during recent years, the Comparative Aging Research Program at the University of Michigan has been organizing symposiums on comparative studies of health and aging at the Annual

Meetings of the Gerontological Society of America. These sessions often involve investigators from Japan, China, and Taiwan. In addition, American investigators have often been invited to participate in conferences in other countries. The other format entails the organization of special conferences. Support for such events can be obtained from the National Institutes of Health, private foundations, and resources in foreign countries. The second approach is much more focused and massive, but requires a considerable amount of resources to implement.

Planning and Execution

In view of the potential returns and risks involved in comparative research with other countries, it may be useful to enumerate some suggestions for successful execution. First, it is important to adopt a long-term perspective. As indicated previously, substantial investment is required and significant return within a short time is unlikely. It takes time and effort to identify and nurture a close working relationship with a dependable and trusted collaborator in a foreign nation. Given the vast differences in terms of culture and social system, it is extremely difficult, if not impossible, to undertake meaningful empirical research without such a contact.

Second, a necessary condition in the successful conduct of cross-cultural comparative research is the development of a collegial group. White (1976) suggests that an international consortium of banks may serve as a useful model for a successful collegial group. In such a group, each member controls its own resources; all are equal partners in the consortium, although their size and resources may vary; and all have a common interest in seeing that each prospers individually and all prosper collectively.

Third, all participants must be prepared to use a common language in the planning and execution of the research. Furthermore, bilingual investigators who have substantial background in at least two cultures are critical for a successful operation. For instance, in the Comparative Aging Research Program (CARP) at the University of Michigan, about one half of the research staff are native speakers of Chinese and Japanese, although English is the common language in planning and execution of the research. In addition, all collaborative investigators in Japan, China, and Taiwan are proficient in English.

Fourth, it is critical to learn about various resources for comparative research with foreign populations. These include established centers of foreign studies, major funding agencies, and the network of investigators undertaking comparative research. In addition, for those who are interested in undertaking cross-cultural comparative research on a long-term basis, it is imperative to mobilize support at their own institutions. Substantial contributions from both U.S. and foreign institutions are signs of strong interest and commitment, which are often required for collaborative comparative research to succeed.

Despite the potential risks, a comparative research initiative can yield quite handsome returns. For instance, one of the most significant potential contributions of a comparative aging research program is that many more initiatives can be built upon the organizational ties and research infrastructures established by the program and its foreign collaborating institutions. Thus, with a very modest additional investment, many important gerontological research questions can be investigated within a cross-cultural context. Furthermore, as the research operations are fully implemented, activities can be extended to additional countries as well as to additional age groups, including middle-aged and young adults, thus incorporating a lifespan developmental perspective.

AGENDA FOR FUTURE RESEARCH

In view of the present state of comparative aging research, an agenda for future research can be outlined. The collection of comparable data and the assessment of equivalence of key measures deserve the highest priority. Without resolving these concerns, cross-cultural comparisons are not justified. Once conceptual and measurement equivalence is demonstrated, equivalence in causal linkages can be properly examined, and substantive explanations for cross-cultural differences can be sought without being confounded by nonequivalent measures. To accomplish this objective, further explication of theories of comparative aging and considerably more empirical research, both cross-sectional and longitudinal, are essential. Finally, given the relatively massive scale and complexity of comparative research, a network of international investigators and research institutions is required to collaborate closely in order to implement such research successfully.

ACKNOWLEDGMENT

Support for this research was provided under grants, R37 AG06643, R01 AG08094, and T32 AG00134 by the National Institute on Aging.

REFERENCES

Angel R, Thoits P (1987). The impact of culture on the cognitive structure of illness. Cult Med Psychiatr 11:465–494.

Blalock HM (1982). Conceptualization and measurement in the social sciences. Beverly Hills, CA, Sage.

Brislin RW (1976). Comparative research methodology: Cross-cultural studies. Int J Psychol 11(3):215–229.

Cogwill DO (1986). Aging around the world. Belmont, CA, Wadsworth.

Davidson A, Jaccard JJ, Triandis HC, Morales ML, and Diaz-Guerrero R (1976). Cross-cultural model testing: Toward a solution of the etic-emic dilemma. Int J Psychol 11:1–13.

Davis-Freidmann D (1983). Long Lives: Chinese elderly and the Communist Revolution. Cambridge, MA, Harvard University Press.

Fry PS, Ghosh R (1980). Attributional difference in the life satisfactions of the elderly: A cross-cultural comparison of Asian and United States subjects. Int J Psychol 15:201–212.

Hofstede G, Bond MH (1984). Hofstede's culture dimensions: An independent validation using Rokeach's value survey. Cross-Cultural Psychol 15(4):17–33.

Hui CH, Triandis HC (1983). Multistrategy approach to cross-cultural research: The case for locus of control. Cross-Cultural Psychol 14(1):65–83.

Iwatt A (1987). Epidemiology of hemorrhoids in the adult Nigerian and English: A comparative study. Central African J Med 33(3):61–66.

Jackson JS, Tucker MB, Bowman PB (1982). Conceptual and methodological problems in survey research on black Americans. In Liu WT (ed), Methodological problems in Minority Research. Chicago, Pacific/Asian American Mental Health Center.

Kalimo E, Bice TW, Novosel M (1970). Cross-cultural analysis of selected emotional questions from the Cornell Medical Index. Br J Pre Soc Med 224:229–240.

Kleinmann A (1978). Concepts and a model for the comparison of medical systems as cultural systems. Soc Sci Med 12:85–93.

Kohn ML (1987). Cross-national research as an analytic strategy, Am Sociol Rev 52:713–731.

Liang J, Asane H, Bollen KA, Kahana EF, Maeda D (1987a). Cross-cultural comparability of the Philadelphia Geriatric Center Morale Scale: An American-Japanese comparison. J Gerontol 42:37–43.

Liang J, Lawrence RH, Bollen KA (1987b). Race differences in factorial structures of two measures of subjective well-being. J Gerontol 42:426–428.

Liang J, Bennett J, Akiyama H, Maeda D (1989). The Philadelphia Geriatric Center Morale Scale: An American and Japanese comparison. Paper presented at the Annual Scientific Meetings of the Gerontological Society of America, Minneapolis, November.

Liang J, Tran TV, Krause N, Markides K (1988). Generational differences in the structure of CES-D in Mexican Americans. J Gerontol: Soc Sci: 43:S1–S7.

Markides K, Liang J, Jackson JS (1990). Race, ethnicity, and aging: Theoretical and methodological issues. In Binstock R, George LK (eds), Handbook of Aging and Social Sciences, 3rd ed. New York, Academic Press.

Miller, J, Slomczynski KM, Schoenberg RJ (1981). Assessing comparability of measurement in cross-national research: Authoritarian-conservatism in different sociocultural settings. Soc Psychol Quart 3:178–191.

Mortimer, JA (1988). The epidemiology of dementia: International comparisons. In Brody JA, Maddox, GL (eds), Epidemiology and aging: An International Perspective. New York, Springer. 1988.

Palmore E (1983). Cross-cultural research. Res Aging 5:45–57.

Palmore E (1975). The Honorable Elders: A cross-cultural analysis of aging in Japan. Durham, NC, Duke University Press.

Pflanz M (1976). Problems and methods in cross-national comparisons of diagnoses and diseases. In Pflanz M Schach E (eds), Cross-National Sociomedical Research: Concepts, Methods, and Practice. Herdweg, Germany, Georg Thieme.

Reed DM, Strong JP, Hayashi T, Newman III WP, Tracy, RE, Guzman MA, Stemmermann GN (1988). Comparison of two measures of atherosclerosis in a prospective epidemiology study. Atherosclerosis 8:782–787.

Schoenberg BS (1986). Descriptive epidemiology of Parkinson's disease: Disease distribution and hypothesis formulation. Ad Neurol 45:277–283.

Schoenborn, CA, Stephens T (1988). Health promotion in the United States and Canada: Smoking, exercise, and other health-related behaviors. Am J Public Health 78:983–984.

Schuman H (1966). The random probe: A technique for evaluating the validity of closed questions. Am Sociol Rev 41:224–235.

Torrey BB, Kinsella K, Taeuber CM (1987). An aging world. International Population Reports Series P-95, No. 78, U.S. Department of Commerce, Bureau of Census, Washington, DC.

Triandis HC, Brislin RW (1984). Cross-cultural psychology. Am Psychol 39(9):1006–1016.

Van Saase JLCM, Van Romunde LKJ, Cats A, Vandenbrouke JP, Valkenburg, HA (1989). Epidemiology of osteoarthritis: Zoetermeer survey: Comparison of radiological osteoarthritis in a Dutch population with that in 10 other countries. Ann Rheum Dis 48:271–280.
White, KL (1976). Planning and execution, cost and benefits of cross-national sociomedical research. In Pflanz M, Schach E (eds), Cross-National Sociomedical Research: Concepts, Methods, and Practice. Herdweg, Germany, Georg Thieme.

IV

ANALYTIC ISSUES IN THE EPIDEMIOLOGIC STUDY OF THE ELDERLY

21

Methodological Issues in a Survey of the Last Days of Life

DWIGHT B. BROCK, MONICA B. HOLMES,
DANIEL J. FOLEY, AND DOUGLAS HOLMES

Mortality is an end point common to many epidemiologic studies, especially those involving older populations. In the past, most studies have dealt with the analysis of mortality in terms of causes of death and risk factors related to the death. In a recent National Institute on Aging (NIA) study known as the Survey of the Last Days of Life, we concentrated our efforts on the study of the circumstances experienced and conditions surrounding the deaths of a sample of older resident decedents in Fairfield County, Connecticut. This chapter describes the methodological issues associated with the planning and conduct of the study.

The Survey of the Last Days of Life was developed to meet the need for descriptive information about death and dying among older persons. At the time it was being planned, an extensive search of the literature on death and dying, conducted for NIA by Bortnichak and Ostfeld (1980), revealed that specific data on basic events associated with dying were lacking—such as who dies peacefully while asleep, who dies in great pain, who dies in the presence of family and friends, who dies after a long illness with full awareness of impending death, and who dies suddenly with no warning. Brody et al (1981) pointed out the need for studying these and other characteristics of older persons near the time of death, especially since the majority of deaths in the United States occur in the population aged 65 and older. In addition to providing answers to the basic questions listed earlier, the knowledge from this study was expected to be useful for informing patients and their families and friends and was especially valuable for planning the most appropriate care for older persons as they approach the time of death.

Indeed, the scope and breadth of the study extended beyond the basic issues discussed in the previous paragraph. Although it was known that older persons often experience a variety of medical conditions and events throughout their lives, the extent to which some of these conditions were present was not known. Thus, we sought to describe the lifetime history of dementia, deafness, blindness, paralytic stroke, hip fracture, and Parkinson's disease, as well as the lifetime history of admissions to nursing homes. We also wished to document the lifetime use of medical aids such as pacemakers and medically produced conditions such as ostomies. Further, because of a strong interest in the issue of pain management, we sought information about the use of pain medications.

We wanted to study two other substantive areas of concern as this survey developed. One involved the provision of sound epidemiologic data on the decline in physical, cognitive, and sensory functioning in the last year of life. The other centered on transitions between residential and care settings during the last three months of the person's life. We wished to document all such transitions that entailed an episode of care such as a hospitalization or a nursing home admission. A data set encompassing all these subject areas would provide a comprehensive picture of the dying process and help to "demystify" (Kübler-Ross, 1969) death for populations of older persons.

SURVEY PLANNING AND DESIGN

Although the most appropriate design was originally believed to be prospective, it was impractical to carry out such a study design with resources available at the time. To conduct the study in that way would have entailed embedding a "last-days-of-life" component into an ongoing epidemiologic study and extending the length of the study to follow the subjects until a large number of deaths of older persons occurred. Instead, we decided that a more practical approach would be to select a sample of death certificates of older persons in a defined community and interview informants about the decedents' last days. Earlier, the National Center for Health Statistics (NCHS) had conducted mail surveys of informants in their National Mortality Followback Surveys during the 1960s (see, for example, NCHS, 1965), but their surveys did not focus on older populations and did not record medical conditions present or immediate circumstances surrounding the deaths beyond those listed as causes of death. In what follows, we describe the definition of the population under study and issues related to the sampling design, including stratification, allocation of the sample over time, and estimation of population parameters.

Population Definition

The target population for the survey was the set of all resident decedents age 65 and older whose deaths were recorded between October 1, 1984, and September 30, 1985, in Health Service Area No. 1 (HSA-1) in Connecticut. The area encompasses a 30-mile strip of eastern Fairfield County abutting New York State. The choice of this region, which includes 14 municipalities and surrounding areas, was based on the demographic characteristics and geographic distribution of its population, the number of deaths of older persons observed there during 1978–1981, and the nature of its health service delivery system. Also pertinent to the choice of the area was the already-existing community relationship with the health care system established by DMH Associates, the fieldwork contractor. A description of the development of community relations is included later in this chapter.

To provide evidence that the population was reasonably representative of older people in the United States, population characteristics of the area were examined from 1980 Census data. These data showed that some 13 percent of the population of HSA-1 was age 65 and older, compared to 11.3 percent in the total United States. The data in Table 21-1 on the age and sex distribution of five important municipalities in the area showed a wide variety of population sizes, but relative uniformity in the proportion that is 65 years old and older. Further, although Bridgeport, Stamford, and Norwalk are urban areas, almost 8 percent of HSA-1 is classified as rural by the Census Bureau. Although breakdowns of the older population by race were not available in 1982 during the planning of the study, it was known that some 3300 black or Hispanic older persons were living in Bridgeport at the time, thus assuring that there would be minority representation in the sample.

Some variation in living arrangements was observed in the area as well, with the percentage of single-person households ranging from a low of 27% in Westport to a high of 42% in Bridgeport. This was an important consideration in the design, since living status was believed to influence the course of action taken by family members of some decedents in their last days of life. Another important consideration in determining eligibility for the study was the location of death of these older persons. Analysis of previous years' mortality data (1978–1981) showed the following categories for place of death:

1. Died in town of residence (59.2 percent)
2. HSA-1 resident who died in other Connecticut HSA (7.7 percent)
3. Other Connecticut resident who died in HSA-1 (4.2 percent)
4. HSA-1 resident who died in other HSA-1 town (23.9 percent)
5. HSA-1 resident who died out of state (2.1 percent)
6. Out-of-state resident who died in HSA-1 (2.9 percent).

In determining the eligible population for the survey, it was clear that categories 3 and 6 would be out of scope. Because the Connecticut mortality data system is quite complete in recording place of death, it was possible to include decedents in categories 2 and 4 as eligible. The individuals in category 5 were included when it was possible to establish contact with an appropriate informant by telephone or through the use of

Table 21-1 Distribution by Age and Sex of Residents Age 65 and Over in Illustrative Study Municipalities

	65–74		75–84		85+			Total community	
Municipality	Male	Female	Male	Female	Male	Female	Total	Male	Female
Bridgeport	4,735	6,581	1,875	3,913	545	1,403	19,052	66,267	76,279
	8%	9%	3%	6%	1%	2%	14%	100%	100%
Fairfield	2,005	2,419	679	1,246	218	563	7,130	26,372	28,477
	8%	9%	3%	5%	1%	2%	13%	100%	100%
Norwalk	2,233	2,964	862	1,584	210	570	8,423	37,182	40,585
	6%	8%	3%	4%	1%	2%	11%	100%	100%
Stamford	3,101	4,338	1,261	2,455	342	815	12,312	48,285	54,168
	7%	8%	3%	5%	1%	2%	12%	100%	100%
Westport	701	812	252	447	50	159	2,422	12,324	12,966
	6%	7%	2%	4%	1%	2%	10%	100%	100%
Total	12,775	20,114	4,930	9,645	1,365	3,510	52,339	190,430	212,475
								Total:	402,905

Source: 1980 Census.

medical records. Overall, approximately 98 percent of all HSA-1 resident decedents were accessible through informants for inclusion in the study.

Sampling Plan

A sample of 1500 death certificates was selected for persons age 65 and older whose deaths were recorded between October 1, 1984, and September 30, 1985. The sampling rate was determined on the basis of the number of deaths of older persons occurring in HSA-1 at the time of the survey. Sampling proportional to the number of deaths occurring each month allowed for the standardization of the time interval between the date of death and the collection of follow-up information.

Stratification and Allocation of the Sample to Months

The analysis of the HSA-1 mortality data for 1978-81 guided the development of the sampling plan. First, substantial monthly variation in the number of deaths was observed, with the average number of deaths being greater in spring and winter than in summer and fall, thus reinforcing the notion of proportional allocation of the sample to months. Also, as expected, there was considerable variation in the number of deaths by age and sex (see Table 21-2). To provide adequate numbers in the younger age groups, it was decided to oversample the decedents aged 65–74, thus allowing for analysis of health conditions and other characteristics of the decedents comparing younger and older decedents. This was believed to be particularly important since the spectrum of health problems confronting older individuals seems to shift at around age 75 (Kovar, 1977). Further, since mortality rates for males are known to be higher than those for females at a given age, it was deemed appropriate to stratify the sample by sex. Stratification by sex would also help account for differences in living arrangements and in health problems experienced by the two sexes. Finally, since maximum power to detect differences among these four groups would be obtained with equal sample sizes in the groups, equal allocation was applied, yielding a sample of approximately 375 decedents per group.

The actual total sample and responding sample are shown in Table 21-3. Variation in the yield per cell was a result of the monthly spacing of the sample to account for seasonal differences in mortality in the study area. Although there was little variation in response rates for three of the cells, clearly the highest response was obtained in the older female group, with a response rate of almost 87 percent. Reasons for nonre-

Table 21-2 Number of Decedents in CT HSA-1 by Year, Age, and Sex[a]

	65–74		75+	
Year	Male	Female	Male	Female
1978	801 (20)	539 (13)	1,153 (28)	1,598 (39)
1979	773 (19)	600 (15)	1,034 (25)	1,658 (41)
1980	825 (19)	581 (13)	1,201 (28)	1,728 (40)
1981	798 (19)	604 (14)	1,183 (27)	1,724 (40)

Source: Connecticut State Department of Health.

[a]Figures in parentheses are percents of decedents 65 and older each year.

Table 21-3 Distribution of Total Sample and Responding Sample by Age and Sex of Decedent, Survey of the Last Days of Life

	Total sample			Responding sample		
Age	Male	Female	Total	Male	Female	Total
65–74	376	375	751	297	302	599
75 and older	371	378	749	300	328	628
Total	747	753	1500	597	630	1227

sponse include both the inability of the interviewers to locate an appropriate informant and refusal of the informant to answer the interviewers' questions. Detailed discussion of these issues follows in the sections on field implementation.

Estimation Procedure

As in any sample survey, to compute estimates to make inferences appropriately from the sample population surveyed, it was necessary to develop an estimation procedure that properly accounted for the design of the sample. This procedure involves the following steps:

1. *Inflation by the reciprocals of the probabilities of selection.* The probabilities varied by stratum: males 65–74, 0.51; males 75 and older, 0.35; females 65–74, 0.66; and females 75 and older, 0.23.
2. *Nonresponse adjustment.* The estimates were inflated by a factor that had as its numerator the number of individuals selected into the sample and as its denominator the number of completed interviews.
3. *Poststratification to known population totals.* The estimates were ratio adjusted to the total number of decedents age 65 and older in HSA-1 for the period of the survey. This total was known from the vital statistics records from the state of Connecticut. The effect of the ratio estimation process was to make the sample more representative of the population of older decedents in HSA-1 during the survey period. The actual production of the estimates was accomplished by constructing a weight for each respondent by multiplying the inflation, nonresponse adjustment, and poststratification factors together and multiplying the resulting weight by the appropriate measure for each individual. Weighted denominators were computed by adding the weights for all respondents. Thus, the estimated total population of decedents for HSA-1 was 3995, whereas the number of individuals in the sample was 1227, yielding an average weight of approximately 3.26 per individual in the sample. This means that on the average each interview in the sample represented more than three decedents in the population.

Development of Community Relations

Because of the intention to collect pain medication data from hospitals, nursing homes, and physicians, and because of the sensitivity of the data to be collected in general, it was necessary to do some basic community organizational work. The purpose was to inform the institutions, physicians, and social service agencies in the community about the legitimacy of the study and to obtain their cooperation and support so that if anyone questioned the study, it would be a recognized professional effort. The latter point should not be overlooked. Contacting relatives of persons who have died is a sensitive effort; invariably, during each month of the study, several informants would ask local organizations (e.g., nursing homes, hospice programs, the visiting nurse association, and so on) about the study.

Following discussions with a local health care consulting group, a study advisory group was established with representation from several hospitals, nursing homes, visiting nurse associations, and human service organizations in the study area. Once the advisory group was established, letters were sent to the chief executive officers of each of the seven hospitals and 26 nursing homes in the study area. These letters were followed by telephone calls and further discussions during which the exact procedures for information gathering were established for each facility. These procedures varied slightly from facility to facility, but the important point was to establish the credentials of the investigators and the legitimacy of the study and its data collection needs. Despite these efforts, it is important to note that one hospital and three nursing homes refused to allow access to their records.

Although the study was not seeking any data from human service organizations, it was particularly important that they be informed about the survey. This was because key informants did contact such organizations to ask whether they knew about the study and because interviewers were given a list of organizations to which they could make referrals should anyone they interviewed inquire about services or seem to be in considerable distress. In fact, interviewers on occasion did make referrals to organizations providing these services to older persons.

Finally, to ensure cooperation of physicians, the study was presented at a meeting of the County Medical Society. This presentation automatically made the investigation a "study of record." Although the County Medical Society did not endorse the study (as they do not endorse *any* study), when individual physicians questioned why the study was being done or who knew about it, it was possible to refer them to the County Medical Society.

Investigators seeking to conduct a "Last Days of Life" study in which relatives are asked to report about the deceased person should be sure that all the appropriate agencies and organizations in the community know about the study. This is necessary even if data will not be gathered from institutions and physicians, because persons in the study sample can be expected to call their doctor, their local hospice program, or the administrator of a nursing home to inquire whether the study is legitimate. When service providers are informed and can refer those who inquire about the legitimacy and importance of the study, the entire control of the field work is much smoother.

DEVELOPMENT OF THE SURVEY INSTRUMENTS

A number of instruments were required to elicit the information collected in the survey. Forms were developed for (1) abstracting information from the death certificates for sampling purposes, (2) screening informants to determine the most appropriate respondent, (3) gathering the principal data about the decedent, and (4) collecting information on hospital and nursing home use and the use of prescription medications for pain. Although the development of these forms required considerable thought and work, the specific methodological issues related to items 1, 2, and 4 were relatively straightforward and will not be discussed in detail here. However, several issues regarding the development of the principal questionnaire are of sufficient interest to merit additional discussion.

Substantive Considerations

As discussed in the introduction to this chapter, the variables of interest in this study could be categorized into four basic groups: the circumstances of death, the lifetime histories of selected diseases and conditions, trends in health status and functioning, and transitions among residential settings related to episodes of care. Each of these areas presented slightly different challenges with regard to the development of survey instrumentation.

The principal difficulty in designing the questions on the circumstances of death had to do with the questions on the respondents' perceptions of the decedents' awareness of impending death. For example, it was learned in the survey pretest that simply asking the respondent whether the decedent was aware that death was approaching yielded a high proportion of missing data and "Don't Know" responses. It was therefore necessary to elicit additional information from the respondent concerning awareness—namely, whether the decedent displayed behavior indicating awareness or whether the decedent's physician had given any indication that the patient was terminally ill.

The questions on lifetime history were designed to gather information about a number of events, diseases, or conditions that are commonly present in older persons near the time of death but are not necessarily related to the cause of death. Items were chosen that would have had a sufficiently high impact on the decedent's life to be reliably recalled by the next of kin. Blindness, deafness, use of a hearing aid, use of a pacemaker, and surgery leading to an ostomy were included in this section of the questionnaire. Among the diseases included in the lifetime history were physician diagnoses of Parkinson's disease, heart disease, cancer, stroke and dementia. The latter was elicited by asking the respondent whether the decedent had been diagnosed with Alzheimer's disease, chronic brain syndrome, dementia, senility, or any other memory or orientation impairment, since at the time of the survey the term *Alzheimer's disease* was not used as commonly as it is now, and it was desired to include other forms of dementia as well. Finally, two other events and conditions were included: whether the decedent had ever had a hip fracture or any other fracture and whether the decedent had ever been admitted to a nursing home.

The third major area of the questionnaire dealt with trends in physical, cognitive, and sensory functioning and symptoms experienced by the decedent at three time points during the last year of the decedent's life. Identical sets of questions were asked concerning the day before death, a typical day one month before death, and a typical day one year before death. These sections of the instrument were color coded to remind the interviewers about the time period to which they were referring. Also, if it was clear from the responses to the questions about the day before death that the individual was functioning well and the death was due to a cause with a sudden onset, the interviewers were instructed to skip out of the repeated questions for the earlier time periods in order to minimize respondent burden.

Many of the questions on physical and cognitive functioning were adapted from similar items used in other NIA studies such as the Established Populations for Epidemiologic Studies of the Elderly (EPESE) (Cornoni-Huntley et al, 1986). Symptom and pain questions were derived from work done by the Hebrew Rehabilitation Center for Aged for the National Hospice Study (see, for example, Morris, et al, 1986).

The final substantive area of interest was the use of health care in the last period of life and the documentation of transitions among residential settings due to episodes of care. The idea here was to gather information about the place of death and the various settings where the decedent was living before death occurred. After much development work and testing, it was decided that the most efficient way to gather this information was to enter it onto a grid that allowed for up to eight places to be recorded. The interviewer began with the location where the death took place and worked backward to previous residential locations that involved episodes of health care. The first page of the grid is shown in Figure 21-1, with the remainder of the grid simply continuing backward in time to as many as eight previous places or three months before death, whichever occurred first. The time period of three months was chosen primarily because of the small number of transitions that occurred in the month before death as measured in the pretest for the survey. The residential grid has been useful in characterizing changes in patterns of health care use in the last days of life.

Definition of the "Last Days of Life"

In the initial phases of the development of this study, when the emphasis was on the circumstances of death, it was believed that a relatively short period of one month was appropriate to define the "last days." Indeed, in the National Hospice Study (Morris et al, 1986) it was found that the quality of life of terminally ill cancer patients declined dramatically between the third and first week before the deaths took place. Further, since many of the items related to the immediate circumstances were of short duration, it was deemed best for the reliability of the data to limit the respondent's recall to the last month of the person's life.

However, for some areas of interest in this study, as further development took place, it became clear that a longer recall period would be necessary to define the last days of life. For example, transitions in residential settings involving episodes of health care were traced back for three months preceding death primarily because there were so few transitions in the last month of life, as observed in the pretest of the survey. By going back the two additional months, we were able to present a relatively clear picture of important transitions that occurred in the use of care.

For persons with a long illness leading to death, it was necessary to extend the recall period regarding trends in functioning and symptoms. By examining the last year of the person's life, we were able to establish points at which changes occurred in physical, cognitive, and sensory functioning as well as the development of symptoms. Finally, for persons whose deaths were a result of illnesses or conditions with a sudden onset, it was necessary to concentrate data collection on the last day of the person's life. Thus, the definition of "last days" depended not only on the type of information that was sought but also on the health characteristics of the individual being studied.

RESIDENTIAL GRID

Place of Death	Place 1			Place 2		
18. Where did death take place? ___ (111)	19. Where did he/she spend the night before that? ___ (112)			23. Where did he/she spend the night before going to ___ (Place 1)? ___ (121)		
9999 ☐ DK 1 ☐ Hospital 2 ☐ Nursing Home 3 ☐ Personal Care Dom Care 4 ☐ Hospice 5 ☐ In Transit to Med Facility 6 ☐ Other, Community (includes on the streets)	9999 ☐ DK 1 ☐ Hospital 2 ☐ Nursing Home 3 ☐ Personal Care Dom Care 4 ☐ Hospice		21. At that time, how many consecutive nights was he/she at this place? ___ ___ Nights ___ ___ Months ___ ___ Years Total Nights ___ (116)	9999 ☐ DK 1 ☐ Hospital 2 ☐ Nursing Home 3 ☐ Personal Care Dom Care 4 ☐ Hospice		25. At that time, how many consecutive nights was he/she at this place? ___ ___ Nights ___ ___ Months ___ ___ Years Total Nights ___ (125)
		FINISH 20. With whom was he/she living at time?	3 MONTHS BEFORE 22. With whom was he/she living at time?		FINISH 24. With whom was he/she living at time?	3 MONTHS BEFORE 26. With whom was he/she living at time?
7 ☐ Own Home	7 ☐ Own Home	___ ☐ (113)	___ ☐ (117)	7 ☐ Own Home	___ ☐ (122)	___ ☐ (126)
8 ☐ Own Apartment	8 ☐ Own Apartment	___ ☐ (114)	___ ☐ (118)	8 ☐ Own Apartment	___ ☐ (123)	___ ☐ (127)
9 ☐ Relative's Home/Apartment	9 ☐ Relative's Home/Apartment	___ ☐ (115)	___ ☐ (119)	9 ☐ Relative's Home/Apartment	___ ☐ (124)	___ ☐ (128)
		(Use relationship code below)	(Use relationship code below)		(Use relationship code below)	(Use relationship code below)

RELATIONSHIP CODE:

(0) Alone
(1) Spouse
(2) Daughter or step-daughter
(3) Son or step-son
(4) Daughter-in-law
(5) Son-in-law
(6) Sister
(7) Brother
(8) Brother-in-law
(9) Sister-in-law
(10) Granddaughter
(11) Grandson
(12) Niece
(13) Nephew
(14) Cousin
(15) Mother(in-law) or step-mother
(16) Father(in-law) or step-father
(17) Grandparent
(18) Aunt or uncle
(19) Other relative
(20) Neighbor
(21) Friend
(22) Agency person
(9999) Don't know

Figure 21-1 Residential grid questionnaire page from the Survey of the Last Days of Life.

CONDUCT AND ANALYSIS OF THE PRETEST

Because of the complexity and sensitive nature of the study, a pretest was planned to resolve several methodological and procedural issues. Although it had been shown in other studies of surrogate respondents that reliable data could be obtained from next-of-kin interviews (see, for example, Pickle, Brown, and Blot, 1983), it was not known how well the respondents would answer detailed questions of the type outlined earlier, nor was it known what was the most appropriate method of approaching the respondents. In particular, the following questions were of specific concern:

1. What is the effect on response of two different time intervals (two months or three months after the death) for contacting the informant?
2. What is the effect on response of sudden as opposed to lingering death?
3. What is the effect on response and data quality of telephone rather than in-person interviews in cases of reluctant respondents?

The hypotheses were that the longer waiting period for contacting the informant would elicit a higher response rate, that respondents for decedents whose deaths were sudden would be more reluctant to participate, and that respondents would not be willing to provide a 45-minute interview on the telephone.

To test these hypotheses and to evaluate the entire survey procedure, a sample of 71 death certificates registered in January and February of 1984 in the study area was selected for interviews with the next of kin. The sample was stratified by time interval and by type of death (sudden versus lingering). Sudden deaths were defined as follows:

- Onset of each contributing cause of death listed on the certificate was listed as less than one week.
- No cancer was listed on the certificate.
- The individual did not die in a nursing home.

All other deaths were considered to be lingering.

Of the 71 cases selected for interview, 60 cases were completed (85%). Ten individuals refused the interview and one person was too ill and an alternative informant could not be found. Interestingly, the difference in response rates for cases of sudden versus lingering death was not statistically significant, and the response rates for the two time intervals were identical. Thus, it appeared that these two factors had little effect on the willingness of a respondent to participate in this study. On the other hand, the use of the telephone turned out to be a much more important factor.

Of 60 completed interviews, 31 were conducted in person, nine were done by telephone because the respondent lived out of the study area, and 20 were completed by telephone because the respondent was reluctant to be interviewed in person. Many of these respondents lived in the inner city area of Bridgeport and were apparently distrustful of strangers coming to their homes. However, they viewed a telephone interview as less invasive and were more willing to talk to an interviewer, in some cases for a considerable length of time—up to an hour and a half in one case! Approximately 25 percent of these telephone "converted refusals" took as long or longer than the average 45-minute interview. Thus, the use of the telephone proved to be invaluable in eliciting responses from reluctant informants with no apparent compromising of the quality of the data.

The other results of the pretest were related primarily to field procedures, wording of questions, skip patterns, and so on. Examples of the kinds of decisions made included the decision to expand the questions about awareness of impending death to include decedent behaviors and physician reporting and the decision to extend the coverage of the health care transition grid to three months before death. Another important decision was to drop the collection of prescription pain medication data from physicians' offices and to include only medication data from hospital and nursing home records. Two other valuable pieces of information were learned from the pretest. First, in a number of cases of reluctant respondents, it was not unusual for the informant to provide answers to some of the questions in the process of refusing. Thus, in some cases, especially cases of sudden death, where most of the questions on the decline in health status and functioning were skipped anyway, it was possible to substantially complete the questionnaire. Second, the most common refuser was the wife of a younger male decedent (i.e., one between the ages of 65 and 74). In some of these cases it was possible to identify another informant to complete that portion of the interview left undone.

FIELD IMPLEMENTATION

Selection and Training of Interviewers

Since the subject matter of this study involved some medical and epidemiologic content, it was thought that the interviewing staff should have some background in nursing, social work, or other human services. In addition, prior to in-person job interviews, prospective interviewers were screened by telephone. Not all persons who initially applied were willing to conduct interviews with bereaved persons. Ultimately, a total of 16 interviewers conducted the study interviews. Among these were four registered nurses and seven persons with advanced degrees in social work, or another human service; several had extensive hospice background as staff or as volunteers.

Study interviewers received extensive training regarding the purpose of each question and its coding, interviewing techniques, the initial presentation of the study to the informant and techniques for insuring a high response rate, and overall study procedures. The interview was mastered initially through role-playing exercises and later through observation of experienced interviewers. More difficult than the study itself was the complexity of study procedures and the sensitivity of the subject matter, which made the initial approach to the informant listed on the death certificate a difficult challenge. The initiative required to track down the key informants who had unlisted or disconnected telephones and the courage required to call a respondent if the previous attempt was made to someone who was hostile or abusive meant that the interviewers needed to be highly motivated and to possess a great deal of self-confidence.

Selection and Abstraction of Death Certificates

As already discussed, the study sample was drawn on a monthly basis. The first month of data collection was for deaths that occurred in October, 1984; the last month was for deaths that occurred in September, 1985. Each month a death certificate abstracter went to each of the 14 towns in the study area and obtained data on age and sex for every resident 65 and over whose death occurred in one of the 14 towns. Depending on the total number of cases in the universe for each of the four study strata (younger females 65–74, older females 75+, younger males 65–74, and older males 75+), the sampling interval for that group was decided for that month. Thus, for example, if the requirement for the month of May was 112 cases in each group, then the sampling interval for any group would depend on the number of cases in the universe for that group. A random sample was then drawn for each of the four groups.

Once all the death certificate information was abstracted for the monthly sample, copies of the death certificate abstracts were distributed to the interviewers. Interviewers were assigned cases on the basis of geography; interviewers generally covered the three or four towns that were closest to where they lived, although care was taken not to assign an interviewer to cases involving personal acquaintances. At the same time that interviewer assignments were made, a letter explaining the purpose of the study and introducing the fact that an interviewer would be calling was sent to the key informant listed on the death certificate. This letter was signed by Dr. T. Franklin Williams, Director of the National Institute on Aging. The letter was then followed by a telephone call from the interviewer assigned to the respondent.

Selection and Screening of Respondents

A brief screening interview was conducted to determine whether that individual was indeed the best person with whom to conduct the full interview. The key informant listed on the death certificate was not always the most knowledgeable person: the principal care person (PCP). In 17 percent of the cases the key informant turned out not to be the PCP but was willing to provide the identity of the person who was the PCP. In those cases the interviewer would contact the PCP, explain the study, and arrange to interview that individual.

Overall, 33 percent of the respondents were spouses, 23 percent were daughters or stepdaughters, and 15 percent were sons. Siblings of the deceased accounted for 9 percent of respondents, and daughters-in-law accounted for another 5 percent. The remaining respondents included in-laws, grandchildren, nieces and nephews, various other relatives, friends, and nursing home staff. Not surprisingly, given the differential death rate for men and for women, whereas 51 percent of respondents for male decedents were spouses, only 16 percent of respondents for female decedents were spouses. Respondents for female decedents were far more likely than those for male decedents to be either daughters or sons. Of course, not everyone selected for the study could be interviewed. As discussed later, in 5 percent of the cases it was impossible to locate or contact a key informant, and in an additional 13 percent of cases the informant refused to be interviewed and would not provide the identity of an alternate.

Tracing Hard-to-Find Informants

In 14 percent of the cases, the key informant listed on the death certificate had an unlisted telephone number or no telephone, and it was necessary to use alternative means for establishing even an initial contact. In the case of unlisted telephones or insufficient information on the death certificate (i.e., address listed by state only), interviewers contacted funeral directors, physicians, and cemetery officials or read obituary notices in the hope of obtaining a full address, telephone number, the name of a relative with a listed telephone number, or the unlisted number itself. Unfortunately, not all funeral directors or cemetery managers were willing to provide such information. Also, physicians listed on the death certificate had such information only if the patient had ever been seen in the physician's office and not if the patient had only been seen in the hospital. In addition, obituary notices often did not provide sufficiently detailed addresses. If it was impossible to obtain a telephone number or if there was no telephone but an adequate address was available or could be obtained, interviewers made up to three house calls and either found someone at home or left letters asking the person to contact the interviewer or the study director. In some cases the person listed as the key informant was already deceased or had moved out of the area and could not be traced.

For patients who died in a nursing home, if it was impossible to find a key informant, a study nurse conducted the interview with a staff person at the nursing home. Ultimately, of the 1500 cases sampled, it was impossible to make contact with any informant in 77 (or 5%) of the cases. Tracking potential informants or dealing with the "detective" aspects of the field work was often arduous and time-consuming.

Interviewing Reluctant Respondents

The reluctance of many persons to allow a stranger into their home for reasons of either security or privacy, and the busy work schedules of many PCPs, which made it hard for them to schedule a home visit, resulted in 55 percent of the interviews being conducted by telephone. Reasons for conducting telephone interviews were out of area PCP (20 percent), reluctant PCP (41 percent), and too busy/other (39 percent). Telephone interviews lasted 31 minutes on average, whereas the average duration of in-person interviews was 46 minutes. Interviewers felt that they received as much information during telephone as during face-to-face interviews but reported that most people interviewed by telephone tended to be more businesslike and less likely to digress or to cause interruptions. It is certainly possible that the same personality traits (e.g., caution, reticence) that would influence someone to choose a telephone over an in-person interview would cause the telephone interviews to be more brief and less expansive.

To control the number of telephone interviews to the extent possible, interviewers were paid at a lower rate for telephone interviews than for in-person interviews. This provided an incentive for the interviewers to strive to complete as many interviews in person as possible.

Despite the option to conduct the interview by telephone, some PCPs refused to be interviewed or to provide the name of another family member who could provide the information. Early in the study, refusals were referred to the project director for attempted conversion, but as interviewers became more experienced in eliciting cooperation, it was found that those who refused the interviewer and could not be persuaded to participate would not change their mind for anyone else and became angry if recontacted, interpreting such further efforts as intrusiveness or harassment. Thus, only where potential respondents themselves expressed reluctance but agreed to a later contact were any further efforts made to persuade participation.

The most frequent reason for refusal (49 percent) was the respondents' assessment that the subject matter was too personal or painful and that they wanted neither to share the details of a loved one's death with a stranger nor to be reminded of their grief. Twenty-four percent of the refusers became quite angry at the idea of the interview and expressed their disapproval in strong terms, including hanging up on the interviewers in midsentence. Other reasons for refusal were the lack of knowledge on the part of the respondent about the deceased's condition and the inability to offer a substitute respondent (5 percent), and the illness/mental frailty of the respondent in the absence of an alternative respondent (14 percent).

The importance of the rapport between interviewer and respondent cannot be overemphasized. In fact, as stated earlier, as the interviewers gained more experience in administering the instruments and interacting with potential respondents, they indeed were the most effective means of obtaining response. This experience reinforced the well-known notion from the survey research literature that well-trained, conscientious interviewers are the most valuable resource in a field effort such as this one.

Collection of Institutional Data

Once the interview was completed, the PCP was asked to sign release forms to be used to obtain pain medication and service use data from hospitals and/or nursing homes if the deceased spent any time in such an institution during the last 30 days of life. In the case of in-person interviews, signed releases were obtained at the time of the interview, although even some persons interviewed in person did not want to grant permission to the study to obtain institutional data. Some refused to sign until they consulted a relative (usually these were widows who wanted to consult a son) or an attorney; many such respondents never returned the release forms. In the case of telephone interviews, the interviewer explained the purpose of the institutional data and let the respondent know that the release(s) would be in the mail with a stamped, self-addressed envelope for their return. If telephone respondents did not return the mailed releases, they were followed up two times, but releases were still not obtained in all cases. Among some respondents, the suspiciousness of strangers that made them reluctant to allow anyone into their home also made them reluctant to sign any paper that appeared "official." There was a total of 697 cases with a hospital stay during some portion of the last 30 days of life; in 191 cases (27 percent) a signed release could not be obtained. Similarly, there were 312 cases with a nursing home stay; in 66 cases (21 percent) a signed release form could not be obtained.

Quality of the Response

Most informants had been close to the deceased and were quite well informed about most of the issues queried. Some of the information was offered with less certainty by some informants because they were unable to respond with the precision required. Thus, for example, not all respondents were able to provide accurate information about the exact number of days that the deceased had spent in a variety of different settings during the entire 90 days before death. Because this seemed to be a particularly complicated requirement, interviewers were asked to provide a rating of their confidence regarding this information. In 83 percent of the interviews the interviewers rated themselves as "very confident" in the information, in 12 percent they stated that they were "somewhat confident," and in 5 percent they rated themselves as "not confident." Not all respondents were able to respond to questions about the deceased's condition one day before death, particularly if the deceased was in an institution and they did not have contact on the last day. Questions about medications that the deceased was taking prior to death were particularly difficult and often could not be answered. In general, however, most questions were answered by most informants with a great deal of thought and effort aimed at providing accurate responses.

SUMMARY OF FINDINGS AND CONCLUSIONS

Findings

As mentioned earlier, several questions were asked in the survey to establish lifetime period prevalence rates for major conditions and events influencing the quality of life in older persons. Table 21-4 presents the lifetime prevalence rates for selected sensory impairments, medical conditions, diagnoses, and nursing home utilization. Blindness was reported for about 7 percent of the decedents and deafness was reported for about 9 percent. Of those reported to be deaf, about 63 percent had used a hearing aid.

Over one fourth of the decedents had experienced a stroke in their lifetime, according to the surrogate respondents and about 11 percent had fractured their hip at some time before death. Large proportions were reported to have diagnoses of heart disease (43 percent) and cancer (34 percent), and Alzheimer's disease or related dementia (as diagnosed by a physician) was reported to have affected more than 11 percent of this population of decedents. Also, some 35 percent were reported to have spent some time in a nursing home.

Questions on the circumstances surrounding death were among those originally proposed by Brody et al (1981) as the basis for conducting the study. Results for some of the circumstances are presented in Table 21-5. The causes of death given in the table are taken from the death certificates as the first-listed causes. The distribution of causes presented here compares reasonably well with the underlying-cause-of-death information published by the NCHS (1986). The published underlying causes for national

Table 21-4 Lifetime History of Selected Disease and Conditions, Survey of the Last Days of Life (in percent)

Blindness	6.5%
Deafness	9.2
Used a hearing aid	(62.9)
Ever had:	
Stroke	27.0
Hip fracture	11.0
Colostomy/ileostomy	4.2
Diagnosis of:	
Heart disease	43.2
Used a pacemaker	(17.2)
Cancer	34.0
Alzheimer's or other dementia	11.2
Ever in a nursing home	35.0

Table 21-5 Circumstances Surrounding Death for Older Decedents in the Survey of the Last Days of Life (in percent)

Causes	
Heart disease	58%
Cancer	10
Stroke	5
Pneumonia/influenza	5
Other	22
Died in sleep	53
Aware of impending death	35
(median duration of awareness—days)	(58)
Death was unexpected (i.e., family and friends surprised)	50
Saw family in last three days	89

mortality for persons aged 65 and over are heart disease, 43 percent; cancer, 20 percent; stroke, 9 percent; pneumonia/influenza, 4 percent; and other causes, 24 percent. Other data on the circumstances of death showed that more than half the decedents were reported to have died in their sleep, although another 20 percent were unaccounted for, in that the respondents did not know whether the decedents had died in their sleep. More than one third of the decedents were reported to have shown awareness that death was approaching, with a median duration of this awareness of approximately 58 days. Half of the families of decedents expressed surprise at the occurrence of the death—that is, the death was unexpected. Finally, it should provide comfort to older persons and their families to know that approximately nine of every 10 decedents in this study saw various members of their families in the last three days of life.

Data from this study provided information about the use of acute and long-term care facilities (i.e., hospitals and nursing homes) in the last three months of life and the transitions among these facilities and community residence. The most recent change in residence prior to death due to an episode of care is presented in Table 21-6. Although one fifth of the deaths occurred at home, about 30 percent of the decedents actually were at home as of the night before death. Similarly, although over half the deaths occurred in hospitals, only about 45 percent were in the hospital as of the night before death.

For those individuals who spent the night before they died in a hospital, 80 percent had been living in a private residence before the hospital stay. For those who spent the night before death in a nursing home, the residential and health care settings were more varied, with 42 percent having been in a hospital and 48 percent having been in

Table 21-6 Most Recent Transition Between Residential and Care Settings, Survey of the Last Days of Life (in percent)

Location the night before death occurred		Prior residence		
		Hospital	LTC facility	Private residence
Hospital	45	1	18	80
LTC facility	25	42	9	48
Private residence	30	26	2	

Table 21-7 Trends in Health and Functional Status in the Last Year of Life (in percent)

Health characteristic reported by the respondent	Day before	Month before	Year before
Excellent/good health	11	24	53
No limitations in moving around	13	30	59
No difficulty with orientation or recognizing family	51	78	87
(with Alzheimer's)	(8)	(24)	(39)
No difficulty with bowel or bladder	30	61	81
(with Alzheimer's)	(5)	(17)	(37)
Able to breathe freely	52	60	76
No pain	61	60	80
No pain medication	69	73	86
No nausea	87	85	96
No diarrhea	90	88	95

a private residence before the episode of nursing home care. Approximately one fourth of the persons who died at home had been hospitalized at least once in the prior three-month period. The remaining home deaths were probably due to causes with sudden onset.

In Table 21-7, changes in several general health characteristics and behaviors of the decedents are reported for the day before death occurred, a typical day one month before death, and a typical day one year before death. More than half the decedents were reported to have been in good or excellent health a year before death, and about 60 percent were freely ambulatory. As the individuals approached the time of death, the rates for good health and mobility decreased substantially to just under 15 percent in both on the day before death. With regard to cognitive function, the demise was not reported to be as great as overall health and mobility, as more than half the decedents were reported to have had no difficulty with orientation or recognizing family as recently as the day before death. Bowel and bladder control were not as favorably maintained as cognition, however, with less than one third reporting no difficulty on the day before death. The latter percentage suggests that if there is a bias toward under-reporting of problems, it is not necessarily due to the sensitive nature of the questions.

Whereas the vast majority of decedents were reported not to have suffered from nausea or diarrhea on the day before death (87 and 90 percent, respectively), only between one half and two thirds of the decedents were reported to have been able to breathe freely, or not to have had pain or not to have received pain medication.

Conclusions

The resolution of a number of methodological, design, and data collection issues was required to determine that it was feasible to conduct a survey of the last days of life in the manner we have described. The level of interview completion rate obtained attests to the thorough preparation, dedication, and persistency of the field staff. The use of a simple but effective sampling design has provided data useful for descriptive analyses such as those given earlier, which allow appropriate inferences to be drawn to the population of decedents from which the sample was selected. These data allow for the examination of a broad variety of issues related to dying in older persons. Some of these concerns involve the "demystifying" of death (Kübler-Ross, 1969) by providing basic descriptive information about the circumstances surrounding death in older persons as well as the course of health status and functioning in the last year of life, transitions among residential and health care settings in the last three months, and the lifetime history of selected diseases, conditions, and events experienced by the decedents. These data can be used to inform patients, family, and friends about the occurrence of death in old age and to provide information about planning and administration of the most appropriate health care for these individuals.

REFERENCES

Bortnichak E, Ostfeld A (1980). Circumstances surrounding death in the elderly—a review of the literature. Unpublished manuscript, Yale University.

Brody JA, Cornoni-Huntley J, and Patrick CH (1981). Research epidemiology as a growth industry at the National Institute on Aging. Public Health Rep. 96:269.

Cornoni-Huntley J, Brock DB, Ostfeld AM, Taylor JO, Wallace RB (1986). Established Populations for Epidemiologic Studies of the Elderly: Resource Data Book. NIH Pub. No. 86-2443. Washington, DC, US Government Printing Office.

Kovar MG (1977). Elderly people: the population 65 years and over. In Health, United States, 1976–1977. DHEW Pub. No. (HRA) 77-1232. National Center for Health Statistics, Hyattsville, MD.

Kübler-Ross E (1969). On Death and Dying. New York, Macmillan.

Morris JN, Suissa S, Sherwood S, Wright S, Greer D (1986). Last days: A study of the quality of life of terminally ill cancer patients. J Chronic Dis 39:47.

National Center for Health Statistics (1965). Hospitalization in the last year of life: United States, 1961. Vital and Health Statistics, Public Health Service Pub. No. 1000, Series 22, No. 1, Washington, DC.

National Center for Health Statistics (1986). Advanced report of final mortality statistics, 1984. Monthly Vital Statistics Report, 35 (Supplement 2). DHHS Publ. No. 86-1120. Public Health Service, Hyattsville, MD.

Pickle LW, Brown LM, Blot WJ (1983). Information available from surrogate respondents in case-control interview studies. Am J Epidemiol 118:99.

22

Grade of Membership Analysis in the Epidemiology of Aging

KENNETH G. MANTON AND
MAX A. WOODBURY

Adequate description of the health and functional status of the elderly and their change in status is often difficult because of the complexity of the health and functional state of very elderly persons. At advanced ages, for example, there is a high prevalence of multiple co-morbid conditions. These co-morbid conditions may interact in a complex way with underlying age-related changes of physiologic function and homeostatic capacity. The functional state of older persons is also complex because of a high prevalence of some degree of impairment in multiple physical and cognitive dimensions of functioning (Manton and Stallard, 1989; Manton et al, 1989).

To describe such complex, multidimensional states, we need models that represent the status of the elderly person on multiple (sometimes self-reported) measures whose relation to the basic physiologic characteristics of the person may be complex and indirect. Furthermore, the type of data that is frequently available is coded only in terms of discrete responses, that is, where the presence of a disease entity or loss of a functional ability is indicated as an event rather than a continuous variable such as systolic blood pressure or blood sugar level. Thus, the underlying continuous state process of physiologic change with age must be described in terms of a multidimensional "jump" or discrete state process. Making the analyses even more difficult is the fact that such data are often generated from either a "select" population or a "complex" sample design. Thus, the statistical variation represented in the sample may be altered in complex ways by the observational plan. Such considerations arise, for example, in certain of NIA's EPESE studies and in most national health surveys.

To deal with these problems we propose the use of analytic procedures based on Grade of Membership (GoM) principles (Zadeh, 1965). These procedures, like many other statistical methodologies, are multivariate. However, they are explicitly designed to deal with discrete response data and to represent the underlying physical status of an individual in terms of multiple "fuzzy" partitions. The fuzzy partitions can be shown to have advantages in describing the complex health and functional status of an elderly person because they can represent individual heterogeneity *within* the health states or dimensions they identify.

It must be emphasized that the description generated by the fuzzy partition–Grade of Membership model is more than the simple identification of multivariate patterns within the data. This is because the estimation of parameters by different Grade of Membership models is done using maximum likelihood procedures so that the parameters estimates have known statistical properties. Furthermore, the model parameters can be shown to be mathematically identifiable (e.g., the parameter estimates *cannot* be rotated as in standard factor analysis) because the parameter estimates have a mathematically unique relation to the data. This identifiability means that multivariate structural hypotheses can be tested about sets of parameters. Furthermore, the maximum likelihood function can be constrained in specific ways to represent different types of hypothetically determined models of "causal" structures. In addition, the procedures can be adapted to deal with the effects of complex sample design and other features of data generation that may cause statistical inference to deviate from the assumptions of random sampling.

In the following discussion we present the basic features of GoM-type models and illustrate how they can be modified to deal with longitudinal data on aging changes. We then describe how the models can be adapted to deal with complex sample design effects. Finally, we illustrate the model using data from the 1982 and 1984 National Long Term Care Survey (NLTCS).

THE GRADE OF MEMBERSHIP IN A FUZZY PARTITION (GoM) MODEL: DEFINITION

The fuzzy partition structure of the GoM model can be described as a set of equations of relatively simple form. The form of these equations is dictated by the assumption that individuals are multidimensional physiologic systems whose complex state can be summarized by some parsimonious set of parameters that depend in number and kind on the breadth and detail of the substantive focus of the analysis. To present these equations let us assume that all data for a set of I ($i = 1, 2, \ldots, I$) individuals or cases is coded into a set of categorical variables (X_{ij}, $j = 1, 2, \ldots, J$), where an individual i has one of L_j responses to the jth variable. It is also useful to define binary variables, y_{ijl}s, which are 1 when $X_{ij} = 1$ ($l = 1, 2, \ldots, L_j$) and 0 otherwise. The requirement that the data be discretely coded does not limit us to dealing only with discretely measured variables or require that our model be restricted to representing only discrete or jump processes. It can be shown that any continuous variable can be well approximated by a relatively small number of discrete categories (Scott, 1985). This is because the information in an empirical continuous distribution is usually summarized (approximated) in a statistical procedure by a limited number of moments. The distribution described by the selected number of moments, if small, can be well represented by a small number of discrete categories. For example, in modeling continuous variables in procedures that assume a multivariate normal distribution, the analysis is restricted to only two moments—the mean and covariance (and variance). Furthermore, the practical limitations of measurement techniques often cause continuous variables to be represented as discrete variables with a relatively small number of values (e.g., income, education, blood pressure).

The discrete response variables available in a data set are predicted in the model by two types of coefficients. The first is made up of the λ_{kjl}, which represent the probability that a person "exactly" like the kth group has the lth response to the jth variable. To be "exactly" like the kth group means that the probability that a person has a given attribute is identical to the probability of that attribute occurring for the kth group.

The second type of coefficients includes the grades of membership (g_{ik}s), which are coefficients that describe the relationship of the individuals to the group profiles described the the λ_{kjl}s. The g_{ik}s are combining weights or mixing coefficients that combine the λ_{kjl}s in the way that "best" (in a likelihood sense) describes the probability that a given $y_{ijl} = 1.0$. The g_{ik}s are *not* probabilities of classification, as is discussed in the next session. The g_{ik}s are estimated under the constraints that $\Sigma_k g_{ik} = 1.0$ and $0.0 \leq g_{ik} \leq 1.0$. Thus, the basic equation is

$$\Pr[y_{ijl} = 1 \mid \mathbf{G},\Lambda] = \sum_{k=1}^{K} g_{ik}\lambda_{kjl} \tag{1}$$

This equation indicates that the probability that a person has any given attribute is the inner product of the K pairs of g_{ik} and λ_{kjl} estimates. Thus, there is an equation like (1) to be estimated for each data element (i.e., for $I \times J \times \overline{L}_j$ terms).The value K describes how many types or dimensions are necessary to explain all nonrandom variation of the y_{ijl}. The substantive nature of the K types is described the the λ_{kjl} in the set of variables and by the g_{ik} in the set of individuals. Both g_{ik} and λ_{kjl} are parameters that must be estimated from the model.

The coefficients g_{ik} and λ_{kjl} are estimated using maximum likelihood procedures. For example, in analyzing the prevalence of attributes (i.e., their probability at a given time) one could use the following multinomial likelihood function

$$L = \prod_{i}\prod_{j}\prod_{l}\left[\sum_{k=1}^{K} g_{ik}\lambda_{kjl}\right]^{y_{ijl}} \tag{2}$$

Estimation of the likelihood involves solving for the set of ($I \times K g_{ik}$) parameters and the $K \times J \times L_j \lambda_{kjl}$ parameters that produces the maximum value of L for the selected number (K) of types. Thus, the solution is computer intensive—especially since both g_{ik}s and λ_{kjl}s must be solved with boundary constraints in order to maintain a substantively meaningful interpretation. Though computer intensive, the advantage of the solution is that it is subject only to very general distributional assumptions, as described in the next section. Other forms of likelihood function can be generated for other types of GoM models applicable to events generated by other types of processes. For example, in modeling the temporal incidence of health events the Poisson form of the likelihood is more appropriate. In this case the λ_{kjl} can be related directly to the time-integrated hazard function for a given outcome.

THE PROPERTIES OF THE GoM MODEL: COMPARISONS TO OTHER ANALYTIC PROCEDURES

Equations (1) and (2) describe the basic structure of the GoM model. To understand its characteristic properties and behavior it is used both to compare the properties of the procedure to the properties of selected other multivariate analytic strategies and to consider certain of its properties in more formal theoretical terms.

A more familiar multivariate procedure that one might apply to data on the elderly is factor analysis. One common form of factor analysis is that based upon maximum likelihood procedures for jointly normally distributed observed variables due to Lawley and Maxwell (1971; Dillon and Goldstein, 1984). Many other forms of principal component and factor analysis (e.g., Harman, 1976) are based upon the use of least squares procedures to calculate the eigenvectors and eigenvalues of a sample correlation (or covariance) matrix. The least square factor analytic procedures have the disadvantage that the coefficients in their solutions are not mathematically identifiable, so that a given solution is not "unique" and thus may be subjected to any rigid rotation. The statistical properties of these models (i.e., of the coefficients estimated), because of their nonidentifiability, are not well defined. The maximum likelihood procedures due to Lawley and Maxwell are identifiable and thus the statistical properties of parameter estimates are known. The maximum likelihood equations first presented by Lawley and Maxwell (1971) are the basis for the confirmatory factor analysis and linear structural relation models for which Jöreskög (1969) and colleagues (e.g., Jöreskög and Sörböm, 1983) have developed computer algorithms. That is, the maximum likelihood equations presented by Lawley and Maxwell were not readily soluble until Jöreskög modified the Fletcher–Powell–Davidson procedure for function minimization. Even with these algorithms, however, the Lawley–Maxwell equations are computationally burdensome and the statistical theory of those procedures is still in evolution (Saris, Satorra, and Sörböm, 1987).

As for the GoM model, we can formally describe the Lawley–Maxwell factor-analytic model in terms of its likelihood function with appropriate attention paid to the problems of the identifiability of parameters. The mathematical and statistical description of a procedure is unambiguously expressed in the likelihood function whose form represents the basic sampling process by which the observed data are assumed to be generated. The log likelihood function used in the estimation of the factor analysis coefficients can be represented as

$$F(\mathbf{S}, \Sigma(\Pi)) = \ln|\Sigma| + \mathbf{Tr}\,(\mathbf{S}\Sigma^{-1}) - \ln|\mathbf{S}| - p \tag{3}$$

(Saris et al, p. 109), where $\mathbf{S}$ is the observed sample covariance matrix for p variables and $\Sigma(\Pi)$ is the covariance matrix generated by the parameter set Π. The minimum of (3) provides the likelihood function value for a given model with the free parameter vector (Π). The likelihood ratio test statistic for nested models is $T = n(F(\Pi_1) - F(\Pi_2))$, where $F(\Pi_2)$ is the more general (i.e., less constrained) model. If the null model is correct and the data have the multivariate normal distribution, then T is asymptotically a χ^2 variable with degrees of freedom equal to the difference in the number of parameter estimated in the two models (Saris, et al, 1987).

There are a number of functional forms used to calculate $\Sigma(\Pi)$, depending on the form of factor analysis assumed—for example, a second-order factor analysis model used by Lawley and Maxwell is $\Sigma = \Psi + \Lambda\Phi\Lambda'$, where Ψ is the diagonal covariance matrix of the unique components (i.e., the "error" structure), Λ is the factor loadings matrix (i.e., the correlation of the observed variables with, for example, the K latent factors), and Φ is the covariance matrix for the common factors. The test of the ability of the model parameters to reproduce the data is based upon the Wishart distribution (Anderson, 1971) for the sample covariance matrix, and it has been said to be very sensitive to departures from multivariate normality (Dillon and Goldstein, 1984; the sample covariance matrix has the Wishart distribution if the data have the multivariate normal distribution).

The likelihood ratio evaluation of the closeness of **S** and $\Sigma(\Pi)$ in (3) makes it clear that only second-order statistical moments are used in parameter estimation (and testing). In the GoM likelihood no specific assumption is made about the distribution of the g_{ik}s over individuals; that is, the multinomial likelihood in (2) refers to the probability distribution of the responses for each individual.

It can be shown that the likelihood estimation for GoM can reproduce up to the Jth order moments of the distribution of the g_{ik}s. Furthermore, for the Jth-order moments that are identifiable, one can show (Tolley and Manton, 1989) first, that the λ_{kjl} are consistently estimated and, second, that up to the Jth-order moments of the g_{ik} are consistently estimated. This is considerably more general than standard forms of maximum-likelihood factor analyses where only information on the second-order moments are used in parameter estimation. Since we expect that much of our data on the elderly population will be coded into discrete categories, and many combinations of events will be rare, we can expect that there will be important information in these higher-order moments; that is, for the type of health and functional data generated in the EPESE studies, multivariate normality is clearly often an inappropriate assumption. Interestingly, although the maximum likelihood computations for both GoM and factor analysis are burdensome, the GoM model actually permits analyses of many more variables than the maximum likelihood factor analysis model.

In addition to the restriction that only the second-order moments are exploited, the parameters of the factor analytic model do not naturally describe discrete events. For example, the factor scores in a factor analytic model can vary between plus and minus infinity and thus are not restricted to a natural range for the probability of event outcomes.

As a consequence, we shall compare the GoM model with a second, less-restrictive type of alternative model. In selecting a second model for comparison several choices were considered and rejected. For example, cluster analyis models are often used to group cases on multivariate responses. These models, generically, do not impose conditions on the overall distribution of cases. However, most cluster analysis procedures do not have well-characterized statistical properties (Dillon and Goldstein, 1984; chap. 5). Those for whom tests have been generated required strong distributional assumptions about the distribution of cases within groups, usually multivariate normality, which is again not appropriate for our data. So-called multidimensional scaling models are also used to describe multivariate data. They involve generating groupings on scales generated by heuristically minimizing some distance or maximizing a similarity measure. The advantage of multidimensional scaling is its ability to reduce the dimensionality of a spatial mapping of data by using nonlinearities. The "scale" can be modified by modifying the exponent nonlinearily in the Minkowski metric (distance) function. In general, except in restricted cases [e.g., where the Mahalanobis D^2 distance function is used—again appropriate for normal variables (Van de Geer, 1971)], the solutions are not mathematically "identifiable" and generally have unknown formal statistical properties. Alternatively, there are forms of factor analysis that are specialized for discrete data. These procedures, often based upon the analysis of tetrachoric correlations (e.g., Muthen and Christoffersson, 1981), still require the underlying factors to be normally distributed.

Thus, the second procedure we selected to compare to GoM was the latent-class model (LCM), originally due to Lazarsfeld and Henry (1968) and Goodman (1978). The LCM was selected both because it is general and because its statistical properties can be well established. In the LCM models a set of latent tables is extracted from the data using maximum likelihood procedures (Clogg, 1981). The latent tables are assumed to be able to reproduce the data except for statistical fluctuations. A problem occurs with these procedures when J, the number of variables, becomes large (e.g., $>$ 10). In these cases the table becomes too sparse for analysis. For example, in a report by Eaton et al (1989) observations of individuals on 33 binary variables symptomatic of psychiatric disorders were analyzed using standard maximum likelihood approaches for the LCM. Those measures define a table with 2^{33} (or 8.6 billion) cells. Thus, the aggregate data procedure was computationally and statistically problematic because of both the large number of terms in the likelihood and the sparseness of the data table; that is, the statistical requirements of the likelihood procedures used for frequency data that there be a reasonable average size cell population would not be met.

To deal with the problems of the estimation algorithm we defined a new LCM estimation strategy for the same data analyzed by Eaton et al (1989). In this procedure we defined a likelihood function dealing only with symptom combinations that appeared in the data sets (Woodbury, Tolley, Manton, 1991, in review). The multinomial likelihood for this model is written as follows:

$$L = \prod_{i=1}^{I} \left[\sum_{k=1}^{K} P_k \prod_{j=1}^{J} \prod_{l=1}^{Lj} (\Lambda_{kjl})^{y_{ijl}} \right] \qquad (4)$$

In this model there are K distinct classes into *one* of which each case is *exclusively* assigned—with probability P_k of being in the kth class. Each class is characterized by the Λ_{kjl}, which are probabilities much like the λ_{kjl} in the multinomial GoM model. The basic difference between the two models is the way in which the K groups or types are defined. In (4) there is *no* within-group heterogeneity; that is, all persons within the group have the same probability profile for all outcomes of all variables and fit exactly into one of the K groups. This could be directly represented mathematically by defining grouping coefficients g^*_{ik} for this model. The g^*_{ik} for this model follows the constraint $\Sigma_k g_{ik} = 1.0$ but has the *additional* requirement that the g^*_{ik}can adopt only the values of 1 or 0. Thus, the LCM model can be viewed as a special case of the fuzzy partition model, where, in contrast, a person may have partial membership in multiple groups.

This point can also be made geometrically. In both the LCM and GoM models, observation x_{ijl} are described by a $K-1$ dimensional K-simplex. For example, a two-dimensional simplex is a triangle that is defined by the three vertices, λ_{kjl} or Λ_{kjl} (hence the logical equivalence of these types of coefficients in the two models). In the LCM model (or in any standard "discrete" classification model) points can be located only at the vertices (because the g^* can only be 0 or 1). In the GoM model, the ability of the g_{ik}s to vary allows data to fall anywhere within (or on) the boundaries of the simplex. Although the requirement that cases fall only at the vertices in the LCM seems restrictive, this is a direct consequence (and requirement) of the mathematical structure of the model (i.e., $g^*_{ik} = 0.$ or 1.0).Thus, the GoM model seems to represent more naturally the nature of complex phenomena in the real world.

In contrast, in the GoM model, as more information is added, the difference between the estimated and true values converges to 0 with probability 1. The estimate converges "in probability" to the true point in the simplex, for example, to the g_{ik} position (0.0, 0.0, 0.5, 0.3, 0.2).

The net effect on parameter estimates of the more general structure of the GoM model is that, whereas the Λ_{kjl}s must explain the variation in the g^*_{ik}s that adopt values other than 0 or 1, the λ_{kjl}s are freed of this heterogeneity because of the simultaneous estimation of the g_{ik}s. As a consequence, the fundamental properties of the underlying psychiatric disorders are more clearly identified in the GoM model. This can be briefly demonstrated in Table 22-1 (Woodbury, Tolley, Manton, 1991, in review), which compares the λ_{kjl}s and Λ_{kjl}s from a six-dimensional analysis (six pure types, six classes) of the data on 33 psychiatric symptoms in the John Hopkins ECA study (Eaton et al, 1989).

In the table we see that the Λ_{kjl}s estimable for the LCM are "fuzzy" with most variables loading, to some degree, on all the groups. This "fuzziness" occurs in the Λ_{kjl} estimates because, since the g^*_{ik}s can only adopt the value 0 or 1, considerable residual within-group heterogeneity must be forced in the Λ_{kjl}s. In contrast, the symptoms identifying the six disorders are clearly represented in the λ_{kjl}s—because the "fuzziness" is represented in the g_{ik}s. Thus, in a fundamental sense, the "fuzziness" is a property of the way in which persons manifest complex disease states; that is, it is *in* the data. The issue left to the analyst is how to best describe the fuzziness. In the GoM model it is attributed to individual variation in disease expression. In the LCM model it is assumed to be a property of the disease definitions.

Conceptually, the GoM representation of individual heterogeneity seems more appropriate. It is, for example, consistent with the analyses of psychiatric disorders in the community, in clinics, and in in-patient facilities where there was increasing differentiation of patient symptom profiles (Strauss et al, 1979). Its advantages can also be demonstrated statistically in several ways. First, the GoM representation describes the data significantly better than the LCM—even after adjusting for degrees of freedom. Second, the LCM shows certain problems when the sample population is altered by only deleting *non*symptomatic cases, that is, by deleting cases where all 33 symptoms are *not* present. Such cases contribute no information to identification of the characteristics of the disease. Yet in the LCM the group profiles (i.e., the Λ_{kjl}) changed when those cases were deleted whereas the λ_{kjl} profiles in the GoM were stable. This sensitivity of the LCM occurs because its likelihood requires that individual information be integrated out before the Λ_{kjl}s are estimated. This makes the likelihood function sensitive to the marginal distribution and to sample fluctuations (whether random or systematic, as when a two-stage sampling procedure is used). The GoM model does not reflect the same degree of sensitivity because those effects can be isolated in the g_{ik}s. Both of these properties of the GoM model are illustrated in Woodbury, Tolley, and Manton (1991, in review).

LONGITUDINAL EXTENSIONS OF THE GoM MODEL

In studies of aging it is important to be able to describe change in health, functional, and social state over time. This can be done in the GoM model by restructuring the multinomial form of the likelihood function to represent the temporal organization of

Table 22-1 Comparison of λ_{kjl} and Λ_{kjl} from Six-Dimensional Analyses of 33 Psychiatric Symptoms in Johns Hopkins ECA Data

	Frequency (%)	Discrete groups 1		2		3		4		5		6	
		λ_{kjl}	Λ_{kjl}	λ_{kjl}	Λ_{kjl}	λ_{kjl}	Λ_{kjl}	λ_{kjl}	Λ_{kjl}	λ_{kjl}	Λ_{kjl}	λ_{kjl}	Λ_{kjl}
Sad for 2 weeks	4.12	100.0	37.9	0.0	34.8	0.0	2.39	0.0	2.57	0.0	16.50	0.0	1.03
Sad for 2 years	1.20	39.6	13.1	0.0	10.4	0.0	0.70	0.0	0.00	0.0	12.92	0.0	0.34
Fainting	0.33	0.0	3.0	30.0	0.9	0.0	3.49	0.0	0.00	0.0	0.00	0.0	0.16
Shortness of breath	1.17	0.0	6.1	100.0	16.0	0.0	17.07	0.0	0.88	0.0	0.00	0.0	0.41
Palpitations	2.12	0.0	12.6	100.0	16.6	0.0	19.63	0.0	1.92	0.0	22.11	0.0	0.76
Felt dizzy	2.30	0.0	12.4	100.0	19.9	0.0	15.20	0.0	2.79	0.0	0.00	0.0	1.05
Feel weak	1.35	0.0	6.11	100.0	18.5	0.0	16.92	0.0	2.48	0.0	1.88	0.0	0.46
Nervous person	23.61	100.0	67.9	100.0	86.2	100.0	68.65	0.0	34.07	0.0	39.02	0.0	16.98
Fright attack	1.83	0.0	7.30	100.0	30.9	0.0	100.00	0.0	0.00	0.0	0.00	0.0	0.00
Phobias													
Eating in public	1.05	0.0	1.94	100.0	25.1	0.0	0.93	0.0	5.27	0.0	0.00	0.0	0.21
Speaking in small group	1.53	0.0	2.41	100.0	18.9	0.0	15.88	0.0	8.14	0.0	0.76	0.0	0.53
Speaking to strangers	1.89	0.0	2.9	100.0	39.7	0.0	4.74	0.0	10.45	0.0	0.00	0.0	0.45
Being alone	1.38	0.0	4.5	80.5	32.0	0.0	5.10	0.0	3.87	0.0	5.38	0.0	0.33
Tunnels and bridges	3.56	0.0	1.8	0.0	50.9	0.0	17.15	100.0	29.96	37.9	0.00	0.0	0.64
Crowds	2.72	0.0	4.4	100.0	48.4	0.0	22.78	0.0	15.99	0.0	0.00	0.0	0.52

Public transporations	4.04	0.0	2.8	100.0	55.6	0.0	17.90	100.0	30.62	0.0	0.00	0.0	0.88
Outside house alone	1.32	0.0	3.7	100.0	23.5	0.0	0.00	0.0	6.76	0.0	0.00	0.0	0.35
Heights	7.69	0.0	5.2	0.0	54.3	0.0	17.09	100.0	47.92	0.0	0.00	0.0	3.39
Closed place	2.88	0.0	2.6	100.0	43.7	0.0	2.91	100.0	17.74	0.0	6.50	0.0	0.88
Storms	4.67	0.0	3.9	0.0	46.0	0.0	22.97	100.0	26.53	0.0	6.08	0.0	1.87
Water	4.42	0.0	4.0	0.0	35.4	0.0	32.73	100.0	30.46	0.0	6.48	0.0	1.43
Bugs	8.99	0.0	13.0	0.0	55.5	0.0	23.92	100.0	52.35	0.0	13.21	0.0	3.72
Animals	2.04	0.0	2.9	0.0	25.6	0.0	0.66	91.6	11.50	0.0	0.00	0.0	0.78
Crying spells	4.88	0.0	22.5	0.0	32.1	0.0	9.15	0.0	5.72	0.0	100.00	0.0	2.22
Felt hopeless	3.99	0.0	29.5	0.0	26.5	0.0	5.58	0.0	3.07	100.0	100.00	0.0	1.08
Change in weight or appetite	6.12	100.0	32.9	0.0	48.4	0.0	26.22	0.0	6.45	100.0	10.98	0.0	2.77
Sleeping more or less	10.74	100.0	52.6	0.0	64.9	0.0	24.92	0.0	16.85	0.0	35.96	0.0	5.21
Talking or moving slower	5.72	100.0	37.8	0.0	72.9	0.0	5.12	0.0	6.39	0.0	5.38	0.0	1.68
Interest in sex much less	2.21	63.0	13.6	0.0	23.3	0.0	9.18	0.0	3.57	0.0	1.36	0.0	0.91
More tired	7.36	100.0	48.7	0.0	61.6	0.0	5.17	0.0	6.83	0.0	2.80	0.0	2.84
Worthless, sinful, or guilty	2.80	100.0	25.0	0.0	32.8	0.0	0.57	0.0	1.61	0.0	16.81	0.0	0.69
Difficulty concentrating or thinking	5.20	100.0	38.9	0.0	53.9	0.0	6.55	0.0	4.22	0.0	11.80	0.0	1.54
Thoughts of death or suicide	9.28	0.0	41.9	0.0	63.3	0.0	24.74	0.0	15.14	100.0	36.44	0.0	4.51

the observation plan. Specifically, a very general longitudinal formulation of GoM may be constructed by separating observations on individuals into the temporal components identified in one's observational plan.

Specifically, let us assume that there are fixed time measurements made on all J variables on each individual at each of $t = 1, 2, \ldots, T$ measurement times. Let us also assume that there are e "episodes" that describe changes in specific health variables between times of measurements that occur continuously over time.

In concrete terms, in the 1982 and 1984 NLTCS (Manton, 1988) the two surveys provide the $T = 2$ sets of measurements on health and functional status. In between the surveys there are changes in the Medicare service "status" of the individual represented by the episode variables. We assume that an episode is terminated (censored) whenever an observation time t occurs. In this case we have $I \times T \times \bar{e}_t$ terms in the longitudinal form of the likelihood. The multinomial form of the likelihood can be written as

$$L = \prod_i \prod_t \prod_e \prod_j \prod_l \left(\sum_k g_{ik \cdot t} \lambda_{kjl} \right)^{y_{ijl \cdot te}} \tag{5}$$

In (5) we describe the temporal structure of the data by a process whose structure is determined by restricting the λ_{kjl}s (i.e., the λ_{kjl}s are assumed to be fixed over time, for each t and e). This requires all temporal variation to be represented by the $g_{ik \cdot t}$ (i.e., we allow the g_{ik} to vary only over time, t; all episodes between times of measurement have the same $g_{ik \cdot t}$s, an assumption we will test in our example). Other patterns of constraints could be imposed on the parameters of the likelihood function depending upon what is assumed about the nature of the underlying stochastic health process (Manton and Stallard, 1988).

Alternatively, we might wish to describe changes in Medicare service use that occur between the T measurements (e.g., the probability of the use of hospitals, home health agencies, or skilled nursing facility, the lengths of stay in those facilities, the types of follow-up services). This might be represented by constructing a multinomial variable that has l_1 ways of exiting a type of service state at each of l_2 times. The $\lambda_{kj(l_1 \times l_2)}$ probabilities estimated for this variable can be used to calculate multiple-decrement life tables—a set of l_1 tables for each of the K types. Generally, the transition variables will not be used to define the K types; that is, its coefficients are estimated in a separate set of calculations conducted conditionally upon the K types defined on health status—conditionally on the distribution of the $g_{ik \cdot t}$. Such transition variables may also be used to test the significance of differences in service use patterns over time if all episodes associated with a given time period are used to construct T independent transition variables. The likelihood function values associated with those T variables may be used to construct multivariate likelihood ratio tests (see Tolley and Manton, 1987).

COMPLEX SAMPLE DESIGN EFFECTS ON GoM

In this section we discuss three effects of complex survey design on the likelihood estimation: (1) the effects of sample weights, (2) the effects of intracluster correlations, and (3) the use of poststratification weights. In this discussion we adopt the perspective of superpopulation modeling because we will wish to use our parameter estimates to extrapolate beyond our sample—over both population and time (Cassel et al, 1977). Standard approaches to dealing with the effects of sample design on inference are based on finite population theory and are not directly applicable to the analysis of longitudinal data (Woodbury et al, 1989).

The Effects of Sample Weights on Likelihood Estimates

To understand how population weighting affects the estimation of coefficients we need to write the likelihood function with sample weights w_i, which are the inverse of the probability of selection. This form of the likelihood function is written as follows:

$$L = \prod_i \prod_t \prod_e \prod_j \prod_l \prod_l \left(\sum_k g_{ik \cdot t} \lambda_{kjl} \right)^{w_i y_{ijl \cdot te}} \tag{6}$$

We see that the (necessarily) nonnegative weights (w_i) appear in each term of the likelihood function. The weights, however, do not affect the estimates of the $g_{ik \cdot t}$s because the w_i represent scaling factors that depend only on i. Thus, they do not affect the values of the $g_{ik \cdot t}$s derived by maximizing L for the individual terms. Substantively this is obvious because the sample weights are determined by the sample design that is under the control of the investigator instituting the survey and is not informed by the data. Thus, they provide *no* new information about individuals in the sample and reduce the efficiency of the estimates of the λ_{kjl}s. A more sensible procedure, then, is to estimate the $g_{ik \cdot t}$ and the λ_{kjl}s and to postweight the $g_{ik \cdot t}$ distribution to generate the population distribution of the original characteristics $y_{ijl \cdot te}$.

This would not be the case *if* the weights were informative about longitudinal changes in the sample, for example, if death and nonresponse factors (i.e., phenomena not controlled by the investigator) were associated with health factors altering the probability of selection, and hence the realized rather than designed weights (Hoem, 1985). The factors in the sample design correlated with transitions have to be explicitly included in the model (Hoem, 1985). If they are not represented, the assumption that individual outcomes are independent when conditioned on the estimates of the $g_{ik}k_{\cdot t}$ parameters is violated. By including the sample factors affecting transition rates in the model, one in effect makes the w_i estimates conditionally noninformative about outcomes.

Intracluster Correlations

In sample design, stratification is used to increase the precision of parameters estimated for rare subpopulation. In addition, in national samples a truly random sample (weighted within strata) would be extremely expensive. To reduce expense, samples are frequently selected from a small number of geographically defined clusters, or primary sampling units (PSU). The problem with the geographic clustering of cases is that, although it is a cost-effective way of interviewing a given number of cases, the effective power of the sample is reduced because of correlations in response within clusters of PSUs. The correlations results because the characteristics of persons drawn from a given area are more likely to be homogeneous than those of a similar number of persons drawn randomly. The correlation might result from either socioeconomic filtering processes affecting the residential grouping of persons or common sociocultural and physical environmental effects. For example, high SES persons may live in a spatially defined area of a large metropolis. Yet, living in that particular metropolitan subenvironment might produce special health characteristics (e.g., chronic respiratory disease due to poorer air quality, poorer cardiovascular functioning due to greater difficulting in getting adequate aerobic exercise; mental problems due to greater stress).

A failure to adjust for clustering effects may affect test procedures because a failure to account for the correlation causes the error degrees of freedom to be overestimated. Approximate adjustments for such effects (e.g., selection on an α level of 0.01 as conservative approximation for 0.05) could waste valuable information. One approach, based on finite population theory, uses Taylor series linearization procedures to adjust variance estimates (O'Brien, 1981). These require assumptions that the population characteristics are a priori fixed. This type of sampling model was developed for surveys that "enumerate" selected characteristics at fixed points in time. This is problematic when systematic nonresponse affects the weighting and is correlated with the attributes causing changes or when the phenomena under study are stochastic processes, such as changes in health and functioning.

In the GoM procedure we take an alternative-model-based approach to deal with intraclass correlations. In this approach we view the likelihood function as "contaminated" by the PSU effect with the degree of contamination being an empirically estimable quantity. The basic principle of this approach can be illustrated in the likelihood GoM procedures applicable to the estimation of responses for twins. Specifically, the modified likelihood can be written, where contamination results from the correlation of responses within twin pairs:

$$L = \prod_{i}\prod_{j}\prod_{l}\left(\sum_{k} g_{ik}(T)\lambda_{kjl}\right)^{y_{ijl}} \tag{7}$$

where $T = 1, 2$ is an indicator defining whether an observation is the first or second member of a given term pair (Manton and Woodbury, 1989). To determine whether the distribution shows evidence of within-twin-response correlation, one can estimate a model where all likelihood elements for $T = 1$ and 2 are constrained to be equal and then reestimate the likelihood allowing the estimates to vary for twin pairs. In the first evaluation, it is assumed that the effect of being a member of a twin pair can be represented by forcing the g_{ik}s for twins to be equal. This constrained likelihood will produce a smaller likelihood value than when allowing the g_{ik}s to be different for twins. The change in the likelihood will give a likelihood ratio test of the homogeneity of twin pairs on the J measures used to define the K type with degrees of freedom equal to $K-1$ times the number of twin pairs.

This procedure could be generalized to represent cluster effects by generalizing t to represent all persons sampled in a PSU and requiring all such persons to have equal g_{ik}s. The change in the likelihood with and without constraints on the g_{ik}s in a PSU is a test for homogeneity within clusters. The problem with this test is its stringency. This can be dealt with by (1) calculating g_{ik} s for the J measure and then (2), conditional on the K_1 types, calculating a set of K_2 constrained measures based on variables representing PSU membership. The significance of the K_2 types represents whether there are variables not represented by the J variables associated with the PSU grouping, which generates a correlation of responses.

This procedure deals directly with intra-PSU correlations. If the intraclass correlations in a PSU approach 0.0, conditional upon the observed variables, the likelihood procedure is no longer "contaminated." These procedures can be generalized to the longitudinal data by using the likelihood function appropriately specified to deal with both the sample design and the temporal structure of the data. Specified in this way the effects of both informative sample factors and intracluster correlations can be dealt with.

The procedure specified earlier can be made both mathematically more elegant and more practical by appealing to empirical Bayesian principles (Morris, 1982). That is, instead of specifying the constraints on an indicator T to represent contamination, one could impose the constraint that the responses be sampled from an underlying distribution specific to a PSU (or a set of PSUs). This would require generalizing the GoM model to an empirical Bayesian form, as shown in Woodbury and Manton (1991). This leads to the following more complex negative binomial likelihood function:

$$L = \prod_i \prod_j \prod_l \left(\frac{\sum_k g_{ik} \lambda_{kjl}}{\Sigma_k g_{ik} \Sigma_l \lambda_{kjl}} \right)^{y_{ijl}} \tag{8}$$

In this model the Poisson parameters, λ_{kjl} are assumed to be distributed according to a multivariate Dirichelet distribution. The variance of that distribution represents the effect of heterogeneity in individual responses that is not described by the observed variables. One source of the additional variation is the effect of the unobserved factors generating the correlation of responses within a PSU. Thus, the generalized likelihood function implicitly adjusts for the effects of clustering.

Poststratification Weighting

Often one wishes to use the likelihood estimates to describe the characteristics of a population with a specific distribution of characteristics. For example, there are community and national studies of long-term care services. In the community studies one may find additional interventions whose impact one would wish to weight up to the national level. The weighted prevalence of attribute x_{ijl} can be calculated for a specified distribution of population characteristics by

$$\sum_i w_i \lambda_{ijl} = \sum_k \bar{g}_k \lambda_{kjl} \tag{9}$$

where

$$\bar{g}_k = \frac{1}{I} \sum_i w_i g_{ik}$$

In these equations the $\bar{g}_k$ are weighted estimates of characteristics (x_{ijl}) where the weights may be specified from a number of sources.

MISSING DATA

One of the major difficulties in longitudinal studies of the elderly is that of systematically missing data; that is, the pattern of nonresponse is informative about the phenomena of interest. To resolve this problem, the missing data must be included as information in the estimation procedure. This can be accomplished by introducing an $L_j + 1$ category for each of the J variables, which is 1.0 if the response to the variable is missing. Analyses with missing data explicitly identified can help to identify types where non-response is a function of associated characteristics. For example, in Berkman et al. (1989) analyses of data from the Yale EPESE project showed that very frail persons with a high likelihood of senile dementia were also likely to have a large proportion of nonresponses.

EXAMPLE: 1982 AND 1984 NLTCS

To illustrate the GoM procedure we draw upon data from the 1982–1984 NLTCS and linked data from Medicare administrative records for the periods September 30, 1982 to October 1, 1983, and September 30, 1984, to October 1, 1985. The periods were selected to test changes in Medicare service use due to the introduction of PPS (Liu and Manton, 1988; Manton and Liu, 1989). These data are detailed enough to illustrate a number of the methodological features of the GoM model and similar in structure to several of NIA's EPESE sites.

The 1982 and 1984 NLTCSs are national surveys where, for elderly Medicare-eligible persons living in the community, a large number of objective health and functional status measurements were made. In the current analysis 56 such measures are used to define K health and functioning dimensions that represent persons in both 1982 and 1984 [i.e., $J = 56$; $\lambda_{kjl}(1982) = \lambda_{kjl}(1984)$]. In addition to the survey data all records were linked to a continuous history of Medicare Part A service use (i.e., acute hospital, home health, and skilled nursing facility service use funded by Medicare). In these records exact dates on which the service was begun, and when the service was discontinued, were available. Thus, continuous data were available to define episodes. This required us to make decisions about the selection of cases for the prespecified goals of different longitudinal analyses of service use.

In a previous analysis, because of computational restrictions, we selected a sample of 6917 episodes for analysis. This sample was weighted so that skilled nursing facility (SNF) episodes were all sampled with decreasing sample proportions for home health, hospital, and community episodes. The oversampling of SNFs and of home health and hospital episodes on a relative base increased the marginal distribution of the severity of disability in the sample (Manton and Liu, 1989). In another set of analyses (Manton et al, 1989) all episodes occurring to persons who were identified as chronically disabled according to the detailed household interview in either 1982 or 1984 were selected—producing a little over 27,000 episodes. In the current analysis, for the purpose of illustrating the methodology and its relative robustness for alternative sample definition criteria, we extended that definition to the broadest extent possible to include all persons with a detailed interview in either year. A comparison of the λ_{kjl} coefficients for the 56 variables used to form the groups for a $K = 4$ type of solution from the three analyses with the different case selection criterion showed that substantially similar function and health status types were identified, that is, that the analysis was reasonably robust to the selection imposed. For the analysis of health services, the selection of persons chronically disabled on the detailed community interview would, in most cases, be preferred because persons disabled in 1982 who became nondisabled in 1984 are eliminated by that criterion, producing a more functionally comparable population than the analysis of the total samples receiving the detailed community survey in the two years.

This meant that the general form of our likelihood function was that shown in equation (5), where $T = 1,2$ (for 1982 or 1984) where $J = 56$ variables were measured on 6088 persons in 1982 and 5932 persons in 1984 (i.e., all persons who responded to the detailed community interview in either 1982 or 1984). This means that all persons had passed a screen in either 1982 or 1984, although there are persons who were disabled in 1982 and who, by 1984, had become nondisabled (and were returned for their illustrative analysis). In the 12 months following the 1982 survey there were 15, 386 service episodes for the 6088 persons. Following the 1984 survey (because of the smaller sampling fraction for nondisabled persons surviving from 1982) there were 14,208 service episodes. The values of the 56 variables were assumed to be chronic health measures that were relatively stable and had a constant effect on each episode occurring in the 12 months following the survey (an assumption tested below).

Considering the likelihood with 29,594 terms one must impose constraints in order to describe specific health and health service processes. The constraints have to be imposed over the time domains, e and t, on the g_{ik} and λ_{kjl} coefficients. In the following analysis we estimated two types of dependent processes. The first described health changes between 1982 and 1984 as changes in g_{ik}s with all individual episode terms set equal but with the g_{ik}s allowed to change between time 1 and 2 (i.e., the $g_{ik \cdot te}$s were constrained over e). To examine these changes the types had to be defined in a common way in both periods. This was done by constraining the λ_{kjl} for the 56 measures to be equal in 1982 and 1984; that is, the λ_{kjl} are held equal across both time and episode. The $g_{ik \cdot t}$s (for persons who survived from 1982 to 1984; the $g_{ik \cdot te}$s were allowed to change over time t, but not episode e) and the moments of the $g_{ik \cdot t}$s, for the populations at the two time points, could be compared and used to describe change in the K-dimensional health process for all persons.

The second type of process describes service episodes. This type of process is represented in a series of λ^*_{kjl} estimates for specific service use variables that we estimated in a separate second conditional calculation. For example, in the 1982 and 1984 NLTCSs, interview records were linked to Part A service use in which were recorded the exact dates of the use of acute care hospitals, home health agencies, and skilled nursing facilities. In addition, the times of death, dates of reinterview, and end of follow-up are recorded. From these records, for 12-month periods indexed at the end of the survey period (to avoid left-censoring from death occurring during the survey process), we can calculate λ^*_{kjl} variables for 1982 and 1984 that, for each of the K health and functioning types, describe the use (duration) and mode of termination of each of four types of episodes (i.e., hospital, home health agency (HHA), SNF, "community"). These λ^*_{kjl} can be tested to see whether the use of any of the different types of services had changed between 1982 and 1984.

In addition, life table parameters can be calculated from the λ^*_{kjl}s to describe this service use. These life tables can be weighted (with the individual sample weights) to reproduce the national volume of Medicare service use (controlled on health and functioning by the K types) for the sample groups selected. These life tables can be adjusted to reflect the effect of systematic missing data (very limited in the NLTCS) and the effects of sample design (again very small in this survey) and they can be used to test the specification of the process (by seeing whether entering the episode process information into the definition of the K types provides significant improvement in the χ^2 for the process). In this example we test for the effects of dependence on prior patterns of service use by defining four additional variables to represent a cross-temporal dependence on type of service episode in order to assess the specification of our process model.

A first step in the analysis is to determine the number of dimensions necessary to describe the data. In prior sections we discussed likelihood ratio tests of the differences between K and $K + 1$ types. In the following example we followed a different decision criteria because the focus of our analysis was the service use transitions. That is, instead of selecting K to best describe the 56 functional status measures, we selected K to allow the transition variables to be reliably determined (Berkman et al, 1989). Because certain transitions were relatively rare (e.g., for SNFs) we selected a smaller number of dimensions than would be the case if one wished to explain all of the systematic variation in the health and functional measures [in the analysis in Manton and Liu (1989) we performed sampling within episode types to increase the information on SNFs]. The number of types that could be supported in the estimation of the transition variables was four. This produced estimates of 4×5, or 20 service use life tables (because there are five ways to end a service episode, for example, for hospital stays discharged to a SNF, home health services, the community, death, or end of follow-up) for both 1982 and 1984.

The λ_{kjl} for the 56 health and functioning variables help describe the substantive nature of the four types. These coefficients are presented in Table 22-2. In the table the variable labels are presented on the left with the frequency of the occurrence of that attribute in the 1982 and 1984 pooled samples represented in the column labeled "frequency." (Because of different sample definitions these vary across the three different samples, i.e., the weighted 6917, the 27,000 persons disabled only sample of episodes, and the total sample.)

The next four columns contain the λ_{kjl}s for the four types. Type 1 has no serious functional limitation and, although clearly subject to multiple health conditions [about 2.6 conditions on average—in the analysis in Manton and Liu (1989) with 6917 episodes the average was 2.4]. Type 2 has limited trouble with ADLs and significant problems with outside mobility. There are problems climbing stairs and holding a package but few problems with handling and grasping objects. This group has fewer medical problems than Type 1, although it has the highest risk of hip fracture. The third type has trouble with mobility and has a number of cardiopulmonary problems. The fourth type has high levels of ADL impairment and, although having many medical problems (though fewer than Type 3), it is most distinguished by cognitive impairment and other neurological problems (e.g., Parkinsonism). These types were substantially similar to the types identified in Manton and Liu (1989) and Manton et al (1989) despite the significant differences in the mode of case selection.

These four types, defined on health and functioning variables, may be assessed for

Table 22-2 56 Health and Functional Variables Measured in the 1982 and 1984 NLTCS Used to Define the Four Health and Functioning Types

	Frequency	Type 1	2	3	4
Eating	7.26	0.00	0.00	0.00	37.58
Get in/out bed	30.46	0.00	21.09	0.00	100.00
Get about inside	44.33	0.00	73.45	0.00	100.00
Dressing	23.81	0.00	0.00	0.00	100.00
Bathing	48.36	0.00	60.09	34.52	100.00
Using toilet	25.28	0.00	0.00	0.00	100.00
Bedfast	1.07	0.00	0.00	0.00	4.75
No inside activity	1.85	0.00	0.00	0.00	8.43
Wheelchairfast	4.43	0.00	0.00	0.00	20.49
Heavy work	79.09	17.70	100.00	100.00	100.00
Light work	28.84	0.00	0.00	0.00	100.00
Laundry	51.05	0.00	65.09	47.75	100.00
Cooking	38.02	0.00	0.00	0.00	100.00
Grocery shopping	67.16	0.00	100.00	100.00	100.00
Get about outside	66.97	0.00	100.00	100.00	100.00
Traveling	65.57	0.00	100.00	100.00	100.00
Managing money	32.32	0.00	24.17	0.00	100.00
Taking medicine	28.38	0.00	0.00	0.00	100.00
Telephoning	18.44	0.00	0.00	0.00	88.82
Climbing 1 flight stairs					
No problem	13.80	45.65	0.00	0.00	0.00
Some difficulty	25.98	54.35	39.37	0.00	0.00
Very difficult	34.00	0.00	43.83	82.81	3.03
Cannot	26.22	0.00	16.80	17.19	96.97
Bend for socks					
No Problem	38.59	90.10	55.34	0.00	0.00
Some difficulty	27.66	9.90	41.92	49.98	0.00
Very difficult	20.07	0.00	2.74	50.02	25.67
Cannot	13.68	0.00	0.00	0.00	74.33
Hold 10-lb. package					
No problem	22.76	74.02	0.00	0.00	0.00
Some difficulty	16.12	25.98	29.93	6.70	0.00
Very difficult	16.84	0.00	28.83	44.82	0.00
Cannot	44.27	0.00	41.25	48.48	100.00
Reach over head					
No problem	50.72	100.00	91.63	0.00	0.00
Some difficulty	22.70	0.00	8.37	55.04	24.62
Very difficult	15.59	0.00	0.00	33.85	32.22
Cannot	10.99	0.00	0.00	11.11	43.16
Combing hair					
No problem	66.38	100.00	100.00	0.00	0.00
Some difficulty	17.83	0.00	0.00	79.55	23.60
Very difficult	8.75	0.00	0.00	20.45	32.24
Cannot	7.04	0.00	0.00	0.00	44.16
Washing hair					
No problem	47.98	100.00	86.56	0.00	0.00
Some difficulty	15.21	0.00	13.44	58.56	0.00
Very difficult	10.52	0.00	0.00	41.44	5.98
Cannot	26.30	0.00	0.00	0.00	94.02

Table 22-2 56 Health and Functional Variables Measured in the 1982 and 1984 NLTCS Used to Define the Four Health and Functioning Types

	Frequency	Type 1	2	3	4
Grasp small objects					
No problem	62.42	100.00	100.00	0.00	27.60
Some difficulty	21.41	0.00	0.00	72.83	22.90
Very difficult	11.53	0.00	0.00	27.17	26.26
Cannot see well enough to read	4.64	0.00	0.00	0.00	23.23
newspaper	71.50	93.25	4.32	73.17	40.84
Rheumatism, arthritis	73.65	60.15	62.12	100.00	69.53
Paralysis	9.66	0.00	0.00	2.67	39.56
Permanent stiffness	25.24	8.03	2.94	64.92	32.58
MS	0.90	0.25	0.27	0.04	3.22
Cerebral palsy	0.42	0.00	0.00	0.41	1.42
Epilepsy	0.98	0.41	0.00	0.78	2.97
Parkinson's disease	3.38	1.62	0.00	1.46	11.11
Glaucoma	8.79	5.21	11.35	5.87	12.98
Diabetes	19.47	9.33	7.98	41.51	23.85
Cancer	6.83	5.99	2.63	10.58	9.02
Constipation	34.58	14.96	0.00	84.68	49.20
Insomnia	42.29	22.85	0.00	100.00	41.21
Headache	18.97	0.00	0.00	75.03	15.65
Obesity	21.99	22.42	6.78	57.47	5.35
Arteriosclerosis	33.46	14.19	0.00	75.90	54.41
Mental retardation	1.72	0.00	0.00	0.00	7.51
Senility	9.54	0.00	0.00	0.00	42.97
Heart attack	8.30	0.00	0.00	31.70	6.23
Other heart problem	33.71	13.05	0.00	100.00	31.25
Hypertension	46.26	34.97	21.27	100.00	36.81
Stroke	8.57	1.64	0.00	8.28	27.64
Circulation trouble	54.85	26.72	8.72	100.00	76.04
Pneumonia	6.99	0.00	0.00	24.11	7.16
Bronchitis	14.07	3.02	0.00	53.29	7.48
Influenza	16.77	10.77	0.00	50.58	12.15
Emphysema	11.54	6.00	0.00	32.86	10.77
Asthma	8.15	2.18	0.00	31.28	3.99
Broken hip	2.35	0.00	6.41	0.00	2.95
Other fractures	5.72	2.57	6.62	6.92	7.45

"predictive" validity by examining the distribution of other types of variables on these types. Demographic variables and their associated λ_{kjl}s are presented in Table 22-3.

We see that Type 3, the most morbid subgroup, is heavily female, as is Type 2. Both the highly functional (Type 1) and frail groups are more likely to be male. Of greatest interest in this table is age, which shows that Types 2 and 4 are very elderly, whereas 1 and 3 are relatively young. Thus, Type 4 represents the frail oldest-old characterized by neurological problems, and Type 2 are relatively healthy but very elderly. Although functional, the two young groups have high levels of morbidity.

A second set of factors that can be used to describe the predictive validity of the four types consists of service use measures. These are presented in Table 22-4. In the

Table 22-3 External Variables Describing Demographic

	Frequency	Type 1	Type 2	Type 3	Type 4
Sex					
Male	34.70	57.94	22.23	4.99	46.97
Female	65.00	42.06	77.77	95.01	53.03
Age					
65–69	18.22	25.98	3.82	31.38	13.37
71–74	21.55	38.13	10.86	32.38	16.00
75–79	22.23	24.43	19.83	28.24	16.83
80–84	19.17	15.50	28.88	6.50	24.07
85–89	12.80	5.50	25.25	1.49	17.63
90+	6.03	0.46	11.35	0.00	12.11
Marital status					
Married	42.88	61.74	19.69	34.25	54.43
Not married	57.12	38.26	80.31	65.75	45.57
Education level					
None	2.26	1.41	2.16	0.41	5.29
Grades	21.17	15.11	15.88	30.87	25.50
Jr. high	34.42	30.62	31.56	45.02	32.13
Sr. high	28.39	35.95	31.36	19.68	23.91
College	11.74	13.38	16.57	3.94	11.71
Graduate	2.01	3.53	2.47	0.07	1.46
Annual income (US $)					
0–4999	17.16	9.10	16.91	38.34	7.20
5–6999	14.54	13.88	14.56	21.69	8.56
7–9999	16.15	16.23	11.82	16.96	20.15
10–14999	15.61	21.73	10.45	9.74	19.55
15–29999	12.49	16.56	10.55	2.40	19.29
30000+	4.86	5.09	6.20	0.05	7.63
Refused	6.52	7.06	10.86	1.81	5.45
Living quarters					
House	67.13	72.17	56.32	58.90	80.71
Duplex	6.87	5.18	9.35	8.50	4.63
Apartment	18.31	13.20	29.54	21.42	9.04
Other	7.69	9.46	4.78	11.19	5.62
Satisfaction in living quarters					
Very satisfied	49.28	55.56	59.09	29.21	49.73
Satisfied	42.95	38.81	36.95	52.96	47.11
Not satisfied	7.78	5.63	3.87	17.82	3.16
Disabled	92.79	69.06	100.00	100.00	100.00
Race of sample person					
White	88.51	91.57	89.18	90.05	82.55
Black	10.57	7.53	9.75	9.87	15.87
Other	0.92	0.90	1.07	0.08	1.58
Metropolitan status					
Metropolitan	65.34	65.6	80.61	45.52	66.31
Nonmetropolitan	34.66	34.4	19.39	54.48	33.69

Table 22-4 Associated Measures of Acute and LTC Service Use; Both Formal and Informal

	Frequency	Pure type I	II	III	IV
Ever a nursing home patient	9.60	1.35	16.60	2.14	18.84
On a nursing home waiting list	1.02	0.07	0.72	0.17	3.30
Had hospital stay in last year	45.59	25.32	33.58	65.53	65.07
Uses catheter or colostomy bag	4.19	2.32	0.56	0.00	15.50
Incontinent	26.84	10.59	5.18	43.19	58.04
Relationship of helper(s)					
Spouse	34.96	41.11	17.69	27.05	53.61
Offspring	42.15	10.97	53.89	52.14	57.51
Other relative	29.49	7.43	44.57	33.83	34.80
Friend	12.88	3.26	21.89	21.59	6.38
Other not related	33.52	6.01	41.91	30.40	60.43
Total out-of-pocket payment to helpers					
None	69.97	93.32	65.01	68.51	48.54
Unknown	14.48	2.16	15.28	12.81	30.24
$1–$39	7.08	3.36	11.49	12.63	1.19
$40–$124	4.13	0.74	3.82	5.00	6.76
$125–$399	2.11	0.39	2.93	0.00	5.30
$400+	2.23	0.03	1.46	0.00	7.96
How many helpers					
0	14.78	40.71	6.58	6.72	1.58
1	43.77	50.78	37.88	41.88	44.12
2	23.87	7.45	33.24	29.29	27.18
3	11.18	0.60	14.41	15.65	15.66
4+	6.40	0.46	7.88	6.46	11.46
How many days per week do they help					
0	23.23	62.30	10.94	13.89	3.34
1–5	18.79	14.32	31.88	29.86	1.50
6–7	32.34	22.18	32.07	37.74	46.27
8–12	11.78	1.03	14.77	12.99	18.72
13+	11.85	0.16	10.34	5.52	30.17
Current Medicaid payment	22.58	11.63	17.01	37.84	28.23
Other health insurance	62.65	72.82	67.14	52.24	54.83
Food stamps	12.07	4.51	5.39	32.13	10.14
Supportive housing	31.81	14.62	40.46	27.36	46.68
Service—home nursing	13.11	0.32	7.22	6.13	43.55
Service—therapist in last month	5.13	1.62	3.23	3.56	13.02
Service—emergency room visit, last month	6.71	3.66	2.42	12.60	9.75
Service—other MD office visit	44.04	36.27	36.90	72.59	33.50
Service—MD home visit	2.41	0.28	2.45	0.52	6.82
Service—RX in last month	79.73	66.50	70.48	97.66	87.77
Subjective Health					
Excellent	10.43	23.06	14.20	0.00	1.75
Good	27.99	48.05	46.04	2.16	10.17
Fair	33.76	28.03	37.59	47.76	20.41
Poor	27.82	0.87	2.16	50.08	67.68

table we see that both Types 2 and 4 were likely to have been in a nursing home, whereas Type 4 was most likely to be waiting to enter a home. Types 3 and 4 had much higher rates of hospitalization. Type 4 also clearly required the most informal and formal care series.

Thus, the four types seem clearly to define health and functional dimensions that describe variation on a number of demographic and service factors. In Table 22-5 we show how the life tables describing hospital service use varied over the four types in 1982 and 1984. In the table we present the length of stay (LOS) for hospital episodes discharged to HHA, SNF, community, or death for each of the four health types. In general, the LOS decreased between 1982 and 1984. For example, for persons discharged to the community, the hospital LOS dropped from 10.2 to 9.5 days. The decline is larger for those discharged to HHA (1.7 days) and those discharged dead (3.8 days). There is, however, variation in these discharges LOS by type. For example, the healthy type shows a consistent decline, as does Type 2. However, for Type 3 the LOS increases for all discharges except to the community. For the frail type (4) there is a more rapid discharge to HHA and to death.

In addition to LOS one can examine the proportion of discharge of different types. For example, there is a 2.8 percent increase in discharge to HHA. This is most evident for Type 3 (7.7 increases to 18.8 percent)—an increase compensated for by the decline in community discharges with home health services.

In addition to these parameter estimates, one can calculate weighted transitions that reflect the total number of transitions or service episodes. These parameters reflect changes in the volume of service use. These calculations would, because of the different populations represented, differ across the three analyses.

The specification of the model of the process can also be tested. This was done by including additional variables describing prior health service use and including it in the set of variables defining the K types. This did not significantly improve the fit of the model to the life tables. This suggests the adequacy of the fit of the model to the data; that is, the 56 variables describe the health state of the person sufficiently well that residual association between episodes does not persist.

Table 22-5 Discharges from Hospital Episodes; Comparisons of Discharge Destinations and LOS for Four Health Subtypes, 1982–1984

	SNF		HHA		Community		Death		All	
	1982	1984	1982	1984	1982	1984	1982	1984	1982	1984
	LOS (days)									
1. Highly morbid	14.0	11.0	17.8	17.6	8.8	8.0	17.4	8.1	10.1	8.4
2. Oldest-old	22.1	11.4	14.9	14.1	11.8	12.2	13.6	12.3	13.5	12.4
3. Highly morbid and impaired	10.9	18.1	8.8	10.7	10.0	8.0	17.2	19.9	10.0	12.4
4. "Frail" oldest-old	16.5	18.1	13.4	9.7	10.7	10.4	14.0	9.5	12.3	10.7
	Proporation of Hospital Episodes Terminating									
1. Highly morbid	1.9	1.7	4.8	4.4	83.6	85.9	7.7	5.1		
2. Oldest-old	8.0	8.4	10.7	12.6	67.4	67.1	9.4	9.3		
3. Highly morbid and impaired	.6	1.5	7.7	18.8	87.7	73.9	1.1	2.9		
4. "Frail" oldest-old	8.4	6.9	23.5	24.2	49.6	51.0	15.1	16.3		

As mentioned, if one wished to perform an analysis of health and functional characteristics, an alternative analysis would be performed. This was done for six pure types. The six-pure-type analysis separated out some distinct subgroups. For example, a relatively physically healthy subgroup was identified that has problems with selected IADLs (managing money, making phone calls, taking medication) and with a significant probability of cognitive impairment. In addition, a primarily hip fracture type was isolated (Manton and Stallard, 1989).

The choice between the four- and six-type description of the 56 health and functional variables depends upon the purpose of the analysis. In assessing changes in the profile of Medicare service use, the $g_{ik \cdot t}$ scores are used to control variation in health state for the service use life tables. Thus, the life tables estimated for the nonimpaired group show shorter hospital stays than for the frail type. The dimensionality of the solution in this case is determined by the amount of information contained on the rarest type of transition. If, instead, the primary focus of analysis is the health and functional status, then the six-type solution is preferred. Additionally, the time frame and sample eligibility criteria could be varied. The analysis showed reasonable robustness to this type of sample selection with the major effect being some rescaling of the λ_{kjl}s in samples with higher marginal rates of occurrence. The λ_{kjl}s for predicted variables and for the life table variables also showed substantial stability.

SUMMARY

The properties and use of GoM models were presented and discussed. It was stated that the distinctive characteristic of a GoM model was the way it described the "state" of an individual in terms of a set of K fuzzy partitions within which individual heterogeneity could be described. This was contrasted to standard classification procedures where health status would be described by a set of K discrete groups. Thus, the term *GoM model* applies to a number of different models that employed the fuzzy partitions state description.

These GoM models, in addition to having a distinctive mathematical structure as a consequence of that definition of state, have distinctive statistical properties because the individual g_{ik} scores are directly estimated by maximizing the likelihood. Other models representing the effects of "nuisance" parameters are based on the Kiefer–Wolfowitz (1956) conditions where individual responses are integrated out once the groups are identified. This was demonstrated for the LCM where an E–M-type algorithm is used to estimate P_ks and Λ_{kjl}s—no individual parameters are estimated directly. This is because the g^*_{ik}s that represent the discrete classification are treated as missing data so that their aggregate effects, rather than their individual values, are estimated. By dealing only with aggregate effects, it was shown, such models are affected by changes in the marginal distribution of outcome.

The *GoM* model did not have these dificulties because the g_{ik}s are directly estimated—a computationally intensive task. Although computationally intensive, the direct estimation of the g_{ik}s produces considerable flexibility and stability in the model. Even though g_{ik}s are estimated (i.e., individual level parameters) the asymptotic properties of the g_{ik} and λ_{kjl}s can be determined by recognizing the constraints on the moment space of the g_{ik} distribution implied by the λ_{kjl}s. In this case the consistency of the λ_{kjl}s and of the up-to-Jth-order moments of the g_{ik} distribution could be proved. The consistency is demonstrated for all identifiable distributions, that is, for all distributions equivalent up to the Jth-order moment. This limitation, which is based on the information in the sample, is considerably more general than in most multivariate procedures where the number of moments considered is limited analytically (e.g., in factor analysis to the second-order moments). The statistical properties of the model were shown to have useful properties in analyses of complex sample surveys.

Thus, the term *GoM* refers to a *class* of models with well-identified statistical attributes. The specific form of the model employed depends upon the nature of the phenomena being analyzed. We illustrated how several different types of GoM models could be developed to model health and functional changes among the elderly and oldest-old.

An important feature of this discussion is that the structure of the GoM is general enough to deal with a type of data found in many studies and surveys of elderly populations. This type of data (i.e., high-dimensional discrete response data measured on longitudinally followed individuals assessed at discrete times) is difficult to analyze using other types of multivariate procedures. The degree of robustness demonstrated between studies of the same data with substantively different sample eligibility criteria is also a useful property of the model—especially in longitudinal surveys where different interpretations of sample eligibility criteria can significantly alter the substance of questions to be addressed.

ACKNOWLEDGMENT

The research for this has been supported by NIH grants from the National Institute on Aging AG 01159, AG07198 and AG 03188.

REFERENCES

Anderson TW (1971). The Statistical Analysis of Time Series. New York, Wiley.

Berkman L, Singer B, Manton KG (1989). Black/white differences in health status and mortality among the elderly. Demography, 26:661–678.

Cassel CM, Särndal CE, Wretman JK (1977). Foundations of Inference in Survey Sampling. New York, Wiley.

Clogg CC (1981). New developments in latent structure analysis. In Factor Measurement in Sociological Research: A Multi-Dimensional Perspective (Jackson DJ, Borgeta EF, eds.). Beverly Hills, CA, Sage.

Dillon WR, Goldstein M (1984). Multivariate Analysis: Methods and Applications. New York, Wiley.

Eaton WW, McCutcheon A, Dryman A, Sorenson A (1989). Latent class analysis of anxiety and depression: Applications to data from the NIMH Epidemiologic Catchment Area Program (Eaton WW, Bohrnstedt G, eds.) Sociol Meth 18:104–125.

Goodman L (1978). Analyzing qualitative/categorical data. Cambridge, MA, Addison-Wesley.

Harman HH (1976). Modern Factor Analysis. Chicago, University of Chicago Press.

Hoem J (1985). Weighting, missclassification and other issues in the analysis of survey samples of life histories. In Longitudinal Analysis of Labor Market Data (Heckman J, Singer B, eds.). Cambridge, MA, Cambridge University Press, pp. 249–293.

Jöreskög KG (1969). A general approach to confirmatory maximum likelihood factor analysis. Psychometrika 34:183–202.

Jöreskög KG, Sorbom D (1983). LISREL V User's Guide. Analysis of Structural Relationships by Maximum Likelihood and Least Squares Methods. Chicago, International Educational Services.

Kiefer J, Wolfowitz J (1956). Consistency of the maximum likelihood estimator in the presence of infinitely many parameters. Ann Math Stat 27:887–906.

Lawley DN, Maxwell AE (1971). Factor Analysis as a Statistical Method. New York, Elsevier.

Lazarsfeld PF, Henry NW (1968). Latent Structure Analysis. Boston, Houghton Mifflin.

Liu K, Manton KG (1988). Effects of Medicare's hospital Prospective Payment System (PPS) on disabled Medicare beneficiaries. Final Report prepared for the Dept. of Health and Human Services, Office of the Assistant Secretary for Planning and Evaluation and the Health Care Financing Administration, February.

Manton KG (1988). A longitudinal study of functional change and mortality in the United States. J Gerontol 43:153–161.

Manton KG, Liu K (1990). Recent changes in service use patterns of disabled Medicare beneficiaries. HCF Rev 11:51–66.

Manton KG, Stallard E (1988). Chronic Disease Modeling. London, Charles Griffin.

Manton KG, Stallard E (1989). Cross-sectional estimates of active life expectancy for the U.S. elderly and the oldest-old populations. J Gerontol (In press).

Manton KG, Woodbury MA (1989). Grade of Membership generalizations and aging research. Exp Aging Res.

Manton KG, Tolley HD, Woodbury MA (1989). Multivariate event history process models based on Grade of Membership principles for the study of service use among the elderly. Presented at the Epidemiology and Public Health Session of the International Statistical Institute, Paris, August 29–September 6.

Morris CN (1982). Natural exponential families with quadratic variance functions. An Stat 10:65–80.

Muthen B, Christoffersson A (1981). Simultaneous factor analysis of dichotomous variables in several groups. Psychometrika 46:407–419.

O'Brien KF (1981). Life table analysis for complex survey data. Department of Biostatistics, University of North Carolina Institute of Statistics Mimeo Series No. 137, Chapel Hill, NC.

Saris WE, Satorra A, Sorbom D (1987). The detection and correction of specification errors in structural equations. In Sociological Methodology 1987 (Clogg CC, ed.) San Francisco, Jossey-Bass, pp. 105–130.

Scott DW (1985). Frequency polygons: Theory and application. J Am Stat Assoc 80:348–354.

Strauss JS, et al (1979). Do psychiatric patients fit their diagnoses? Patterns of symptomatology as described with the bilot. J Nerv Men Dis 167:105–112.

Tolley HD, Manton KG (1987). A Grade of Membership approach to even history data. Proceedings of the 1987 Public Health Conference on Records and Statistics. DHHS Pub. No. (PHS) 88-1214, USGPO, Hyattsville, MD, pp. 75–78.

Tolley HD, Manton KG (1991). Large sample properties of a fuzzy partition. J Statistical Matematics (In press).

Van de Geer JP (1971). Introduction to Multivariate Analysis for the Social Sciences. San Francisco, Freeman.

Woodbury MA, Manton KG (1991). Empirical Bayes approaches to multivariate fuzzy partitions. Multivariate Behav Res 26:291–321.
Woodbury MA, Manton KG, George LK (1989). Calculation of equivalent sample size for probability samples: Estimated error variance for rates and averages. Center for Demographic Studies. Durham, NC, Duke University.
Zadeh LA (1965). Fuzzy sets. Inf Control 8:338–353.

23

Issues in Handling Incomplete Data in Surveys of the Elderly

JON H. LEMKE AND GREGG A. DRUBE

Nonresponse biases are often more serious than other possible biases (Little and Rubin, 1987). In surveys of the elderly this is likely to be especially important. In this chapter we focus on the two main problems of item nonresponse when there are actual values underlying the nonresponse. First, we discuss the difficulty in identifying comprehensive explanations of item nonresponse; second, we discuss some analytic options.

By item nonresponse we are referring to incomplete responses to individual questions or blocks of questions by participants in a single survey or a sequence of follow-up surveys in a cohort study. Item nonresponse is in contrast to unit nonresponse, which occurs when sampled subjects are unable or unwilling to participate in the study.

We include as item nonresponse a participant response of "don't know," a refusal to answer a question, an inadvertently skipped question not corrected during edit procedures, individual questions or blocks of questions skipped because the participant was unable to complete the entire interview or was screened by the interviewer as being cognitively impaired, and follow-up survey questions of participants lost to follow-up after one or more interviews. It is not uncommon in studies of the elderly for participants to rejoin the study after being lost to follow-up for a year or two.

Because the terminology in missing-data research has evolved and is sometimes inconsistent, we will summarize the current terminology consistent with that presented by Little and Rubin (1987).

Missing-data mechanisms are the sets of underlying probabilities that determine whether or not each variable will be observed. Each type of incomplete data has a different missing-data mechanism.

The missing-data mechanism for a variable is either *nonignorable* or *ignorable* based on whether or not the distribution of the missing-data mechanism does or does not depend, respectively, on the missing values. Any variable that is missing as a function of its values has a nonignorable missing-data mechanism.

If a variable is missing independently of all variables, then it is said to be *missing-completely-at-random* (MCAR). If a variable is missing as a function of other variables but not itself, then the variable is *missing-at-random* (MAR). A variable does not need to be MCAR to have an ignorable missing-data mechanism. If a variable is not MCAR or MAR, then its missing-data mechanism is nonignorable. Even though a variable with a nonignorable missing-data mechanism can be missing as a function of other variables as well as of itself, it is important to consider the special case where the variable is missing as a function of its own value independent of all other variables. A variable with a missing-data mechanism that is ignorable does not imply that subjects with that missing variable can be excluded from analysis.

The examples of this chapter are all chosen from the Iowa 65+ Rural Health Study, a population study of 3673 rural elderly from Washington and Iowa counties of Iowa. This study is one of four companion studies jointly referred to as Established Populations for Epidemiologic Studies of the Elderly (EPESE), sponsored by the National Institute on Aging (National Institute on Aging, 1986 and 1990).

Before December 1, 1981, 4600 subjects were enumerated as being 65 or older for the Iowa 65+ Rural Health Study. Of the 3673 interviewed from December 1981 through October 1982 there were 1418 males and 2255 females. Of these interviews, 3217 were face-to-face with the study participant; the remainder were proxy and telephone interviews. Annual follow-up surveys (Follow-ups 1–6) were conducted for each of the next six years. Follow-ups 3 and 6 were personal interviews. Follow-ups 1, 2, 4, and 5 were telephone interviews.

INFLUENCES ON MISSING-DATA MECHANISMS

The search for missing-data mechanisms is often restricted to study population characteristics alone. Yet much of the variability in item nonresponse rates in surveys of the elderly can be attributed to study design, protocol, and implementation. These issues make it impossible for one to obtain a comprehensive explanation of nonresponse patterns within a study and prohibit one from extrapolating nonresponse patterns to other populations.

Order of Questions

For each participant some questions are more sensitive than others, and for some interviewers there are uncomfortable issues to discuss. Even though these questions may vary among participants and interviewers, some areas are more likely to generate item nonresponse. The Iowa 65+ Rural Health Study baseline questionnaire was designed so that sensitive questions were asked as late as possible without disrupting the flow of the questionnaire. Asking sensitive questions too early can create excessive incomplete data for questions that would otherwise be answered. For example, bowel and bladder questions were asked at the end of the health history. Cognitive functioning issues were not addressed until after all physical functioning questions, unless the interviewer deemed a cognitive function test necessary to justify proceeding with the interview or terminating the interview after an abbreviated set of questions. The last questions asked related to respondent income, which were the most sensitive and generated the most missing data. To have begun the interview with variables such as income would have encouraged the participants to refuse other questions more freely.

Length of Questionnaire

The length of a comprehensive interview may create a response burden so that there is more nonresponse at the end of the interview. More questions are skipped inadvertently or intentionally because the participant was unable to complete the entire interview. In addition, the length of the interview may influence whether respondents will participate in future follow-up surveys.

The leisure and income questions at the end of the baseline survey of the Iowa 65+ Rural Health Study had the greatest number of inadvertently missed items. Lemke et al (1983) detected a significant increasing linear trend with age in inadvertently missing responses to the income question by using the weighted least squares (WLS) procedure for categorical data (Grizzle et al, 1969) as detailed in Brock et al, (1986).

Categories of Item Nonresponse

Each type of nonresponse has a different missing-data mechanism and requires a different code. If one fails to recognize the type of incomplete data, one will often fail to identify the underlying missing-data mechanisms.

A good example is the role of education on income nonresponse. If one ignores the type of nonresponse, education appears to have little relationship to income reporting. This is definitely not the case. "Don't know" is significantly more common among those with less than 12 years of education than those with at least 12 years (males: 5.6 percent versus 2.4 percent, females: 14.5 percent versus 8.9 percent); whereas refusals are significantly less common among those with less than 12 years of education (males: 6.4 percent versus 8.7 percent, females: 8.0 percent versus 10.5 percent) (Lemke et al, 1983). If one pools the "don't know" responses and the refusals, one cannot understand the role of education in the missing-data mechanism for the income variable.

Protocol Variation

The EPESE study sites had somewhat different protocols and were designed based on regional experiences with securing optimal local study participation (National Institute on Aging, 1986 and 1990). A study protocol includes survey logistics such as interviewer training, procedures to contact possible respondents, procedures to enroll initial nonparticipants, field coding procedures, procedures to recover inadvertently missed questions or questions with inconsistent responses, reliability tests, assignment of interviewers to respondents expected to be difficult to interview, possible alternative phrasing of questions not understood by participants, and more. Most of these can influence the amount of item nonresponse.

Even when protocols are identical there are different levels of aggressiveness within the personalities and commitments of the interviewers. Other studies on other elderly populations will have different protocols as each tries to learn from the experiences of previous studies. Even within studies, it is difficult to convey equivalent messages to all interviewers, particularly if they are not all trained at the same time or if the answers to any one interviewer's questions must be relayed to all interviewers.

Sparseness of Incomplete Data

There are many difficulties in statistical analyses of sparse data, including lack of power to detect relationships and restricted ability to use large-sample asymptotic theory. Given that one of the goals when planning a survey is to minimize the amount of incomplete data for each participant, analyses of nonresponse patterns are unlikely to detect patterns and reasons for item nonresponse. The greater the success in obtaining complete information, the more difficult it becomes to detect the patterns.

Surveys of the elderly must have an honest approach to item nonresponse and not just seek to minimize it. If participants don't know the answer to a question, they should be encouraged to say "I don't know." If an area of questioning is sensitive to a participant, they must be given the opportunity to refuse. When interviewers are trained to force responses, respondents will create answers when they actually do not know the answer and misclassification biases will become a problem. If participants are pressed for answers they do not want to give, they are more likely to lie, and reporting biases will become a problem. Thus, no incomplete data may be as bad as substantial amounts. In addition, a relentless pressing for answers may increase loss to follow-up for later surveys.

Planned Omissions and Skip Patterns

Many factors may influence whether or not an interview can or should be completed. Since inconsistent responses occur with poorer physical, cognitive, and psychological functioning (Colsher and Wallace, 1989), it may be preferable to have missing data than possibly false information.

Frail respondents may not be able to complete an extensive interview session. The attentiveness of a respondent can be altered by medication. The most problematic of all are the cognitively impaired, who are not only likely to not know an answer or refuse an answer, but will contribute to misclassification biases so that the characteristics being studied do not represent the truth.

Every study of the elderly has to specify clearly under what circumstances the survey will be terminated, what blocks of questions can be skipped, and whether or not proxy information will be sought. The incomplete data generated by screening participants out of parts of a survey is not MCAR or MAR.

Reliability of Incomplete Data

Reliability studies completed within a short period after initial interviews do not confirm incomplete data. A "don't know" is often accepted as a challenge to find out, if at all possible. Participants will find out whether they can walk half a mile, whether they can count on their social support network, what familial traits exist, or what they have for an income.

Even initial refusals may disappear when the interview has been completed and participants no longer distrust the objectives of the study and the interviewer. However, reliability studies also generate new refusals to questions previously answered, because some participants may regret previously answering a question.

Reliability studies do not have the same response burden as the original interviews and do not use the same interviewers. The interviewer–participant rapport cannot be replicated and the nonresponse patterns cannot be replicated.

Follow-up Surveys

Over the course of a cohort study of the elderly, tremendous changes occur in the nature of nonresponse across follow-up interviews. In Figure 23-1, we present the self-reported ability to walk half a mile three years after having an incomplete response to the same question. Note that only 4.1 percent of those with incomplete data at baseline had incomplete data at follow-up 3 whereas, 54.2 percent of those at follow-up 3 were repeated at follow-up 6. Also, notice the low three-year mortality rates. Missing-date mechanisms can change substantially at different follow-up surveys.

Period of Study

The time period in which a survey is performed plays an important role. If the Iowa 65+ Rural Health Study baseline survey was conducted earlier or later, we expect we would have different item nonresponse patterns. The respondents would have had different experiences with respect to World War I, the Depression, and World War II; and they would have been exposed by health professionals and the mass media to different attitudes toward physical exercise, nutrition, smoking, and alcohol consumption. Cohorts from different time periods should be expected to have different nonresponse patterns and different missing-data mechanisms.

Population Location

Population location can have a strong influence on nonresponse patterns. Nonresponse rates and patterns varied by EPESE study site (National Institute on Aging, 1986 and 1990). Consider the differences between urban and rural populations. Some

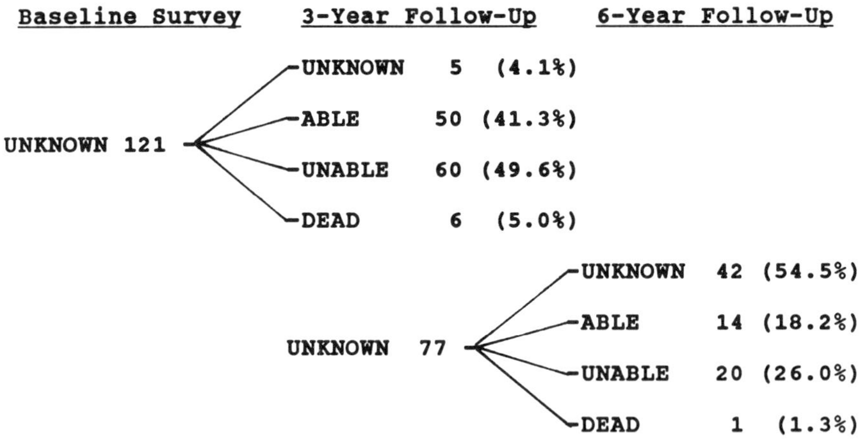

Figure 23-1 Self-reported ability to walk one-half mile by the Iowa 65+ RHS females three years after an unknown ability.

questions are not oriented to rural farm living, such as "Are you able to walk a half mile without help? That's about eight ordinary blocks."

Females from Iowa 65+ Rural Health Study were more likely to say "don't know" to this question than females at the other study sites. However, this is not a sign of poor health; they had a significantly lower 3-year mortality rate than the Iowa females, who reported that they could walk half a mile. They also knew whether or not they could walk half a mile at follow-up 3.

Interviewer–Participant Interaction

One of the more important sources of variability in refusal rates is the rapport established between the interviewer and the participant being interviewed. No matter how extensive the interviewer training, the personality of the interviewer affects how comfortable the participants are when answering sensitive questions.

In Fig. 23-2 we present the distribution of income item refusal rates by interviewer. Of the 3217 face-to-face interviews, 270 (8.4 percent) participants refused to answer this question. The refusal rates by interviewer are marked by the number of interviews conducted by each interviewer. Pearson's χ^2 test statistic for homogeneity of refusal rates across interviewers has a value of 71.47 with a P-value = 0.00003. The distribution appears to be bimodal. Compared to the interviewer with the most interviews (210), with a 3.4 percent refusal rate, nine interviewers had refusal rates at least three times greater.

Income Refusal Rate	Number of Interviews per Interviewer					
20%)	40					
19%)						
18%)						
17%)	167					
16%)						
15%)						
13%)	156	151	144	56		
12%)	141	90				
11%)	85					
10%)	50					
9%)	92	85	44			
8%)	156	83				
7%)	181	137	123	43	43	29
6%)	181	83				
5%)	155	115				
4%)	161	28				
3%)	207	32	116[a]			
2%)						
1%)						
0%)	43					

Figure 23-2 Interviewer-specific income question refusal rates for face-to-face interviews. Interviewers are marked by the number of face-to-face interviews they conducted. Pearson's χ^2 = 71.47 for homogeneity of refusal rates to the income question across interviewers, *df* = 30, *p*-value = 0.00003. Twelve interviewers, each with less than 24 interviews, had a combined refusal rate of 3.45 percent (4/116).

Whether or not one can detect a lack of homogeneity in interviewers' incomplete-data patterns, one must assume the patterns are heterogeneous. Interviewer performance must be monitored during any survey, but additional pressure on interviewers beyond the training sessions to eliminate nonresponse may force some interviewers to contrive answers.

Study Participant Characteristics

Incomplete data are usually attributed to the characteristics of the study participants, ignoring such factors as the type of nonresponse and interviewer–participant interactions. Study participant factors cannot be dismissed as not having a role in the missing-data mechanism, particularly without stratifying analyses by interviewer.

In large surveys of the elderly many patterns of incomplete data can be found by studying participant characteristics alone. For the Iowa 65+ Rural Health Study, some other factors also significantly associated with the income question include marital status and medical history. For women in this cohort, marital status accounts for much of the variability in "don't know" rates (Lemke et al, 1983). This "don't know" rate for income is greatest for presently married women (15.6 percent) and is least for never married women (6.9 percent). For previously married women the rate is 9.1 percent. These differences may reflect their perceptions on need to know. Future studies of the elderly may find these rates changing dramatically.

One composite medical history variable associated with refusals for men combined self-reported histories of cardiovascular disease and high blood pressure. Male participants with a self-reported history of a heart attack are less likely to refuse answering the income question (7.0 percent) than males with a history of high blood pressure and no heart attack (10.2 percent) and males with a history of neither (7.8 percent) (Lemke et al, 1983). Some chronically ill participants are both grateful for the social contact and comfortable answering medical history questions. They will often attempt to discuss much more than is even desired.

ANALYTIC OPTIONS

Studies of nonresponse patterns still leave investigators with the problem of analyzing the original objectives of the study. We have provided substantial evidence that when one analyzes surveys of the elderly, one must choose techniques that assume as little as possible about the missing-data mechanisms.

The analytic methods used in the absence of complete data can be grouped into six categories:

1. Complete-cases-only analyses.
2. Single imputation methods.
3. EM-algorithm.
4. Multiple imputation.
5. Problem-specific methods.
6. Indicator variable procedures for incomplete covariates.

We shall dismiss options 1 and 2, briefly describe methods 3–5, and detail method 6. The appropriateness of methods 3–6 depends upon the extent of understanding of the missing-data mechanisms, the objective of the analysis, and whether the incomplete variables are response variables or explanatory variables.

Complete-Cases-Only Analyses

The most common approach in the applied literature is to ignore subjects with incomplete data. These analyses will often dismiss large proportions of the original study sample for the convenience of using software packages that can handle only complete data sets. There are two primary problems with this approach. First, there is a loss of power accompanying the loss of sample size. Second, there are probably nonresponse biases forcing conclusions that are less likely to represent the study population. In general, complete-case-only analyses are not considered acceptable (Orchard and Woodbury, 1972; Dempster et al, 1977; Rubin, 1978; Whittemore and Grosser, 1985; Lemke and Brock, 1987; Little and Rubin, 1987; and Rubin, 1987).

Single Imputation Methods

Single imputation methods create a value for each missing observation by either imputing a mean value or randomly selecting a value from an underlying distribution of values. This option has two major problems. First, variances are underestimated; thus, standard errors are inappropriately decreased and power is unreasonably increased. Second, nonresponse biases can be exaggerated. Single imputation is no longer acceptable, given its problems and the recent development of multiple imputation (Rubin, 1978; and Rubin, 1987).

EM-algorithm

The EM-algorithm was developed by Orchard and Woodbury (1972). With further development by Dempster et al (1977), it became known as the EM-algorithm. It is an excellent procedure when the objective of the study is to obtain maximum likelihood estimates in the presence of incomplete data with known missing-data mechanisms. It is not as appropriate for comparing and testing nested models, because the likelihood ratio statistics typically cannot be partitioned into components with χ^2 distributions.

The EM-algorithm is an iterative procedure used to obtain maximum likelihood estimates in the absence of complete data. It iterates across cycles, where each cycle includes two different steps: the expectation (E) step and the maximization (M) step. The purpose of the E-step is to allocate proportionately the subjects with incomplete data across the joint distribution of the variables. Then the M-step is used to refit the model of interest. After the first cycle the refit model changes the joint distribution of the variables and the E-step is required to allocate the incomplete data proportionately to the new joint distribution. Again the M-step is required for the fit of the model. Typically, few cycles (3–6) are required until the estimates converge to the maximum likelihood estimates. Even though it is typically assumed that the data are MCAR, this assumption is not required. However, the missing-data mechanisms do have to be specified. Whittemore and Grosser (1985) present how this is done when covariates have missing values.

Multiple Imputation

Rubin (1978, 1987) introduces and thoroughly details multiple imputation. Multiple imputation was developed to maintain the variance–covariance structure of the underlying complete-data set. Single imputation does not provide an accurate assessment of the variability within a data set. To apply multiple imputation, one creates multiple data sets by randomly generating values for the incomplete data from the estimated joint distribution of the variables. This does require a thorough investigation into possible missing-data mechanisms. Analyses are then performed separately on each of the data sets. The estimates from each analysis are then combined, using the variance in estimates to make the inferences. Even though multiple imputation is proposed for the creation of several complete-data sets, it may be preferable that multiple imputation be problem specific when dealing with surveys of the elderly. Indicator variables must be maintained in the data sets so that secondary data users can recognize the extent of the original incomplete data and use alternate methods whenever they consider it necessary.

Problem-Specific Methods

Some specific statistical problems with specific incomplete-data assumptions have been solved, and some are discussed by Little and Rubin (1987). Each method cannot be generalized beyond the scope of the problem it solves. Unfortunately, these procedures are not being incorporated into the applied statistics books with the relevant topics, but exist primarily in the statistical journals.

Indicator Variable Procedures for Incomplete Covariates

The indicator variable models for regression analyses are designed to retain participants in analyses who have incomplete uncorrelated covariates (Cohen and Cohen, 1983; Lemke and Brock, 1987). These models are nonhierarchical and require caution in interpretation. The coefficients of the indicator variables in general should not be tested, but they are nuisance parameters that are the conditions for conditional tests. Whether the regression analysis is a least squares regression, logistic regression, or a Cox regression, the following parameterization permits an interpretation of the parameters compatible with complete-case-only analyses.

Consider the indicator variable regression model for two incomplete uncorrelated covariates. With a complete-response variable Y, the simplest least squares regression model is

$$\begin{aligned} E(Y) = {} & \beta_0 + \beta_{10}Z_1 + \beta_{20}Z_2 + \beta_{120}Z_1Z_2 \\ & + \beta_1(1 - Z_1)X_1 + \beta_2(1 - Z_2)X_2 \end{aligned}$$

where

$$Z_i = \begin{cases} 1 & \text{when the value of } X_i \text{ is unknown,} \\ 0 & \text{when the value of } X_i \text{ is known, } i = 1, 2. \end{cases}$$

These models are most easily understood when the $E(Y)$ is presented for the possible values of the Z_i's and when this response surface, $E(Y)$, is viewed geometrically. In this case, when the X_i's don't interact and are uncorrelated, the expected values of Y are

Z_1	Z_2	
0	0	$E(Y) = \beta_0 + \beta_1 X_1 + \beta_2 X_2$
0	1	$E(Y) = (\beta_0 + \beta_{20}) + \beta_1 X_1$
1	0	$E(Y) = (\beta_0 + \beta_{10}) + \beta_2 X_2$
1	1	$E(Y) = (\beta_0 + \beta_{10} + \beta_{20} + \beta_{120})$.

The intercept β_0 can only be estimated from the complete data. The slope parameters β_1 and β_2 are estimated using all participants that have a known value for X_1 or X_2, respectively. A different model for each subsample with a different nonresponse pattern takes whatever information is available from that subsample.

The increments β_{10}, β_{20}, and β_{120} are nuisance parameters, which cannot be zero if the corresponding slopes are not zero and zero is not in the range of the X_i's. When both covariates are missing, $\beta_0 + \beta_{10} + \beta_{20} + \beta_{120}$ is the $E(Y)$ for the subsample with only knowledge of the value of Y. If no one is missing both covariates, $\beta_{120}Z_1Z_2$ should be dropped from the model. If subjects are missing both covariates and $\beta_{120}Z_1Z_2$ is not included in the model, then the subjects missing both covariates should be dropped from the analysis or one alters the interpretation of the intercept and the increments. Standard regression diagnostics should be employed just as one would when there is complete data. However, the subjects with incomplete data can be expected to highly influence the nuisance parameters. Significance tests of β_{10}, β_{20}, or β_{120} equal to zero are essentially of little value because they reflect the differences between the range of the X_i's and the Y-axis. A geometric perspective highlights these points.

Let the $E(Y) = 1 - ½X_1 - ½X_2$, $0 \leq X_1 \leq 1$ and $0 \leq X_2 \leq 1$. The projection of the response surface on the X_1-plane is a parallelogram with β_0 at the upper extreme corner on the Y-axis. β_{20} is between 0 and $-½$. If X_2 can only be missing when it is 0, β_{20} can be 0. If X_2 can only be missing when it is 1, β_{20} can be $-½$. Setting $\beta_{20} = 0$ is equivalent to substituting 0 as actual values for all missing values of X_2. If the distribution of X_2 is symmetric about ½, it would be informative to test whether $\beta_{20} = -¼$. This would be a test of X_2 being missing as a symmetric function of itself rather than as an asymmetric function of itself. The $-¼$ was known because we knew the actual parameter values of the underlying model. If 0 is not included in the range of X_2, then β_0 is not in the parallelogram and β_{20} cannot be 0, since it also reflects the minimum value of X_2. If X_2 is MCAR, then $\beta_{20} = E(Y|X$ is the mean of all X_2 both known and unknown$) - \beta_0$. If the distributions of X_1 and X_2 are symmetric and their values are MCAR, then β_{120} cannot be 0.

If X_1 and X_2 interact, the fully parameterized interaction model is

$$\begin{aligned} E(Y) = {} & \beta_0 + \beta_{10}Z_1 + \beta_{20}Z_2 + \beta_1(1 - Z_1)X_1 + \beta_2(1 - Z_2)X_2 \\ & + \beta_{120}Z_1Z_2 + \beta_{11}Z_2(1 - Z_1)X_1 + \beta_{22}Z_1(1 - Z_2)X_2 \\ & + \beta_{12}(1 - Z_1)X_1(1 - Z_2)X_2 \end{aligned}$$

where

$$Z_i = \begin{cases} 1 & \text{when the value of } X_i \text{ is unknown,} \\ 0 & \text{when the value of } X_i \text{ is known, } i = 1, 2. \end{cases}$$

For each subsample designated by response pattern, the expected values of Y are

Z_1	Z_2	
0	0	$E(Y) = \beta_0 + \beta_1 X_1 + \beta_2 X_2 + \beta_{12} X_1 X_2$
0	1	$E(Y) = (\beta_0 + \beta_{20}) + (\beta_1 + \beta_{11}) X_1$
1	0	$E(Y) = (\beta_0 + \beta_{10}) + (\beta_2 + \beta_{22}) X_2$
1	1	$E(Y) = (\beta_0 + \beta_{10} + \beta_{20} + \beta_{120})$

The projection is no longer a parallelogram and the slopes for the subsamples are expected to vary arbitrarily so they also contain nuisance parameters β_{11} and β_{22}.

Acceptance of indicator variable models hinges on (1) the explanatory variables being uncorrelated, (2) the correct parameterization of the indicator variables, (3) conditioning on the indicator variables not testing them, (4) recognition of the required interaction structure, (5) a completely specified X-matrix, and (6) an accurate interpretation of the nonhierarchical models. One cannot expect the same significant factors in complete-case-only analyses and indicator variable analyses even if the data are missing completely at random. In the results of a Monte Carlo study with uncorrelated covariates (Lemke and Brock, 1987), the odds always favor the indicator variable procedure over a complete-case-only analysis when they disagree on which variables are significant. This happened whether each variable was MCAR, MAR, or missing as a function of itself.

We propose indicator variable approaches are possible for incomplete uncorrelated covariates but not for incomplete response variables. The value of this method when the covariates are correlated requires further study. One can fit indicator variable models with existing statistical software for least squares regression, logistic regression, or Cox regression subroutines. As in any regression analysis, diagnostics are essential.

SUMMARY

Incomplete-data patterns in comprehensive health studies of the elderly provide fascinating studies in themselves (Brock et al, 1986; Colsher and Wallace, 1989; Lemke et al, 1983; National Institute on Aging, 1986, 1990). Even though one cannot expect to extrapolate specific inferences about item nonresponse to other populations, two general conclusions are easily supported. First, nonresponse biases are serious problems which must be dealt with in all analyses of surveys of the elderly. Second, the missing-data mechanisms are not MCAR or MAR, and the true missing-data mechanisms will remain unknown. We presented a wide range of issues to challenge everyone to analyze data from surveys of the elderly making as few assumptions about the incomplete data as possible.

For either incomplete explanatory variables or response variables, the EM-algorithm (Dempster et al, 1977; Orchard and Woodbury, 1972; Whittemore and Grosser, 1985) and multiple imputation methods (Rubin, 1978, 1987) are possible given that the missing-data mechanisms are assumed to be known. In the case of incomplete, uncorrelated explanatory variables, the indicator-variable procedures (Cohen and Cohen, 1983) can be used to retain all subjects in an analysis.

Given both incomplete explanatory and response variables, it is possible to combine methods by using the indicator variables for the incomplete explanatory variables and either the EM-algorithm or multiple imputation for the incomplete response.

The indicator-variable models can be conveniently performed using existing linear model packages; whereas the EM-algorithm and multiple imputation methods usually require that programs be specially written for the problem at hand. How robust the EM-algorithm and multiple imputation procedures are when the missing-date mechanisms are not MCAR or MAR or are misspecified remains to be studied.

Although the study of incomplete data has become popular, we are seeing little motion in the applied literature to accommodate participants with incomplete data. This is due to many problems, including the unavailability of general statistical packages with incomplete-data options and the lack of statistics and epidemiology textbooks at both the introductory and advanced levels that discuss what to do when data is incomplete. The exceptions include texts dedicated to incomplete-data analysis (Little and Rubin, 1987; Rubin, 1987), survival texts that address censoring, one type of incomplete data not addressed in this chapter, and complex sample survey texts that address survey nonparticipation (unit nonresponse).

ACKNOWLEDGMENTS

Supported in part by contract N01-AG2106 and grant AG-07094 from the National Institute on Aging, and grant CA39065 from the National Cancer Institute. Completed at the Center for Advanced Studies, University of Iowa.

REFERENCES

Brock DB, Lemke JH, Woolson R (1986). Identification of nonrandom item response in an epidemiologic survey of the elderly, ASA Proceedings of Survey Research Methods Section, Alexandria, VA, pp. 430–434.

Cohen J, Cohen P (1983). Applied Multiple Regression/Correlation Analysis for the Behavioral Sciences, 2nd ed. Hillsdale, NJ, Lawrence Erlbaum.

Colsher PL, Wallace RB (1989). Data quality and age: Health and psychobehavioral correlates of item nonresponse and inconsistent responses. Gerontol (Psychol Sci) 44:2,45–52.

Dempster AD, Laird NM, Rubin DB (1977). Maximum likelihood from incomplete data via the EM algorithm (with discussion). J Roy Stat Soc Ser B 39:1–39.

Grizzle JE, Starmer DG, Koch GG. (1969). Analysis of categorical data by linear models. Biometrics 25:489–504.

Lemke JH, Wallace RB, Kohout F, Drube GA, Morris MC (1983). Informative incomplete responses in a survey of the elderly, Abstract in Program and Abstracts of the 1983 American Public Health Association, Dallas, Texas p. 152.

Lemke JH, Brock DB (1987). Retention of survey participants with item nonresponse, Abstract in Program and Abstracts of the 1987 Joint Statistical Meetings, San Francisco, California p. 209.

Little RJA, Rubin DB (1987). Statistical Analysis with Missing Data. New York, Wiley.

National Institute on Aging (1986). Established Populations for Epidemiologic Studies of the elderly. Resource Data Book, Cornoni-Huntley J, Brock DB, Ostfeld AM, Taylor JO, Wallace RB, eds. NIH Pub. No. 86-2443. National Institutes of Health, Bethesda, MD.

National Institute on Aging (1990). Established Populations for Epidemiologic Studies of the Elderly, Vol. II. Resource Data Book, Cornoni-Huntley J, Blazer DB, Lafferty ME, Everett DF, Brock DB, Farmer ME, eds. NIH Pub. No. 90–495. National Institutes of Health, Bethesda, MD.

Orchard T, Woodbury MA (1972). A missing information principle: Theory and applications. Proceedings of the Sixth Berkeley Symposium on Mathematical Statistics and Probability. Berkeley, University of California Press, pp. 697–715.

Rubin DB (1978). Multiple imputations in sample surveys—a phenomenological Bayesian approach to nonresponse. ASA Proceedings of the Survey Research Methods Section, Alexandria, Va, pp. 20–34.

Rubin DB (1987). Multiple Imputation for Nonresponse in Surveys. New York, Wiley.

Whittemore, AS, Grosser S (1985). Regression methods for data with incomplete covariates. In Modern Statistical Methods in Chronic Disease Epidemiology. Moolgavkar SH, Prentice RL, eds. New York, Wiley, pp. 19–34.

24

Utility of Logistic Regression Analysis in Epidemiologic Studies of the Elderly

PETER A. LACHENBRUCH

In many epidemiologic applications, the response variable is a dichotomous (two-state) variable. Let us assume that the variable is coded 0 or 1. Examples include "subject has lung cancer or not;" "subject was exposed to asbestos fibers or not." These variables are frequently assumed to have a Bernouilli distribution. The Bernouilli (or point-binomial) distribution has probability function

$$P(y;\mu) = \mu^{y}(1 - \mu)^{1-y}$$

where μ is the probability that the response is 1. This model serves as the basis for the technique known as logistic regression analysis, which estimates the probability that the response is 1 as a function of one or more predictor variables. Let us assume that the response we are interested in is presence of Alzheimer's disease ($y = 1$ if Alzheimer's disease, 0 if normal), and the predictor variable is presence of more than 10 tangles per 1000 fields in the hippocampus ($x = 1$ if present, 0 if not) as observed at autopsy. A hypothetical data set might look like Table 24-1. We observe that there are five Alzheimer's disease cases and five controls; four of the five Alzheimer subjects have tangles, and four of the five controls do not. Thus, the 2×2 contingency table looks like:

	Tangles	
Alzheimer	No	Yes
No	4	1
Yes	1	4

Table 24-1 Alzheimer's Disease and Tangles

Subject	1	2	3	4	5	6	7	8	9	10
Alzheimer	N	N	N	N	N	Y	Y	Y	Y	Y
Tangles	N	Y	N	N	N	Y	Y	Y	N	Y

The odds ratio is 16 ($4 \times 4/(1 \times 1)$) with log(OR) = 2.7726 with standard error of 1.58 [$\sqrt{(1/1 + 1/4 + 1/4 + 1/1)}$]. The logistic regression model may be written as

$$\log\left(\frac{\mu}{1-\mu}\right) = \alpha + \beta x$$

where the logarithm is taken to the base e (i.e., natural logarithms). Note that $\log(\frac{\mu}{1-\mu})$ is the log of the odds of occurrence. This relationship can be translated into

$$\mu = \frac{1}{1 + e^{-(\alpha+\beta x)}}$$

The usual linear regression programs cannot be used to estimate the parameters since the y variables are 0 or 1, and thus $\log[y/(1 - y)]$ is undefined. A number of special-purpose programs are available for this purpose (e.g., GLIM, SAS PROC LOGIST, BMDPLR).

Fitting the hypothetical data using the logistic regression model gives estimates $\hat{\alpha} = -1.386$ and $\hat{\beta} = 2.773$. The standard error of $\hat{\beta}$ is 1.58. The identity of the estimate of β and the log of the odds ratio is no coincidence. Since μ is the probability of response, logistic regression is fitting models of the log-odds of occurrence, $\log[\mu/(1 - \mu)]$. The difference of the estimates of the log-odds when $x = 0$ and $x = 1$ is the log of the odds ratio. In general, the logistic regression coefficient is the log of the odds ratio for a one-unit increase in the predictor variable. Table 24-2 contains the (briefly annotated) output from the GLIM (Payne, 1985) program I used to analyze this data. The change in the scaled deviance is a χ^2 variable with degrees of freedom equal to the change in degrees of freedom. This χ^2 (=3.85 in this case) is used to test the null hypothesis of no effect of the added factor(s).

The natural extension of the ideas of logistic regression to multiple predictor variables is straightforward. The model now is given by

$$\log\left(\frac{\mu}{1-\mu}\right) = \alpha + \beta_1 x_1 = \cdots + \beta_k x_k$$

The interpretation of the parameters must be modified in a manner analogous to multiple regression. The coefficients are now *partial* coefficients: $\hat{\beta}_1$ now is the estimate of the change in the log-odds ratio for a one-unit change in x_1 *given* that the remaining x's are held fixed.

There are many computer programs that compute logistic regression parameter estimates. GLIM (Payne, 1985), developed as a project of the Royal Statistical Society, provides a unified method for analyzing data that arise from a class of distributions known as the exponential family. This family includes the normal, binomial, and Poisson distributions, so the program permits one to analyze multiple regression models,

Table 24-2 GLIM Output

```
? $units 10$data tngl [Tells GLIM that there are 10 cases, and that I will enter the variable tngl]
? $cal case=%gl(2,5) [This declares the first five cases as non-Alzheimer's disease, and the second
five as Alzheimer's]
? $read
0 1 0 0 0 1 1 1 0 1 [1 if tangle present, 0 if not]
? $cal n=1$err b n$ [declares a binomial model]
? $yva tngl$fac case 2$
? $fit $d e$ [fits model with only the constant term and displays the estimate]
scaled deviance =  13.863 at cycle 4
        d.f. = 9
        estimate        s.e.        parameter
  1 4.768e-07      0.6325       1
  scale parameter taken as 1.000
? $fit +case$d e$ [adds the variable "case" to the model and displays estimates]
scaled deviance =  10.008 (change =  -3.8549) at cycle 4
        d.f. = 8          (change =  -1      )
        estimate            s.e.              parameter
  1       -1.386      1.116       1
  2         2.773     1.580      CASE(2)
  scale parameter taken as 1.000
? $cal %exp(2.773)$ [calculates odds ratio]
        16.01
```

logistic regression models, and log-linear models. BMDP (Dixon, 1988) offers a program to perform stepwise logistic regression. It provides selection of variables, tests of goodness of fit, the ability to handle matched data, and plots of data. SAS (SAS Institute, 1983) offers the LOGIST procedure, which computes stepwise logistic regression, as well as backward elimination. It computes maximum likelihood estimates and test statistics for assessing lack of fit.

There are at least two alternative models for this kind of data: the linear probability model and the probit model. The linear probability model is

$$\mu = \alpha + \beta_1 x_1 + \cdots + \beta_k x_k$$

(recall that μ is the probability of response). This model suffers from several drawbacks. First, it can give estimtes that are greater than 1 or less than 0, which are nonsensical estimates for probabilities. Second, if the probabilies are quite different for different x values, the lack of constant variance can increase the variance of the parameter estimates. Third, the assumption of linearity imposes constraints on the parameters that often are unwanted. For a further discussion of these issues see Aldrich and Nelson (1984). The probit model is

$$\mu = \Phi(\alpha + \beta_1 x_1 + \cdots + \beta_k x_k)$$

where $\Phi(\cdot)$ is the cumulative normal distribution. This model is quite close to the logistic model. GLIM, BMDP, and SAS have programs that permit the analysis of Probit models.

Further information at a beginning level may be found in Adena and Wilson

(1982), Aitkin et al (1989), Aldrich and Nelson (1984), and Kleinbaum et al (1988). An advanced treatment is given in McCullagh and Nelder (1983).

COMBINING LOGISTIC REGRESSION AND MULTIPLE REGRESSION

In many problems in biometry, there may be a mechanism that determines whether a response will occur and a generation of the level of the response given that the response does occur. This can lead to data that have a large fraction of observations tied at 0. One of the obvious problems of this type of data is nonnormality of the distributions. This leads to serious problems of estimation of regression relationships if one does not account for the excess zeros. A similar problem was studied by Lachenbruch (1976) for a two-sample testing problem in which a two-degree-of-freedom test was developed. It has also been studied in the econometric literature, especially by Duan et al (1982), in connection with the Rand Health Insurance study.

Four examples of this sort of data-generating mechanism are presented here. In a study of arthritis (Furst, personal communication, 1984), certain measurements could not be obtained because it was not possible for the patient to walk a required distance, or because the patient's joints were swollen on the measurement day, making it impossible to determine a ring size. The data were "not obtainable" rather than "not measured" or "refused." We needed to model the factors related to the "not obtainable" status. In the study of health care expenditures, 30 percent of the population had no annual expenditure for health care (Cave, 1988). The remaining 70 percent had an expenditure that was approximately log normal. The transformation log (expenditure + 5) seemed to work well. The addition of $5 reduced skewness. Duan et al (1982) used this transformation for the Rand Health Insurance Study data. In cloud-seeding experiments the treatment may have an effect on the probability of measurable rainfall and on the quantity of rain if some rain occurs (e.g., Neyman and Scott, 1967). Of course, other factors might be included in any statistical models of rainfall induction.

M. J. Ball (1987) autopsied the brains of 33 Alzheimer's disease patients and nine "normal" subjects and provided counts of various lesions and "tangles." The number of fields counted were different for each patient, so the data were converted to counts per 1000 fields. (In further correspondence, I have learned that the rate is computed by a slightly different and more complex procedure. This does not affect the example.) In some cases the rates were quite low (under 10 per 1000 fields), and in others fairly high (in the hundreds). The tangles data were clearly nonnormal even after logarithmic transformation. If I eliminated the counts below 10 per 1000 fields from the data, then a log-normal distribution seemed to describe the data adequately. Various models could be used to study the relation between the number of tangles and the number of granulovacuoles. A linear regression gave different results if one used only those subjects with counts greater than 10 rather than the full data set. There was no relation between the predictor, log(tangles + 1), and the dependent variable, granulovacuoles, in the conditional (given count > 10) regression. It is possible to predict $P(\text{count} < 10)$ using logistic regression or a similar technique. Other models that have been proposed for this sort of data include the Tobit (Tobin, 1958), which is a left-censored normal distribution. The "selection model" (Heckman, 1974) uses a probit model to predict whether a positive expenditure occurs, and an unconditional, uncensored linear model of expenditures for nonzero expenditures. Duan et al note that there are difficulties with the selection model in their context: negative predicted expenditures are possible; although some individuals have zero health care costs, these are treated as "censored" in the selection model. It is important in some situations to account for 0 values explicitly. A final model that I have not found in the literature is a mixture-of-distributions model. That is, the probability distribution has the form $f(y) = p(0) + [1 - p(0)]*h(y)$, where $h(y)$ is the distribution of y for $y > 0$. This is similar to the two-part model, but the likelihood is more complicated because of the mixture problem. We shall not consider this model further.

THEORETICAL DEVELOPMENT

Let the dependent variable be denoted by y (which is positive or zero), and define $y_1 = 1$ if $y > 0$, $y_1 = 0$ if $y = 0$; and $y_2 = g(y)$ if $y_1 = 1$ and otherwise undefined (for computing purposes it may be useful to set y_2 to the missing value code when $y_1 = 0$ or to use a weighted analysis that gives the y_2 values the weight y_1). The transformation $g(y)$ should be chosen so that a linear model is appropriate. It is important that no zero or negative values of y be predicted. For example, a common function might be the log of the variable. We assume there is a set of predictor variables $\mathbf{x}$, and we wish to determine a model for $g(y)$ or (y_1,y_2). The least squares regression model will fit the model $E(g(y)) = \mathbf{x}\beta$ but an analysis of residuals is likely to demonstrate a clump of peculiar residuals for the cases in which $y = 0$. More importantly, if distinct mechanisms generate the $y = 0$ values and the $y > 0$ values, two different models should be used. One set of predictors might be used for a logistic or probit model of y_1 values and another used for the model of the y_2 values. An obvious pitfall to avoid is predicting nonpositive y values when $y > 0$. Inclusion of the $y = 0$ cases could suggest a spurious relationship with the $\mathbf{x}$ variables. We let $p(\mathbf{x})$ be the probability of $y_1 = 0$ when $\mathbf{x}$ is the covariable vector.

The likelihood may be written as

$$L(y_1,y_2) = \Pi(p(\mathbf{x}))^{1-y_1}\{(1 - p(\mathbf{x}))f(y_2;\mathbf{x})\}^{y_1}$$

We can separate the terms with $p(\mathbf{x})$ and $f(y_2;\mathbf{x})$ to find distinct parts of L for determining the parameters of $f(\cdot)$ and p. We shall fit a logistic model for $p(\mathbf{x})$. Thus, the likelihoods can be solved separately for the equations predicting $y_1 = 0$ (= no response) and those predicting y_2. In particular, the log-likelihood for a logistic model for $P(y_1 = 0 \mid \mathbf{x})$ and a normal model for $E(y_2 \mid \mathbf{x})$ is

$$\log L = \Sigma\{y_1(\alpha + \beta\mathbf{x}) - \log(1 + \exp(\alpha + \beta\mathbf{x})) + y_1(0.5 \log(2\pi\sigma^2) - 0.5[y_2 - \gamma\mathbf{x})/\sigma]^2\}$$

It is easy to see that the solutions for α, β, and γ do not involve terms from the other part of the likelihood. (This also shows that the estimates for the parameters will be asymptotically normal and independent, since the information matrix is a block diagonal matrix.)

One should examine the residuals as a matter of good statistical practice. There are two sets of residuals to be examined: the studentized logistic regression residuals for the y_1 data and the studentized residuals for y_2 data. The joint behavior of such bivariate residuals is not known. An example of the plot of the fits and the residuals is given later.

In both the logistic and least squares regression relationship, testing may be accomplished by using the difference of the likelihoods under the models with and without the effect(s) of interest. Such testing may be done separately within the logistic model and the "normal" model or may be done jointly. I find the interpretation simpler when the testing is done separately within models.

Fitting the models in the example was done using GLIM. This permitted both binary and least squares models to be fit by the same program. They were fit separately since the likelihood factors into two parts whose parameters are distinct. Because of this fitting procedure, the overall likelihood is not computed by the GLIM models. The full model, using both the normal and logistic portions, can be computed using an OWN model within GLIM, but the increase in overall understanding of the model did not seem as useful as the basic idea of the two-part model.

Example

The data in Table 24-3 are a portion of a set collected by MJ Ball (1987). They consist of the counts per 1000 fields of the number of tangles and the number of granulovacuoles in the hippocampus. In the regression analyses we treated tangles below 10 per 1000 fields as if they were zero. Table 24-4 gives some descriptive statistics for the granulovacuoles and tangles overall and by disease status.

The skewness of the tangles variable in the combined data suggested the need for the log transformation. Possibly the new variable, log (tangles + 1), could be improved upon since its skewness indicates it is long-tailed to the left and has a high kurtosis. Normal plots clearly indicated the non-normality of tangles. Residual analysis after fitting the regression on granulovacuoles also indicated substantial normality problems. All linear regressions used log(tangles + 1) as the dependent variable (if tangles were <10 they were recorded to 0). In considering the use of the conditional model, similar statistics were found. For those 28 observations, the skewness of log(tangles + 1) was 0.047, whereas the skewness of the tangles variable was 0.777. The normal plot of the log(tangles + 1) appeared to be close to a straight line.

The first regression used granulovacuole count as the independent variable for the full data set (Tables 24-5a and 24-6a). For this model we find that the number of granulovacuoles is a strong predictor of the log of tangles. The examination of studentized residuals shows five large (>2.8 in absolute value) residuals. These all corresponded to Alzheimer's disease patients for whom the tangle count was less than 10.

The second regression model is the conditional model for y_2 = log(tangles + 1) given tangles more than 10 (Tables 24-5b and 24-6b). In GLIM, this can be fit by using y_1 as a weight. The model contains only the granulovacuole density. There is no conditional relationship between granulovacuole density and tangles. There are no large studentized residuals: the maximum residual is about 1.25 in absolute value.

The relationship of the number of granulovacuoles to y_1, the indicator for tangles

Table 24-3 Alzheimer's Autopsy Data[a]

Granulovacuoles	Tangles	Status	Y_1
18.700	1.375	1.000	0.000
1.541	0.203	1.000	0.000
10.890	0.385	1.000	0.000
80.000	2.974	1.000	0.000
3.390	0.000	1.000	0.000
6.573	0.381	1.000	0.000
10.842	0.261	1.000	0.000
0.000	0.577	1.000	0.000
1.225	0.394	1.000	0.000
35.503	8.848	2.000	0.000
244.864	109.780	2.000	1.000
94.448	47.870	2.000	1.000
408.205	50.674	2.000	1.000
34.146	4.761	2.000	0.000
318.939	23.373	2.000	1.000
402.025	36.277	2.000	1.000
272.031	3.490	2.000	0.000
306.712	101.940	2.000	1.000
59.859	17.167	2.000	1.000
171.006	13.326	2.000	1.000
138.848	5.270	2.000	0.000
189.569	20.065	2.000	1.000
308.211	18.248	2.000	1.000
150.826	49.619	2.000	1.000
243.229	113.736	2.000	1.000
337.024	136.753	2.000	1.000
196.594	67.160	2.000	1.000
72.102	26.170	2.000	1.000
139.122	34.189	2.000	1.000
190.476	52.952	2.000	1.000
86.674	3.065	2.000	0.000
161.567	67.285	2.000	1.000
441.841	38.129	2.000	1.000
68.027	24.050	2.000	1.000
12.613	33.871	2.000	1.000
88.977	19.399	2.000	1.000
34.183	25.244	2.000	1.000
196.950	50.794	2.000	1.000
54.077	109.497	2.000	1.000
59.375	90.693	2.000	1.000
125.160	137.127	2.000	1.000
149.551	81.163	2.000	1.000

Source: Ball (1987).

[a]Granulovacuoles and tangles units are counts per 1000 fields; Status: 1 = Normal, 2 = Alzheimer's disease; Y_1 = 1 if tangles are more than 10, 0 otherwise.

Table 24-4 Description of Alzheimer's Data[a]

	Granulovacuoles	Tangles	ln(Tangles + 1)
Normals (n = 9)			
Mean	14.8	0.73	0
S.D.	25.2	0.93	0
Skewness	2.22	1.81	0
Kurtosis	3.37	1.99	0
Alzheimer (33)			
Mean	175.5	49.15	3.26
S.D.	119.4	39.91	1.53
Skewness	0.639	0.83	−1.29
Kurtosis	−0.574	−0.45	0.54
Combined (n = 42)			
Mean	141.1	38.78	2.56
S.D.	125.4	40.59	1.92
Skewness	0.790	1.03	−0.45
Kurtosis	−0.370	−0.035	−1.49

[a]Tangles are coded as the raw data values; log(tangles + 1) is set to zero if tangles are less than or equal to 10.

Table 24-5 Analysis for Full Data Set, Tangle >10, and Logistic Models

a. Full Data Model

Analysis of Deviance

Model	Deviance	df	Difference
Intercept	150.47	41	
Intercept + granulovacuole	108.47	40	42.00

Analysis of Variance

Source	SS	df	MS	F
Regression	42.00	1	42	15.49
Error	108.47	40	2.711	

b. Tangles >10 Model

Analysis of Deviance

Model	Deviance	df	Difference
Intercept	12.46	27	
Intercept + granulovacuole	12.23	26	0.23

Analysis of Variance

Source	SS	df	MS	F
Regression	0.228	1	0.228	0.484
Error	12.228	26	0.470	

Analysis of Deviance for Logistic Model

Model	Deviance	df	Difference
Intercept	53.47	41	
Intercept + granulovacuole	37.79	40	15.68

Table 24-6

Model	Estimate	S.E.	Parameter
a. Coefficients and S.E. for E(y) Models			
Intercept + Granulo	1.424	0.385	Intercept
	0.00807	0.00205	Granulovacuole
b. Coefficients and S.E. for $E(y_2)$ Model			
Model	Estimate	S.E.	Parameter
Intercept + Granulo	3.704	0.241	Intercept
	0.000759	0.00109	Granulovacuole
c. Coefficients and S.E. for $P(y_1 = 1)$ Models			
Model	Estimate	S.E.	Parameter
Intercept + Granulo	−1.016	0.5965	Intercept
	0.017	0.00606	Granulovacuole

Note: Status (normal or Alzheimer's disease) was modeled as a two-level factor in these models.

more than 10, was fit by a logistic model with GLIM (Tables 24-5c and 24-6c). The effect of granulovacuoles is clear: it is very important in predicting tangles >10 with a $\chi^2 = 15.68$. In Fig. 24-1 $P(y_1 = 1 \mid \text{granulovacuole})$ is plotted against $E[\log(\text{tangles} + 1) \mid \text{granulovacuole, tangles} > 10]$; and in Figure 24-2 the studentized residuals from the logistic model for $P(y_1 = 1)$ are plotted against the studentized residuals from the conditional model. The first plot is of interest if one is primarily concerned with the effect of this variable on the probability that the tangles are greater than 10 and the expectation of the number of tangles given that the number of tangles is greater than 10. There are no negative residuals for the logistic model plotted in this picture. All negative logistic residuals occurred for cases with tangles less than 10, and these are eliminated in the plot. There was one large negative residual (not shown) that occurred for a subject who had no tangles and a low granulovacuole count. Note that $E(y_2)$ is simply the mean of the observations since the regression coefficient is very small. The full effect of granulovacuoles is in predicting $y_1 = 1$.

We have described a two-part model for regression with excess zeros. The advantages of the model include better fits to the least squares regression component and a structure that specifically accounts for the zero values. In the econometric literature there is often a strong emphasis on a single equation to model the overall data, with specific emphasis on determining the expectation of the dependent variable at a given value of **x**. Greater understanding is often possible if one uses the two models separately since different mechanisms may lead to zero values and the level of the nonzero values. Different predictors may be used in the logistic and normal parts of the model. In our example, we found that if one used only the granulovacuole variable, a fairly strong relationship with log(tangles + 1) might be inferred (although a hard look at the residuals should alert the user). However, when the model is separated into the distinct parts, we find an altered picture: there is no relationship between granulovacuoles and log(tangles + 1) when the tangles are greater than 10. However, the granulovacuole density is important in predicting "under 10" versus "over 10." Com-

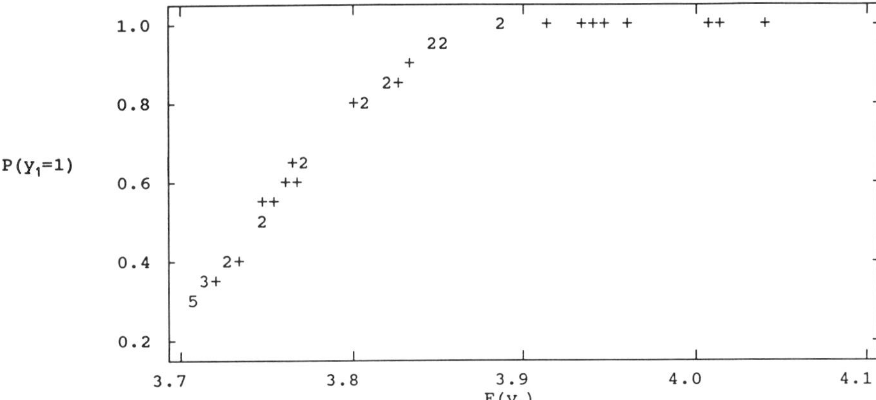

Figure 24-1 Plot of $P(y_1 = 1)$ vs. $E(y_2)$. (Model for logistic includes granulovacuoles.)

menting on an earlier version of this manuscript, Dr. Peter Fewster, an associate of Dr. Ball, notes the following:

> At disease onset we can assume that tangles or granulovacuoles begin to appear within the nerve cells. As the disease progresses more of these lesions will appear within the nerve cells. At the same time nerve cells (probably those cells which have been damaged by such lesions) begin to fall out. Hence the numerical response of these 2 lesions to disease progression is most likely unimodal rather than linear. Now, all our data comes from post-mortem patients. While some of the Alzheimer patients may have died at an early stage, many (most) of them will have died as a result of the severity of their long-standing dementia. Consequently, these very demented brains may in fact be more similar morphometrically (except for nerve cell density counts) to the normal control brains than those which were less demented. (Fewster, 1988)

Thus, some of the results we have noted here may be due to the fact that nerve cells "fall out" as the Alzheimer's patient ages.

The two-part model presented here has the advantage of directly modeling the

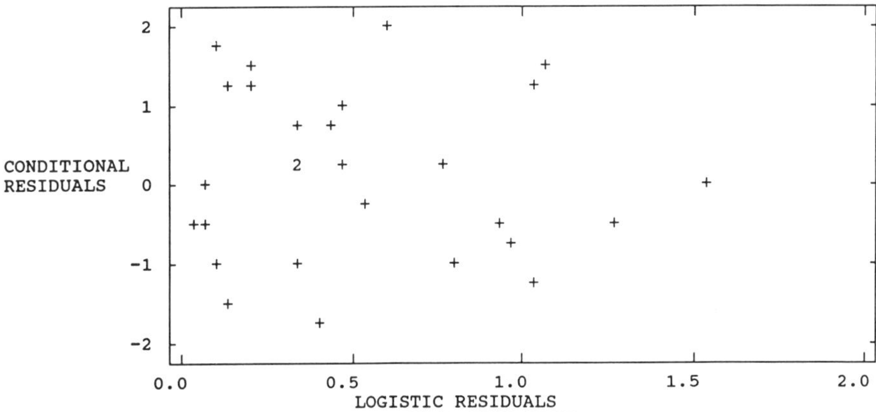

Figure 24-2 Residuals from logistic and from conditional regressions. (Model for logistic includes granulovacuoles.)

properties of interest: the chance of "no response" and a linear model of the level of response given that there is a response. The inclusion of "no response" cases in a linear model has the drawback of using points with a large chance of affecting any linear relationships. Therefore, the two-part model seems a sensible choice. Testing and estimation are easily carried out using generalized linear models. For example, a covariance analysis is handled identically for the logistic and the conditional regression models by examining the deviances with and without various covariates, factors, and interactions.

Two-part models are simple, interpretable, and easily fit. They are fit with a two-step procedure. First, do a logistic regression on the zero versus positive response. Next, do an ordinary regression for the nonzero responses, taking care that the regression does not predict nonpositive numbers. This might be done with transformations or with a restricted prediction equation.

ACKNOWLEDGMENT

I wish to thank Dr. M. J. Ball of the University of Western Ontario for permission to use data he collected and Dr. Peter H. Fewster of the same institution for his comments on the manuscript.

REFERENCES

Adena MA, Wilson SR (1982). Generalised Linear Models in Epidemiological Research. Sydney, The Instat Foundation for Statistical Data Analysis.

Aitkin M, Anderson D, Francis B, Hinde J (1989). Statistical Modelling in GLIM. Oxford, Clarendon Press.

Aldrich JH, Nelson FD (1984). Linear Probability, Logit, and Probit Models. Beverly Hills, Sage Publications.

Ball MJ (1987). Personal communication.

Cave DG (1987). Ph.D. dissertation, University of California at Los Angeles.

Dixon WJ, ed (1988). BMDP Statistical Software Manual, Vol 2. Program LR: Stepwise Logistic Regression. Berkeley, University of California Press.

Duan N, Manning WG, Morris CN, Newhouse JP (1982). A comparison of alternative models for the demand for health care, Rand Corp. Pub. R-2754-HHS.

Fewster P (1988). Personal communication

Furst D (1984). Personal communication

Heckman J (1974). Shadow prices, market wages, and labor supply. Econometrica 42:679–694

Kleinbaum DG, Kupper LL, and Muller KE (1988). Applied Regression Analysis and Other Multivariable Methods, 2nd ed. Boston, PWS-Kent.

Lachenbruch PA (1976). Analysis of data with clumping at zero. Biometr J 18:351–356.

McCullagh PM, Nelder JA (1983). Generalized Linear Models. London, Chapman and Hall.

Neyman J, Scott EL (1967). Some outstanding problems relating to rain modification. Proceedings of the Fifth Berkeley Symposium on Mathematical Statistics and Probability, vol. 5. Berkeley, CA.

Payne CD (1985). The GLIM System Release 4.77 Manual. Oxford, Numerical Algorithms Group.

SAS Institute (1983). SAS User's Guide: The LOGIST Procedure, Cary, NC.

Tobin J (1958). Estimation of relationships for limited dependent variables. Econometrica 26:24–36.

Index